W. Wenz

Abdominal Angiography

In collaboration with
G. van Kaick, D. Beduhn and F.-J. Roth

With 183 figures, some in color,
comprising 351 radiographs and 34 drawings

Springer-Verlag
Berlin · Heidelberg · New York 1974

Priv.-Doz. Dr. D. Beduhn, Dr. G. van Kaick, Dr. F.-J. Roth
Prof. Dr. W. Wenz,
Röntgenabteilung der Chirurgischen Universitätsklinik Heidelberg

ISBN-13: 978-3-642-93027-0 e-ISBN-13: 978-3-642-93025-6
DOI: 10.1007/978-3-642-93025-6

Softcover reprint of the hardcover 1st 1974

Preface

The brilliant yet simple idea of introducing a catheter percutaneously into an artery, without first dissecting it free, using a flexible guide wire, has led to a truly revolutionary breakthrough in abdominal x-ray diagnosis (SELDINGER, 1953).

In the meantime, methods and techniques for injecting contrast media into various vessels have become largely standardized; innumerable publications have appeared which deal with every conceivable aspect of angiographic technique and interpretation.

This volume is designed to present our experience with abdominal angiography. We deliberately refrained from any systematic discussion of the genitourinary tract, which has been adequately dealt with in the literature, also with respect to angiographic findings. Our interest in the retroperitoneal region is based mainly on its significance in differential diagnosis.

In ten years of angiographic activity, our Department had made successful use of a simple technique which appears suitable also for smaller hospitals. We wish to point out its diagnostic potential and, at the same time, to outline its limitations.

Our experience embraces 2804 abdominal angiograms, which we have classified according to clinical and morphologic anatomical criteria. Their diagnostic interpretation has been compared with the surgical or histopathological results. This may help others to avoid errors of the type which we discovered in our own work.

Angiographic diagnosis requires not only familiarity with normal radiographic anatomy, but also specific knowledge of angiographic pathomorphology. We have tried to identify those features which typify the individual findings and to derive therefrom valid generalizations with the aid of simple sketches.

We consider the introduction of subtraction and color subtraction, which facilitates the visualization of epigastric organs and the differentiation of various vascular systems, another contribution to the field of visceral angiography. A number of our findings were made possible by electronic subtraction techniques and are displayed accordingly.

Some of the more recent indications for human angiography are founded on experience gained in animal experimentation. Results we obtained in the angiographic diagnosis of gastrointestinal bleeding of undetermined origin and during shock are included in the appropriate chapters.

The book unquestionably bears the stamp of a surgical university clinic, notably in the composition of the patient population. We are indebted to the Director of our Clinic, Professor Dr. F. LINDER, for his immediate, unstinting support and his contribution to the advancement of abdominal angiography.

Our thanks extend not only to our colleagues at the Clinic, but to all those who have frequently referred patients to us for angiographic examination from outside. We wish to thank Doctors H. CZEMBIREK, H.-J. ENCKE, and H. LOHÖLTER, former scientific assistants at the Department of Radiology, for their active collaboration in screening the patients, and our secretarial staff and technicians without whose devotion and enthusiasm the performance of the numerous angiographic examinations would not have been possible.

We are indepted to Dr. D. KAUFFMANN for his assistance in the English edition.

Credit for the drawings goes to H. HEINRICH, who showed uncommon skill in giving graphic expression to our ideas. Thanks are also due to Mr. KRAMER, our photography expert, for his untiring cooperation in the preparation of color radiographs.

The publishers, Springer-Verlag, have been extremely cooperative and liberal in their production of the book, and we are sincerely grateful.

Last but not least, we also want to express our appreciation to our patients! We endeavored to arrive at the correct diagnosis with the use of a new radiographic technique and so to open the way for a specific, goal-directed therapy. Without their "passive" cooperation, involving some unavoidable discomfort, this book could never have been written.

Heidelberg, November 1973 W. WENZ

Table of Contents

I Introduction and Historical Review

In contrast to the rapid progress of other methods of radiologic diagnosis, much time elapsed between the first angiographic demonstration of intra-abdominal changes by Dos Santos (1931) and the worldwide use being made today of radiologic techniques in the examination of abdominal vasculature.

No doubt the routine performance of abdominal angiography was considerably delayed by the fear of complications due to puncture of the abdominal aorta, as well as by a series of incidents occurring during studies by Ichikawa (1936) involving the surgical exposure of arteries for catheterization. It should be recognized, too, that leading scientists failed to grasp or at least misconstrued the clinical implications of the procedure.

Paul Lecene, for example, has been quoted as follows in the monograph published 1966 by Cormier and associates: "Reynaldo dos Santos' radiographs are very pretty and most certainly of interest to an anatomist, but I question that they would ever be useful to a surgeon."

This completely erroneous appraisal by a notable contemporary is by no means an isolated instance. Even in Germany, well into the fifties, there were still prominent clinic directors who strictly banned angiography, particularly of abdominal vessels.

What are the factors that ultimately led to a breakthrough in roentgenologic angiography?

Three important events should be cited:

1. The first translumbar aortography by direct puncture, proving the feasibility of radiologic visualization of abdominal vessels (Dos Santos et al., 1929).

2. Percutaneous catheterization with the aid of a cannula and a guide wire, without exposure of the artery (Seldinger, 1953).

3. Efforts by three independent research groups to make it possible for a catheter introduced into the vessel lumen to be passed into any of its branches (Oedman; Morino et al.; Tillander, 1956).

In the last analysis, it is to these authors that we owe our knowledge of the course of the celiac and superior mesenteric arteries.

Various methodological way stations still had to be passed before the present-day standardized technique could be developed.

Development of angiography

1928	Forssmann	Catheterization of the human vascular system
1928	Moniz	Carotid angiography
1929	Dos Santos	Translumbar aortography
1936	Ichikawa	Catheter aortography by way of surgically exposed peripheral artery
1951	Abeatici and Campi	Splenoportography
1951	Peirce	Percutaneous catheterization through cannula
1951	Bierman	Selective visceral catheter arteriography via surgically exposed carotid or brachial artery with topical injection of chemotherapeutic agents
1952	Kinmonth	Lymphangiography
1953	Seldinger	Percutaneous catheter aorto-arteriography using cannula and a guide wire
1956	Oedman; Tillander; Morino	Selective arteriography with curved plastic catheters
Further advances:		Superselective arteriography Pharmacoangiography Stereoangiography Magnification techniques Electronic optimization of angiograms Color subtraction Therapeutic use of visceral angiography

Still, the breakthrough to clinical application did not occur until after the routine use of visceral angiography by the Radiodiagnostic Department of the University Clinic in Lund,

Sweden, by OLLE OLSSON and his associates. The technique elaborated by his department was not only adopted by the other Scandinavian clinics but found acceptance throughout the world; it has also influenced the premises underlying this book.

Nevertheless, the technique would not have developed into a routine radiologic procedure had the equipment technology failed to keep pace. It took serial film changers, TV image-amplifying fluoroscopy, cinematography, and video tape recorders to make this success possible. The same is true of the development of less toxic contrast media which do not provoke adverse reactions except in very rare instances.

Countless authors, building systematically upon the state of the art attained, have proposed further improvements and modifications. These pertain to instrumentation, fluoroscopic and intensification techniques, photography, programming, access routes, and pharmacologic management, and, in no small measure, too, evaluation of angiograms by subtraction and color subtraction.

Abdominal angiography was given a further decisive impetus by radiologic research, which achieved significant advances in pharmacoangiography and in the study of tumors, hemorrhages, states of shock, and traumatic changes.

The following pages will report on the evolution to date and on the procedures followed at a clinic which has liberally fostered visceral angiography from the very start.

II Radiologic Anatomy of Abdominal Blood Vessels

The dominant vessel in the abdominal cavity is the abdominal aorta with its branches. Its diagnostic significance far surpasses that of the veins, including the portal vein. However, under certain circumstances, even these vascular regions may become important diagnostic routes as, for example, in portal hypertension (Fig. 1,2)[1].

1 Abdominal Aorta

In the absence of pathologic changes of the vascular wall, the abdominal aorta is a taut, smooth-walled vessel which drains rapidly and is, therefore, on occasion seen in poor contrast on the angiogram. Its branches arise at an acute angle and collaterals develop sparingly or not at all.

The caliber of the abdominal aorta decreases distally. In the adult, it averages 1.5 cm, but it may be as wide as 4 to 5 cm in the elderly (Fig. 10).

MERCIER and VANNEUVILLE (1968) draw a distinction between a "rectilinear" and a "sinuous" type, which they associate with a variety of vascular diseases in the aged. The numerous curves of the abdominal aorta continue into the pelvic arteries and are referred to as "kinking" in the Anglo-American literature (Figs. 22, 23). In these tortuous segments of the vessel, the flow rate of the blood is reduced, which not infrequently results in aortograms of particularly high contrast. As a rule, the angle of bifurcation is obtuse and numerous collateral vessels can be visualized. These are particularly marked in the presence of stenosis or occlusions.

1 Figs. 1–183 appear at the end of the text, on p. 115, beginning with the color photographs, in a separate section of illustrations.

The course of the abdominal aorta in relation to the vertebral column is of very special significance for lumbar aortography. The two French authors just cited found the abdominal aorta located medially in front on the vertebral column in 44% of cases, to the left alongside the column in 50% of cases, and to the right in just 6%. These data, however, are applicable only to a non-scoliotic lumbar column. In the presence of pronounced axial deviations—notably in kyphosis—the abdominal aorta will often extend in tendon fashion across the curvature, as exemplified in Fig. 98.

The level of the bifurcation is of special interest with regard to any direct puncture of the aorta, since variations are far from uncommon. According to PATURET (1951), the bifurcation is located at the level of the lower third of the fourth lumbar vertebra in 70% of all cases; less frequently it is at the level of the fifth lumbar vertebra (low bifurcation) or the upper third of the fourth lumbar (high bifurcation). In relation to the promontory, it may be assumed to be located 6 cm cranially. In three of our own patients, we observed an aortic bifurcation at the level of the third lumbar vertebra, so that for lumbar aortography, with the needle in typical position, iliac puncture proved possible at the level of the third or fourth lumbar vertebra.

While the angle of bifurcation is normally about 70 degrees, it may be different if the aorta and the pelvic arteries follow a tortuous course. With the so-called eccentric sinuous type (MERCIER and VANNEUVILLE, 1968) especially, angles between 10 and 20 degrees may be observed or, at the other extreme, nearly rectangular bends. Occasionally, they represent an insurmountable obstacle to passage of the catheter through the femoral artery. Experience has shown that access from the left pelvic artery is generally less difficult than from the right.

1.1 Symmetric Branches of the Abdominal Aorta

The first pair of symmetrical branches to arise from the abdominal aorta, just below the diaphragm, is composed of the right and left phrenic artery, at the level of the twelfth thoracic vertebra, just above the celiac trunk. Both arteries follow a steep craniolateral course. Two to three branches are distributed in the concavity of the diaphragm. Not infrequently, both arteries arise from a common trunk; they invariably give off branches to the adrenal glands (superior adrenal arteries).

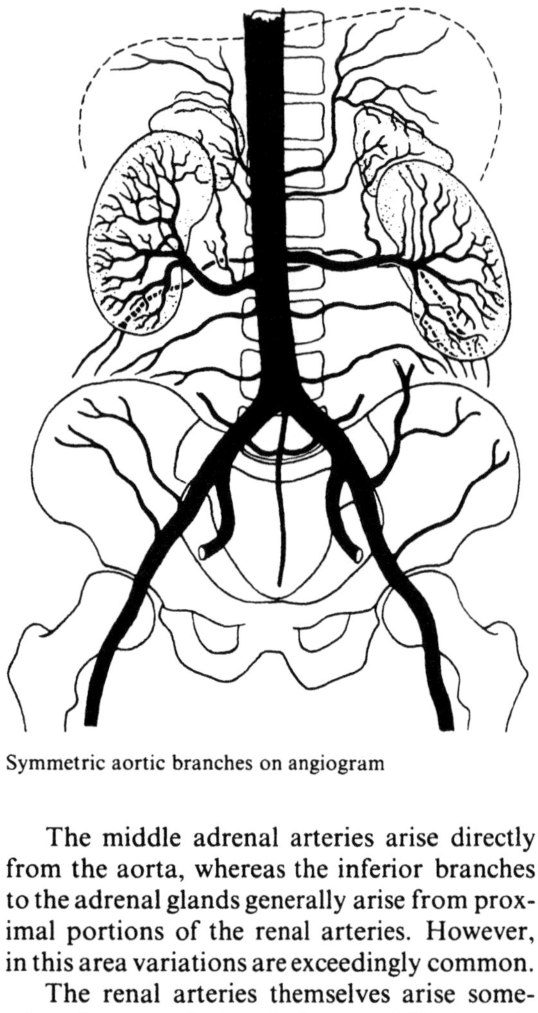

Symmetric aortic branches on angiogram

The middle adrenal arteries arise directly from the aorta, whereas the inferior branches to the adrenal glands generally arise from proximal portions of the renal arteries. However, in this area variations are exceedingly common.

The renal arteries themselves arise somewhere between the level of the twelfth thoracic vertebra and the second and third intervertebral disks. In the great majority of cases, they arise between the first and the second lumbar vertebra.

Merklin and Michels (1958) examined more than 11 000 kidneys and found one renal artery on each side in 72% of the cases, while in the remaining 28% of the kidneys there were multiple renal arteries, usually bilaterally. The symmetrically disposed metameric lumbar arteries arise mostly from the posterior or lateroposterior aspect of the abdominal aorta at the level of each lumbar vertebra; they usually extend no further than $^1/_2$ to 1 cm lateral to the margin of the psoas muscle, but they first give off branches to the spinal canal.

The spinal cord below C4 or C5 is supplied via the branches of the intercostal, lumbar, and sacral arteries, as well as by numerous anterior radicular arteries of varied configuration. The lowest radicular artery is nearly always the one with the largest caliber and is, therefore, also called the greater radicular artery (or Adamkiewicz artery). Its origin varies irregularly between D8 and L3, but more commonly between D9 and D11. Injury to this artery usually leads to severe neurologic disturbances, and for this reason special attention should be paid to this region in lumbar aortography as well as in selective explorations.

1.2 Visceral Branches of the Abdominal Aorta

1.2.1 Celiac Trunk

The first visceral branch of the abdominal aorta is the celiac trunk, arising just below the diaphragm, mostly at the level of the twelfth thoracic to first lumbar intervertebral disk. It arises ventrally and typically divides into three large branches: the hepatic, the splenic, and the left gastric artery (Fig. 24). Of all the visceral arteries, these show the most common anatomic variations and the most numerous anastomoses with other visceral and systemic arteries.

In 1965, Boijsen and associates catalogued the major variants involving the celiac trunk which in 2% of the cases (Paturet, 1951) shares a common origin with the superior mesenteric artery, forming the celiac-mesenteric trunk.

Generally, the trunk measures no more than a few cm in length, arises from the aorta at an acute angle of about 20°, initially keeps close to the anterior aspect of this vessel and

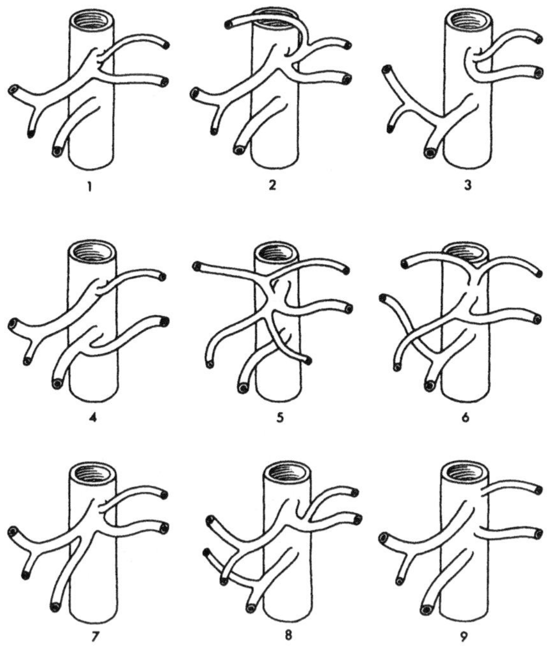

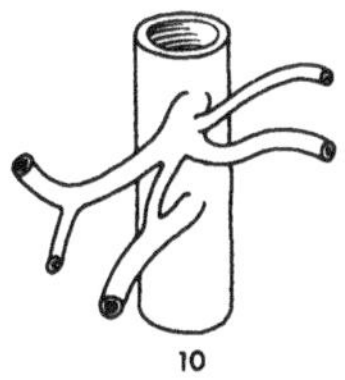

Normal variations of the celiac trunk, the superior mesenteric artery and its branches (according to BOIJSEN, 1965).

1. Normal branching of celiac trunk to the left into the left gastric artery (top) and the splenic artery (bottom). To the right is the common hepatic artery, which continues upward and laterally into proper hepatic artery and downward into the gastroduodenal artery. Caudal to the celiac trunk lies the superior mesenteric artery.
2. The left hepatic artery arising from the left gastric artery.
3. The common hepatic artery arising from the superior mesenteric artery.
4. Splenic artery arising from the superior mesenteric artery.
5. Middle colic artery arising from the celiac trunk.
6. Isolated origin of left gastric artery and left hepatic artery from the aorta. Right hepatic artery arising from superior mesenteric artery.
7. Celiac-mesenteric trunk.
8. Right hepatic artery arising from superior mesenteric.
9. Isolated origin of all celiac branches from aorta. No trunk.
10. Shunt between celiac trunk and trunk of superior mesenteric artery via dorsal pancreatic artery.

courses in a caudal direction, mostly somewhat to the right. In the adult, its caliber varies between 5 and 8 mm.

Instead of all three of these major branches sharing a common origin, the splenic and hepatic arteries alone may arise from a common trunk, while the left gastric artery arises separately from the aorta (as in 10% of cases examined by PATURET, 1951).

Angiographic differentiation of the trunk in an anteroposterior projection is extremely difficult because it appears punctiform if it follows a precise dorsoventral course and is largely concealed by the aorta when slightly inclined unless the examination is carried out in a selective manner. This explains why it is virtually impossible to visualize a stenosis of the celiac trunk except in lateral projection.

The branches arising from the trunk will be discussed when reference is made to the specific organs. They supply the major epigastric organs as well as the stomach and the duodenum.

1.2.2 Superior Mesenteric Artery

This artery, called "grande mésenterique" by the French, supplies by far the largest portion of the intestine (Figs. 2, 25), and is derived from the omphalomesenteric artery of the fetus.

It originates on the anterior aspect of the abdominal aorta, just below the celiac trunk —approximately at the level of the isthmus of the pancreas—is generally situated within the range of the upper third of the first lumbar vertebra, and has a caliber of 8–10 mm in the adult. It runs for a distance of 3 cm in a vertically caudal direction, then deviates from the aorta toward the uncinate process of the pancreas and along the ascending portion of the duodenum, and upon reaching the mesentery divides into numerous branches.

The anatomic location of the superior mesenteric artery also depends on the position of the spinal column. As a rule, the vessel runs left or right of the aorta, usually curving slightly to the right. Among the individual branches arising from the superior mesenteric artery, the retropancreatic segment lying close to the aorta is almost never identifiable in the angiogram. Collateral vessels in this area are inconsequential. The first ramifications ventral to the pancreas include the two pancreatico-duodenal arteries, the most important connecting passages to the celiac trunk, and the first two jejunal arteries. The right colic artery—the only one branching off to the right—is the first one to originate within the mesentery. On the left, another four to five jejunal and ileal branches extend to the small intestine. Between them and the ileocolic artery lies an area of peculiarly low vascularization.

Viewed laterally, there is an angle of 30–50° between the trunk of the superior mesenteric artery and the aorta, which plays an important role in arteriomesenteric compression of the duodenum.

Particular mention should be made here of the anastomosis between the right and left colic arteries which runs on a virtually horizontal plane from the right to the left side and assumes vital significance when one of the two mesenteric arteries is occluded; when this happens, its caliber increases considerably, and a so-called Riolan anastomosis is produced.

1.2.3 Inferior Mesenteric Artery

This artery, which supplies the left colon only, likewise arises from the ventral aspect of the abdominal aorta, 7 to 8 cm below the superior mesenteric and 4 to 5 cm above its bifurcation (Figs. 2, 26). Projected in relation to the lumbar column, its point of origin lies at the level of the lowest segment of the third lumbar vertebra, corresponding to the inferior (horizontal) part of the duodenum. In the aortogram, its origin may be found anywhere between the second and the fourth lumbar vertebrae. Its course nearly always slants downward to the left, so that in anteroposterior aortography its origin is even more difficult to discern than it is in the case of the superior mesenteric artery. The trunk of the vessel has an average length of 3.5 cm and a caliber averaging 5 mm. However, both the length and the caliber are subject to considerable variation. Its major branches are the left colic artery communicating with the right colic artery via RIOLAN's anastomosis; more distally, the sigmoid artery; and lastly, the superior hemorrhoidal artery, a particularly long vessel branching off at the level of the fifth lumbar vertebra and descending to the rectum. This branch forms anastomoses with the middle sacral artery, which arises directly from the bifurcation of the aorta, as well as with the inferior hemorrhoidal artery, hence the internal iliac artery.

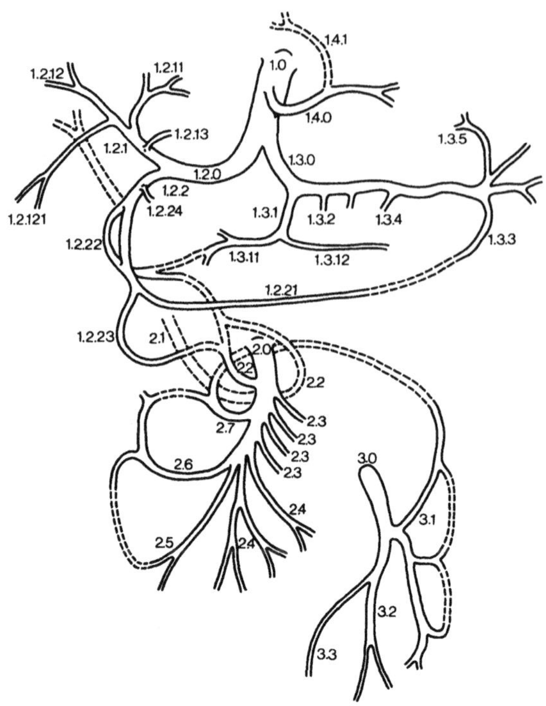

1.3 Nomenclature of Arterial Branches of Celiac Trunk and Mesenteric Arteries

(as proposed by RÜTTIMANN and BEELER, 1970)

1.0	*Celiac trunk*
1.2.0	Common hepatic artery
1.2.1	Proper hepatic artery
1.2.11	Left branch of proper hepatic artery
1.2.12	Right branch of proper hepatic artery
1.2.121	Cystic artery (in 75% of cases) Variant of 1.2.2 or 2.1
1.2.13	Right gastric artery
1.2.2	Gastroduodenal artery
1.2.21	Right gastroepiploic artery (anastomosing with 1.33)
1.2.22	Posterosuperior pancreaticoduodenal artery (forming an arcade with 2.2)
1.2.23	Anterosuperior pancreatico-duodenal artery (forming an arcade with 2.2)
1.2.24	Supraduodenal branches
1.3.0	Splenic artery
1.3.1	Dorsal pancreatic artery (anastomosing in 5% of cases with 1.0 and 2.0)

1.3.11 Right branch of dorsal pancreatic artery (forming KIRK's arcade with 1.2.23)
1.3.12 Transverse pancreatic artery (variant of 2.0, 1.2, 1.2.2)
1.3.2 Pancreatic branches
1.3.3 Left gastroepiploic artery (anastomosing with 1.2.21)
1.3.4 Arteria pancreatica magna
1.3.5 Short gastric artery

1.4.0 Left gastric artery
1.4.1 Left hepatic artery

2.0 *Superior mesenteric artery*

2.1 Right hepatic artery (variant in 25% of cases)
2.2 Inferior pancreaticoduodenal artery
2.3 Jejunal arteries
2.4 Ileal arteries
2.5 Ileocolic artery
2.6 Right colic artery
2.7 Middle colic artery

3.0 *Inferior mesenteric artery*

3.1 Left colic artery
3.2 Sigmoid artery
3.3 Superior rectal (hemorrhoidal) artery

2 Inferior Vena Cava

The inferior vena cava is formed by the confluence of the right and left common iliac veins at the level of the lower margin of the fourth lumbar vertebra. The confluence is situated caudad and to the right of the aortic bifurcation. In cranial direction, the inferior vena cava follows the aorta on the right side up to the level of the second lumbar vertebra, where it deviates ventrally and to the right leading into the foramen of the vena cava within the diaphragm (Fig. 31).

Along its path, the vena cava is in close contact with the right side of the lumbar column, the root of mesentery, the sympathetic trunk, the head of the pancreas and adjoining duodenum, as well as the right kidney and adrenal gland.

Inasmuch as the portal vein carries the blood of the entire gastrointestinal tract and the spleen into the liver, only the hepatic veins, being unpaired, open into the inferior vena cava within or just below the diaphragm. The paired roots of these hepatic veins match the configuration of the aortic branches to the gastrointestinal tract.

A lengthwise anastomosis connecting the four lumbar veins is known as the ascending lumbar vein. It derives from the common iliac vein and ascends in the iliopsoas muscle to the side of the lumbar column in a craniad course. From the abdomen, each ascending lumbar vein runs through a cleft in the medial crus of the diaphragm into its thoracic continuation as the azygos and hemiazygos vein.

3 Portal Vein

The portal vein arises behind the head of the pancreas by the union of its three roots: the superior and inferior mesenteric veins and the splenic vein (Fig. 32). Behind it lies the inferior vena cava in the retroperitoneal cavity. Craniad, the portal vein is crossed ventrally by the superior portion of the duodenum and so reaches the hepatoduodenal ligament; close to the porta hepatis it divides into the right and the left branch.

The tributaries of the portal vein in this region are small veins, such as the gastric veins, and, in the immediate vicinity of its bifurcation, the cystic vein. In addition, minute paraumbilical veins coursing alongside the obliterated umbilical vein in the ligamentum teres hepatis drain into the portal venous system of the liver.

III Angiographic Technique

1 Basic Considerations

For the patient, angiography is invariably a stressful procedure owing to both the manipulation of the vascular system and the injection of a contrast medium. Discriminating use of the technique is, therefore, imperative. It is indicated only in situations in wich less drastic measures prove diagnostically or therapeutically unsatisfactory.

The conventional examination of the gastrointestinal tract with a barium meal permits visualization of the interior surface of the lumen but provides no information about the bowel wall or the interior of parenchymatous organs. Angiography, on the other hand, makes it possible to visualize the intestinal wall itself, to collect information about the major abdominal organs and, last but not least, to visualize the vascular network down to its smallest ramifications.

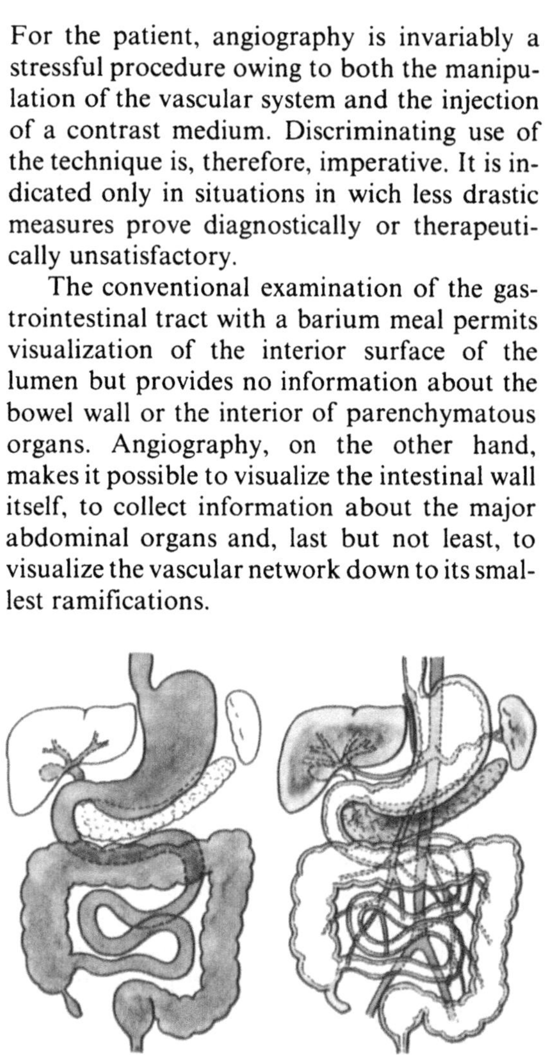

Therefore, the first prerequisites for angiography are consultation with the referring physician, familiarity with clinical and laboratory test data previously obtained, and a critical review of available x-ray studies (plain films, upper GI series, barium enema, cholecystography, and excretory urography).

As a rule, these examinations provide little, if any, information about the abdominal vascular system, with the exception of readily defined, dense soft-tissue "tumors" in the presence of a circumscribed aneurysm of the abdominal aorta, or widening of the aortal segment extending from the thorax into the abdomen in dissecting aneurysm, which may sometimes be visualized even more readily by tomography.

Calcium deposits in Mönckeberg's medial sclerosis, arteriosclerosis, aneurysms, and angiomas at times produce impressive findings.

We should mention, in particular, the recurrent finding of calcified deposits within the splenic artery, recognizable by its typically tortuous course, which are revealed by the contrast medium. Not infrequently, there is a marked disproportion between the spherically disposed calcific shells of the outer strata of an aneurysm—ranging up to a child's head in size—and the often extremely narrow, open internal lumen which is evaluable only by contrast radiography.

2 Patient Preparation and Contraindications

Just as the anesthetist makes his rounds on the eve of the operation, the radiologist, too, should examine the candidate for angiography beforehand and plan his strategy in advance.

In the final analysis, it is the condition of the peripheral vessels which determines the best possible access route. The same applies to the pelvic veins or to a projected splenoportography (determination of size and position of spleen).

A calm and factual explanation to the patient is of considerable importance for the success of the angiographic examination. Even children that are shown how to follow the procedure on the TV screen become cooperative partners in angiography. We try in every case to convince the patient of the need for radiography of his vessels, except of course in acute emergencies, in young children, or in patients who are in very poor general condition.

It is advisable to prescribe a mild sedative or hypnotic on the eve of the angiography. *Premedication* is administered thirty minutes before the operation. We have obtained good results with 0.0005 g of atropine and 0.05 g of intramuscular meperidine.

The recommended premedication for abdominal catheter procedures in children at the Boston Children's Hospital Medical Center comprises a cocktail of 6.25 mg promethazine, 6.25 mg Thorazine, and 25 mg of Demerol in 1 ml. The volume administered is 1 ml per 15 kg of body weight, but never more than a total of 2 ml. Children weighing more than 40 kg received Demerol and Nembutal. In the case of minors, we should not neglect to secure the parents' written consent as well as to explain to the children, just as to the adults, the nature and justification for the procedure. Contraindications to angiography include severe kidney disease, particularly multiple myeloma or other dysproteinemias with renal damage; serious manifestations of cardiac or hepatic insufficiency; hemorrhagic diathesis (Quick value at least 60%, platelet count more than 50000/cu.mm); heparinization. Other contraindications are infections at the puncture site and fever.

3 Equipment

The most important requirement is a room in which the radiologist can work under sterile conditions and perform the angiographic examination without any distractions or interference; next, efficient x-ray equipment with image amplifier circuits and film changers (Fig. 38) is required.

The description of our equipment is in no way intended to imply that it represents the optimum selection and arrangement, but over a number of years it has proved to be a workable system in spite of the considerable turnover of technicians and trainees as well as of visiting radiologists.

The equipment should be ready for use at a moment's notice, particularly with a view to emergency angiography. We use metal cases to store a complete set of instruments for:

1. Translumbar aortography, direct puncture arteriography, and venography.
2. Arterial or venous catheter angiography.
3. Pediatric catheter angiography.
4. Splenoportography.

The details are indicated in Fig. 39. Each case contains several 30–50 cc syringes with the Luer-Lock attachment for saline solution or contrast medium, cannulas for direct puncture or for the SELDINGER catheter, one wide cannula for aspiration of contrast medium and, in the case of direct puncture, connecting tubes. Disposable syringes are used for local anesthesia. 1% novocaine is kept in a measuring cylinder, small bowls are provided for the heparinized saline solution, and an enamelware dish holds the same solution for catheters. One sterilized incision scalpel and two drape sheets, one of them with a long slit, complete the kit.

Catheters and guide wires, arranged according to length and purpose, are kept in a mesh-type holder in glass tubes sealed at one end, for easy removal of catheters from sterilizing fluid with forceps. We use Johnson & Johnson's *Alhydex* for sterilization.

4 Contrast Media and Adverse Reactions

For abdominal angiography contrast media are available which couple high-contrast density with very fast renal elimination and low toxicity. These are water-soluble tri-iodated compounds suitable for fast injection in relatively high doses (the ones most commonly used in Germany are Schering's *Urografin* and Byk-Gulden's *Conray*).

Injection of the contrast medium causes a transient burning sensation of rapid onset, notably in the area supplied by the arteries of the limbs. In the case of visceral arteries, the patient experiences a sensation of heat which is not particularly troublesome as a rule. As long as the patient is properly forewarned, he will not overreact to the sensation of heat with any abrupt movements that might spoil the angiogram.

Systemic reactions are infrequent, but caution is in order in patients with a known history of allergy. The best safeguard against unpleasant surprises is slow injection of 2 to 3 ml of contrast medium through a cannula or catheter and close observation of the patient. Erythema of skin and mucous membranes, taste sensations, headache, dizziness and circulatory reactions are all warning signs of a possible pathologic response. In such cases, before proceeding with the angiography, we give the patient an intravenous injection of 50–100 mg Solu-Decortin Merck, and an antihistamine or calcium preparations if skin wheals or mucosal edema develop (use caution in digitalized patients).

A test for hypersensitivity to the contrast medium affords no protection against untoward incidents and is, therefore, no longer required prior to angiography.

The dosage of the contrast medium depends upon the vascular region to be studied. As little as 3–5 ml may suffice for selective angiography of a suprarenal artery or the inferior phrenic artery; on the other hand, an average 50 ml of a highly concentrated medium is needed for survey aortography.

The examination may be repeated without any hazard. Similarly, it is permissible to make repeated injections of contrast medium into different visceral arteries; as a rule of thumb, we recommend adult doses not exceeding 100 ml of a 76% or 80% tri-iodated contrast medium. In tracing the source of unexplained bleeding, we have used on our patients doses as high as 160 ml of 76% Urografin without provoking any clinically detectable reaction.

In children, the manufacturer's directions should be followed. Not more than 2 ml/kg of a 60% contrast medium should be used in children weighing less than 40 kg, except that for survey aortography we use 15–25 ml of 76% Urografin even in young children.

Anyone performing angiography must be prepared for the possibility of contrast medium incidents.

Precautionary measures for administration of contrast media (as suggested by JUST, 1972)

1. Obtain specific history (allergy?)
2. Inject into supine patient
3. Leave the cannula i. v.
4. Keep the patient under close observation, particularly after the injection
5. Allergic individuals receive prophylactically
   a) antihistaminics i. v.
   b) cortisone derivatives i. v.
6. Keep apparatus, instruments, and drugs handy for immediate use

Allergic skin reactions

Symptoms	*Therapy*
Erythema	Calcium i. v.
Urticaria	Antihistamines i. v.
Pruritus	Cortisone derivatives i. v.
Wheals	
Palpebral edema	

Mild systemic side effects

Symptoms	*Therapy*
Nausea	Provide fresh air
Vomiting	Apply oxygen
Heat sensations	Keep under medical supervision
Sneezing	Valium i. v.
Coughing	

Severe systemic reactions

Respiratory symptoms	*Cardiovascular symptoms*	*Neurologic symptoms*
Tachypnea	Pallor	Trousseau's phenomenon
Dyspnea	Oppressive feeling	Convulsive states
Bronchospasm	Hyperhidrosis	Syncope
Asthmatic attacks	Hypotension	Tonic-clonic spasms
Edema of the glottis	Feeling of annihilation	
	Shock	

Therapy in contrast medium incidents

Respiration

Keep respiratory passages open
Check spontaneous respiration
Supply oxygen
Provide artificial respiration
 a) Mask
 b) Tracheal tube

Circulation

Volume replacement
6% Macrodex

Haemaccel
Gelifundol (plasma substitute)

Corticosteroids

Urbason Soluble
Dexa Scheroson

Sedatives

Valium
Meperidine
Droperidol

Vasopressors

Novadral
Norepinephrine
Hypertensin

Barbiturates

Hexabarbital
Thiopental sodium

Clinical symptoms in contrast medium incidents

System	Stage 1 (excitation phase)	Stage 2 (paralytic phase)
Central nervous system	Drowsiness, restlessness, heat sensations, nervousness, anxiety, dilatation of the pupils, disorientation, tremor, dizziness, spasms, tinnitus, deafness	Unconsciousness, coma, complete sensorimotor paralysis
Autonomic system	Excitation, pallor, hyperhidrosis, salivation or dryness of mouth and throat, nausea, vomiting	Blockage of impulses, profuse perspiration, incontinence, sphincter paralysis
Cardiovascular system	Convulsive hypertension, bradycardia or tachycardia	Abrupt blood pressure drop to shock level, tachycardia followed by cardiac failure (myocardial insufficiency and conduction disorders)
Respiratory system	Increased respiratory rate, hyperpnea and agitated respiration	Cyanosis, increasing respiratory paralysis to respiratory standstill (of central and peripheral origin)

Equipment for management of contrast medium incidents (as suggested by Just, 1972)

Essential	+ Optional	+ Optimal
Guedel tubes	Intubation kit	Anesthesia set
Bottled oxygen	Suction machine	Respirator
Ambu bag	Bellows respirator	
Respirator masks in assorted sizes		
Braun cannulas	ECG scanners	Cardioverter
Disposable syringes	Long needles for i.c. injections	Cardio-resuscitators
Plasma expander	Cardiotonics:	Lung resuscitators
Circulatory stimulants	Epinephrine	
	10% calcium	
	Alupent	
Sedatives		
Cortisone derivatives		
Barbiturates		

5 Aorto-Arteriography

To visualize the aorta and its abdominal branches, the following access routes are technically available:

1. Translumbar aortography.
2. Catheter aorto-arteriography.
3. Retrograde arteriography.
4. Intravenous aortography.

At our clinic, the catheter method is by far the most common. It enables us to probe and visualize selectively from the femoral or brachial arteries the entire aorta, including individual branches of the first and second order.

Conversely, translumbar aortography is limited to the visualization of aortic alterations and lesions of its major branches, while the finer details of peripheral vessels and the parenchyma, the filling of the intestinal wall and the venous system remain hidden by the superimposition of numerous vascular branches of different origin and the excessive dilution of the contrast medium.

Nevertheless, translumbar aortography is the preferred procedure in states of advanced vascular obstruction or tortuosity, in which this technique, applied in tiers, is eminently useful in answering the question whether or not to attempt surgical reconstruction of the vessel. In Scandinavian countries, where the incidence of arterial occlusive diseases is far lower, subdiaphragmatic aortography is seldom employed.

Among our patients, the only indication for retrograde aorto-arteriography was occult aneurysm in the abdominal cavity in persons of advanced age whom we wished to spare the hazards of anesthesia; the primary question in such instances is whether or not to operate. Apart from that, the procedure was also applied in kidney transplants (Fig. 34).

Intravenous aortography is hardly a promising procedure for the detection of pathologic changes in the abdominal area on account of the excessive dilution of the contrast medium on its way through the pulmonary vascular system.

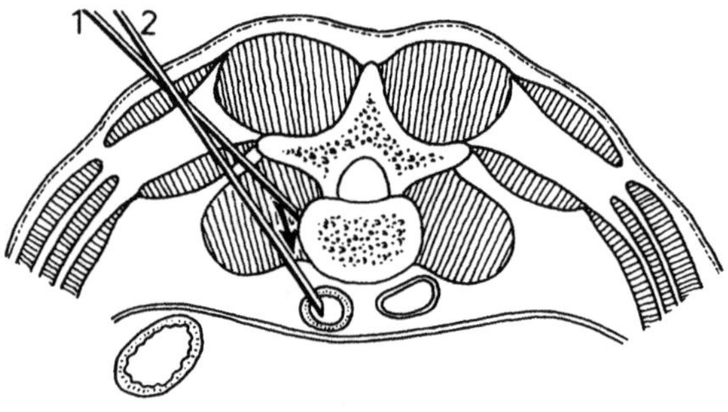

Puncturing technique for direct aortography

5.1 Translumbar Aortography

This technique calls for sturdy needles with an outside diameter of 2 mm and a length between 12 and 18 cm. (Once we had a special 28-cm needle made to order for translumbar aortography of an obese cook who weighed nearly 300 lbs.). The bevels of the needles are ground short; an obturator with the fitted bevel is used during the puncture. As a rule, translumbar aortic puncturing is done under anesthesia, but some authors prefer local anesthesia for this procedure.

The patient is positioned prone on the table. The needle is introduced at a hand's breadth to the left of the medial line, midway between the lower margin of the costal arch and the iliac crest. Next, for subdiaphragmatic or "high" aortography, the tip of the needle is pointed in the direction of the 12th thoracic vertebra, while for low translumbar aortography the target is the third lumbar vertebra.

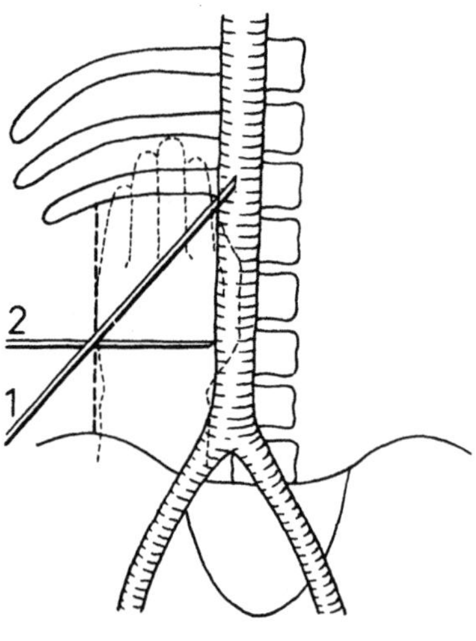

Puncture site for direct aortography

Blunt obturators may be inserted to check for proper positioning of the tip of the needle inside the aorta. We have dispensed with this procedure, preferring instead to inject a few ml of the contrast agent and check the location of the tip with the aid of TV image amplifiers.

In puncturing the aorta, one should bypass the region between the first and second lumbar vertebrae because of the large arteries that originate at this level.

Further, as we shall have occasion to discuss in greater detail in connection with neurologic complications of aortography, there are hazards involved in direct puncture of major lumbar branches of the artery.

Ventral to the transverse processes of the vertebrae, the needle is passed up to the lateral aspect of the vertebra; once there, the needle is placed at a somewhat steeper angle so that the tip will move past the body of the vertebra toward the aorta. With some experience, it is possible to detect the pulsations with the tip of the needle.

In puncturing the vessel itself, it is necessary to overcome a slight resistance, but care must be taken not to perforate the opposite wall. If the obturator is withdrawn from the needle early enough, that is, prior to actual puncture of the aorta, blood will gush out of the cannula in a strong stream synchronous with the pulse once the lumen of the vessel has been penetrated. If the blood drips from the needle under no great pressure, it must be assumed that the position of the needle is faulty. More than once we have found the tip of the needle resting in a lumbar artery or in one of the larger veins. In such cases it is always advisable to withdraw the needle immediately and repeat the puncture, changing the direction of the needle. Of course, the weak stream of blood may also be due to circulatory depression associated with anesthesia.

The contrast medium may be injected manually, but serial films are needed for simultaneous visualization of the abdominal aorta, the pelvic arteries, and the vessels in the extremities. The timing of such exposure must be necessarily brief, so that the films are usually exposed at 70 to 90 kv. In the majority of visceral angiographies, a sequence of two pictures per second is sufficient to visualize all opacifications over a span of some 15 seconds. It is advisable to take a delayed picture as long as 25 seconds after the injection in order to assess venous filling via the mesenteric veins and the splenic vein.

In uncomplicated situations, we follow a routine which comprises exposing two films per second in the first few seconds, followed by three pictures at one-second intervals, and another three at 3-second intervals. This routine has enabled us to prepare satisfactory angiograms in the majority of cases. Of course, extra pictures may be needed, with the filming time extended to 25 seconds, in attempts to localize bleeding sites or to ensure visualization of the splenic vein and the portal vein in portal hypertension.

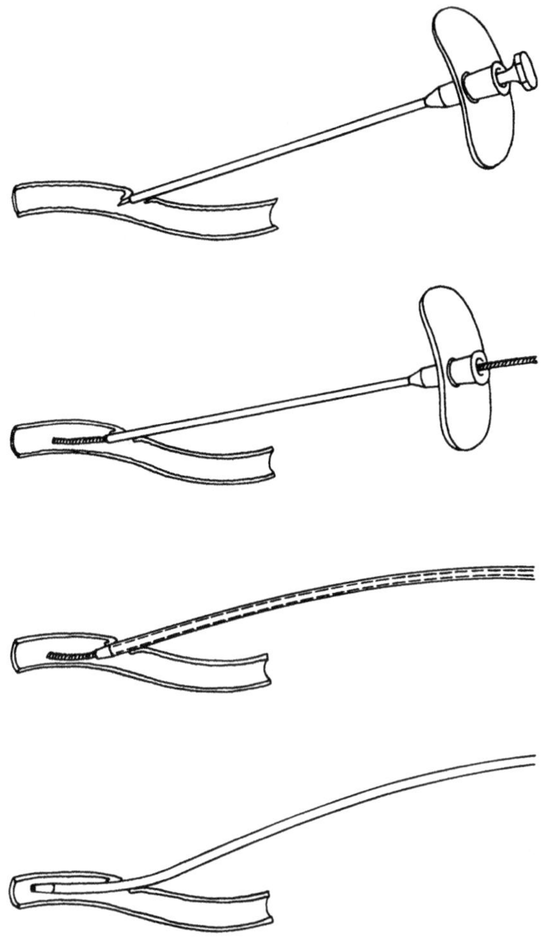

Principle of Seldinger technique

5.2 Indirect or Catheter Aorto-Arteriography

Indirect aorto-arteriography by the method of Seldinger calls for insertion of a catheter into the aorta via a peripheral vessel. For this, special radiolucent polyethylene catheters as well as radiopaque catheters of different diameters are available (Oedman, Judkins, etc.). As a rule, the catheter is inserted into the femoral artery and advanced upstream to the blood flow in the aorta. In the presence of occlusion or severe »kinking« of the pelvic arteries and aorta, the catheter may also be inserted through a brachial or axillary artery. According to Boijsen (1966), this access route is particularly advantageous for superselective visceral arteriography since the tip of the catheter is moved in the direction of flow in the unpaired aortic branches.

The femoral artery is punctured with a needle according to Seldinger (P.E. 160) under local anesthesia. General anesthesia is occasionally required in youngsters. The youngest child ever examined under local anesthesia at our clinic was seven years old. Typically, the cannula is inserted retrograde into the artery by puncturing the femoral artery two fingerbreadths below the inguinal ligament, a site that readily lends itself to compression during and after the angiography. Puncturing the artery at a higher level might result in considerable undetected bleeding into the retroperitoneal region.

Once the cannula has been inserted and the obturator removed, a guide wire (P.E. 160) is carefully threaded through its lumen, flexible end first. The cannula must be held flat and parallel to the course of the artery. The flexible wire must slide without any resistance; in most cases it is possible to negotiate even fairly sharp vascular bends with the aid of a J-shaped guide wire suggested for this use by Baum (1964). If force is used, one risks perforating the vascular wall, detaching a clot or breaking off the tip of the wire.

When the tip of the guide lies above the bifurcation of the abdominal aorta, the cannula is withdrawn and the catheter is inserted into the aorta over the guide wire.

In order to minimize vascular trauma caused by the catheter and avoid an excessively wide puncture hole, the catheter tip is carefully tapered before use over a flame or with the aid of hot air, so that it may closely adjoin the guide wire for a short distance.

Inasmuch as most catheters are used repeatedly and the tip is subject to very rapid fraying, it is advisable to cut off the worn portion before use with a sharp scalpel. The curvature of the tip of the catheter used in selective arteriography is adapted to the shape of the particular branch of the aorta. For example, the renal arteries can be readily explored as a rule with a catheter in the shape of a shepherd's staff. On the other hand, a much sharper curvature is needed for the celiac and superior mesenteric arteries. More difficult explorations, e.g. of the inferior mesenteric artery or the lumbar branches and minor ramifications such as the inferior phrenic arteries and the adrenal arteries, require an S-bend in the catheter end. Care must be taken that the curvature is somewhat greater than the anticipated width of the aortic lumen; what this means in practice is that for younger individuals the curvature must be relatively narrow, while in older patients with signs of generalized arteriosclerosis the radius of curvature should be greater.

The catheters proposed by JUDKINS are easily maneuverable, but their tip has a relatively low taper and therefore needs an adapter for dilation of the opening into the punctured vessel. An example of superselective arteriography of a minor vessel branching out from the arterial trunk is shown in Fig. 28.

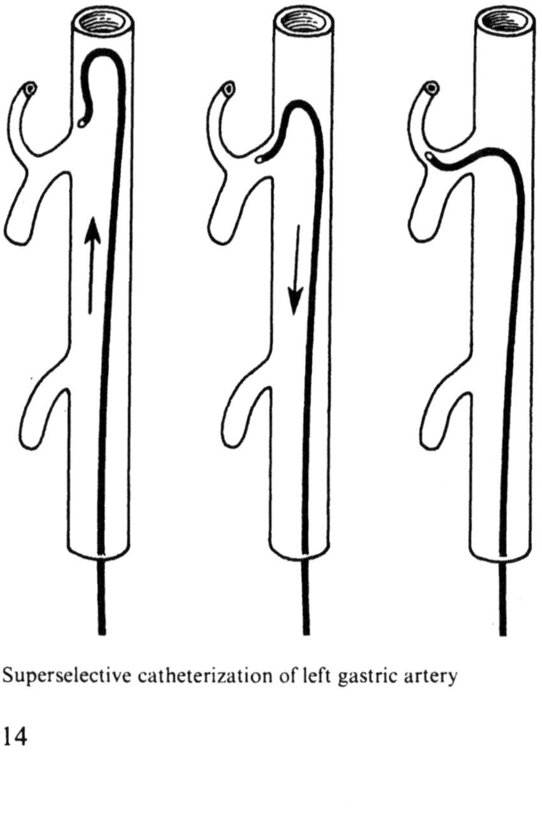

Superselective catheterization of left gastric artery

As soon as the catheter tip has reached the desired arterial level, the guide wire is removed, the catheter is connected to a stopcock and rinsed with heparinized saline solution (1 ml in 1000 ml of physiologic saline). We have the impression that this procedure, suggested by OLSSON's Radiologic Institute in Lund, Sweden, has been very valuable and has minimized the development of blood clots at the catheter tip.

The contrast medium should not be injected unless there is good backflow of blood from the catheter. Before injection of the diagnostic dose of the radiopaque material, a few ml should be injected on a trial basis to monitor the position of the tip with the aid of a TV image amplifier.

Fully automatic contrast medium injectors make it possible to adapt the flow of the medium to specific conditions and to inject an adequate dose of contrast medium in unit time even with a small-bore catheter that is apt to be far less traumatic to the artery (Fig. 38a: *Contrac* Automatic Contrast Medium Injector, Siemens-Erlangen).

Serial films can be prepared in any sequence during injection of the radiopaque substance. For example, to pinpoint a stenosis at the origin of a major aortic branch, 2 to 3 roentgenograms a second are needed from the very start of the injection.

Following the examination, the catheter is slowly withdrawn, while 15–20 ml of heparinized saline solution is continuously administered, to prevent dislodging platelet clumps at the puncture site that might cause local thromboses. The puncture site is compressed by hand for about 10 minutes until bleeding has stopped. In hypertensive patients, compression is performed for half an hour. A compression bandage is then applied and left in place for one or two days. The puncture site is weighted down with a sandbag for 4 to 6 hours. The patient must be transported in a supine position and kept in bed for 24 hours.

The distal end of the catheters normally used in SELDINGER's technique may be occluded by passing tiny spheres suspended on a thin wire through the catheter as far as the tip so that the contrast medium can only escape through the side holes.

One disadvantage is the resultant constriction of the lumen which retards the flow of the contrast material per unit time.

In elderly patients, arteriosclerosis may make it impossible to pass the catheter through the narrowed vessel; in such cases, one may nevertheless obtain good definition of the abdominal aorta down to the renal arteries with the aid of so-called retrograde aortography.

5.3 HETTLER's Percutaneous Catheter Method

The method devised by HETTLER (1960, 1969) adapts to percutaneous catheter procedures the advantages of the closed-end catheter with side holes which have long been known in the angiographic study of the heart and the aorta. With the aid of a specially constructed insertion cannula, a thin-walled teflon-coated external cannula is inserted into the femoral artery and through it the closed-end catheter can be effortlessly introduced into the vascular lumen.

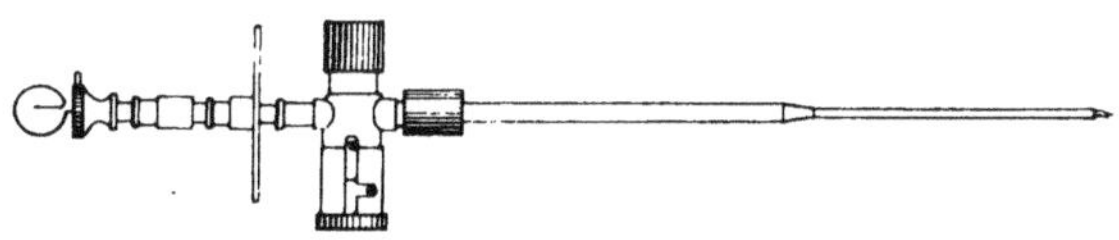

Hettler sheath

Important advantages of this method are the facility with which catheters can be interchanged (e. g. for superselective angiography), the use of closed-end catheters for semi-selective aortography, and the avoidance of excessively sharp catheter tips that can cause intimal lesions.

A disadvantage is seen in the fact that the teflon sleeve always produces a somewhat larger opening in the vascular wall than is produced with SELDINGER's technique. However, comparative investigations (HETTLER, 1969) have shown that complications are no more frequent than with the usual SELDINGER method.

We have no personal experience with this technique but believe that it is an excellent one. However, one should primarily familiarize oneself with *one* technique and try to master that one to perfection.

5.4 Retrograde Arterio-Aortography

Retrograde aortography is based on the principle of introducing into the lumen of the femoral artery a needle (SELDINGER's cannula) of sufficient caliber and injecting a highly concentrated radiopaque material at a rate of 10–20 ml/sec, extending the radiopaque column as far as the origin of the renal artery. In lieu of a cannula, some authors employ a teflon catheter needle, the needle being withdrawn again and the contrast medium injected through the catheter. The level to which contrast reaches is, of course, determined by the existing blood pressure, by curvatures and stenoses of the vessel, as well as by the position of the cannula. This method affords the great advantage of obviating the need for long catheters and at the same time sparing the patient the discomfort of a translumbar puncture. LUDIN et al. (1965) recommend retrograde aortography particularly for outpatients, who only need to rest for a few hours after the examination and may then be sent back home. The method is especially suited to unilateral obliterative changes in the area of the pelvic arteries: the contrast medium is injected from the healthy contralateral side and as a rule the distal portion of the abdominal aorta and its bifurcation can be visualized in such a way that a bilateral peripheral angiogram can be obtained in the same session.

5.5 Intravenous Aortography

In exceptional cases in which the aorta is inaccessible to exploration by any of the techniques described, the aortography may be undertaken by the intravenous route; this procedure is particularly recommended when dissecting aneurysms of the aorta are suspected. It yields a fairly good definition of the thoracic aorta, whereas the abdominal segment and its branches are usually poorly defined owing to the diminishing contrast. Prerequisites for satisfactory radiographs are the availability of a high-speed serial film changer as well as bilateral injection of 30–50 ml of a highly concentrated contrast medium into the median cubital vein (STEINBERG, 1965) or injection of the agent via a catheter introduced into the right heart from the cubital or femoral vein.

5.6 Special Techniques

The angiographic techniques mentioned so far have been improved by different authors or expanded by combination with other methods. Thus, NORDENSTRÖM (1962) utilized a percutaneously introduced balloon catheter, temporarily occluding the aorta.

HERNANDEZ and associates (1965) enhanced the quality of their roentgenograms by injecting physiologic saline and Xylocaine immediately after the radiopaque medium, enabling more rapid and clearcut separation of the individual phases ("embol pulsé").

For better assessment of abdominal neoformations, O'HALLORAN and KAHN (1969) suggest concomitant aortography and cavography, with insertion of separate catheters into the femoral artery and the femoral vein of the same leg. The method is designed to identify the impressions of the aorta or major arterial branches on the vena cava and to differentiate them from tumor impressions.

6 Portography

Numerous methods have been proposed for the visualization of the portal vein. The following access routes have found acceptance:

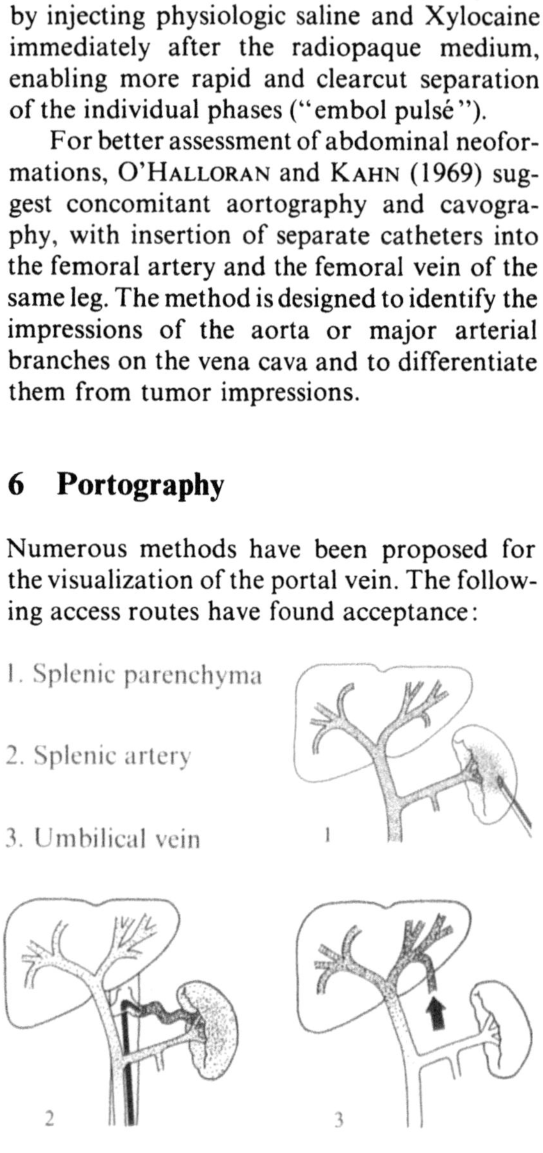

6.1 Splenoportography

This technique has remained essentially unchanged since its initial description by ABEATICI and CAMPI (1951): Fluoroscopy and localization of spleen. Local anesthesia in the 10th or 11th left intercostal space after premedication as described for aorto-arteriography. Stab incision of the skin and insertion of a teflon needle (Long-Dwel catheter, Becton, Dickinson & Co.).

For the examination, the patient holds his breath for a short time until the tip of the needle approaches midpoint in the shadow of the spleen. The needle is removed, leaving the plastic catheter *in situ*, and the patient is allowed to resume breathing. If the catheter is properly positioned, blood will drip out profusely.

With the aid of a graduated manometer filled with heparinized saline solution a pressure reading is taken after which a test injection of about 5 ml Urografin 76% is given. If one of the major branches of the splenic vein fills up immediately, the tip of the catheter is positioned correctly.

We have found in comparative tests in 36 patients studied before and during surgery that the intrasplenic pressure is normally less than 20 cm water column and conforms at a variance of ± 5 cm H_2O to the pressure in the portal vein. Readings above 25 cm H_2O signify portal hypertension.

Serial angiography requires the injection of 30 ml Urografin 76%—at a rate of 10–12 ml/sec—to obtain 8 films at one-second intervals, followed by two films every three seconds (Fig. 32a).

According to the method proposed by WANNAGAT (1959), the spleen is punctured during laparoscopy and application of a pneumoperitoneum. This *laparoscopic splenoportography* combines the advantages of laparoscopy with those of direct catheterization of the spleen.

One of the possible complications of this method is bleeding, especially from the puncture channels created by repeated puncture attempts. Among the first fifty splenoportographies performed at our clinic under anesthesia and with rigid cannulas, we had one instance of severe intraperitoneal bleeding necessitating removal of the spleen. No such complications have occurred since the introduction of plastic catheters.

BOIJSEN (1968) has called attention to the possible development of aneurysms of the splenic artery as a late complication of splenoportography.

The indication for splenoportography is closely related to the possibility of measuring intrasplenic pressure. Consequently, it is the technique of choice in the presence of suspected or clinically established portal hypertension suggesting surgical intervention.

6.2 Arterioportography

BOIJSEN and associates, in 1963, were the first to call attention to the possibility of visualizing the splenic vein, hence indirectly the portal venous system, by injection of the contrast medium via the splenic artery. Utilizing this method, WENZ (1965) was able to visualize selectively an arterioportal shunt of the vessels at the hilus of the spleen with giant aneurysms (Fig. 138).

It is a simple technique in selective visceral arteriography, utilizing the celiac, or superior or inferior mesenteric artery, as an approach in splenectomized patients.

In splenic arteriography, the concentration of the radiopaque material achieved in the splenic, hence the portal vein, is a function of the size of the organ. In splenomegaly, the contrast medium is absorbed as by a big sponge. Initially, poor filling of the efferent veins had led us to assume that there was an obstruction of the splenic vein, but subsequent splenoportography showed this to be incorrect.

In any event, therefore, approximately 40 ml of radiopaque material is required, but this cannot be injected at a rate faster than 6 to 10 ml/sec since greater pressure may cause the catheter tip to snap back into the aorta.

In cases of *postsplenectomy bleeding*, visualization of the portal vein via one of the mesenteric arteries is of considerable importance. This examination is indispensable when a shunt operation is planned.

The indications for arterioportography are:

1. *Postsplenectomy bleeding*. Once the spleen has been removed, there can be no splenoportography.
2. *Unsuccessful splenoportography*—very small spleen or atypical location.
3. *Splenic puncture contraindicated because of inflammatory or malignant spleen changes.*
4. *Arteriovenous fistula*. Arterioportography alone makes it possible to differentiate fully between the arterial and the venous network.

6.3 Omphaloportography (Umbilical Venography)

Portography by way of the open umbilical vein is a simple procedure in the newborn but very rarely necessary in these cases (liver tumor, occlusion of portal vein).

Lately, it has been applied to adults as well, an incision being made over the ligamentum teres which is dissected free. This is followed by re-establishing the patency of the vessel, which may be probed past its opening into the left portal vein. An injection of contrast medium (40–50 ml Urografin 76%) yields angiograms of exceptional quality (Fig. 32b). The portal vein pressure can be measured directly.

Nevertheless, the considerable operative effort required to visualize the ligamentum teres and the occasional failures associated with attempts to reopen the umbilical vein militate against routine employment of this method.

The indication of choice for omphaloportography in the adult is continuous perfusion of the liver with a chemotherapeutic agent, in other words, a therapeutic goal. When all other methods have failed to visualize the intrahepatic portal venous system, one can resort to this technique for diagnostic purposes as well. (For details on the diagnostic and therapeutic significance of transumbilical catheterization of the portal vein, see WIRBATZ, 1971).

7 Cavography

Nowadays the method of choice for the contrast radiography of the inferior vena cava is the simultaneous injection of both femoral veins, readily accessible from the region of the inguinal ligament. Puncture is facilitated if the patient is instructed to execute the Valsalva maneuver; under these conditions, the needle – identical to the one used for femoral arteriography – enters medially to the palpable femoral artery. The tip of the needle is then threaded a few cm craniad with the aid of a flexible guide wire (Fig. 31).

Other authors essentially rely on plastic catheters, introduced in the manner proposed by SELDINGER. Inasmuch as one occasionally finds a so-called pelvic venous spur on the left side, just below the confluence of the two iliac veins, we prefer to inject the contrast medium into both femoral veins for cavography.

Amount of contrast medium: 30 ml each of Urografin 76%; ten films taken at the rate of two per second for the first three seconds, and then one film per second.

If flow is obstructed at an undetermined location, a pelvic approach is used to begin with and after 4 films the x-ray fild is moved craniad far enough to visualize the entire inferior vena cava up to the point where it empties into the right artrium of the heart.

Here and there, one reads of transosseous cavography with injection of the contrast medium via the spinous process (ANACKER, 1964), but this procedure is now considered obsolete.

To define the ascending lumbar veins, the preferred access route is by way of the left lumbar vein. A red Oedman catheter slightly angulated at the tip is inserted into the iliac vein and the tip is rotated slightly to the left (Fig. 30). Since the ascending lumbar vein arises from the iliac vein in a straight line, the catheter tip will usually slip into the lumen with ease, and the vein can be visualized by careful manual injection of 20 ml Urografin 76%. (For details of this technique, cf. BÜCHELER et al., 1971.)

8 Pharmacoangiography

The poor filling of certain vascular regions and the difficulty of differentiating between neoplastic and inflammatory changes prompted a study of the effects of drugs on radiopacified vessels and their utilization for diagnostic purposes.

Starting with ABRAMS (1964), who investigated the effect of epinephrine on kidney tumor tissue, numerous authors concerned with visceral angiography have studied its effect on abdominal vessels. They were interested initially in enhancing the visualization of tumor tissues with epinephrine-type vasoconstrictors (BOIJSEN and REDMAN, 1966; BOIJSEN and REUTER, 1967; KAHN et al., 1967).

In addition, the effects of a number of vasodilators including bradykinin, histamine, tolazoline and glucagon on visceral vessels were investigated. They were found to enhance the visualization of poorly vascularized areas or pathologic changes and to accentuate the definition of mesenteric and portal veins in the late phases of visceral arteriography (BOIJSEN and REDMAN, 1966; CHOU et al., 1965; DANFORD and DAVIDSON, 1969; KAHN and CALLOW, 1965; RÖSCH et al., 1969; STECKEL and GROLLMAN, 1968).

An effect of epinephrine bordering on the paradoxical was reported in 1969 by KAHN and his associates: Improved visualization of the portal vein in the late stages of celiac and mesenteric arteriography, presumably owing to delay in washout of contrast medium during the venous phase.

The list of drugs which have meanwhile been tested in animal and clinical trials for the enhancement of visceral angiography is quite lengthy; in Germany alone, a great many publications have appeared on the subject of pharmacoangiography. We may mention only the attempts to improve visualization of the pancreas by means of secretin (ROSENBUSCH and CEN, 1969). However, any enumeration would be incomplete because new studies on the subject keep appearing. The incessant stream of experimental and clinical reports also shows, however, that results so far obtained have not been satisfactory and the search for the ideal drug in visceral angiography continues.

A balanced account by STECKEL et al. (1971) based on numerous animal experiments provides an overview of current capabilities in pharmacoangiography.

The authors examined the following problem areas:

Vasoconstrictors

1. Possible effect on vascular neoformations.
2. Improved outlining of heavily vascularized tumors.
3. Possible drug reaction of vessels believed to be tumorous.
4. Enhanced filling of duodenal and pancreatic vessels when superselective angiography is not possible.

Vasodilators

1. Enhanced definition of poorly visible tumors.
2. Possible reaction of suspected tumor vessels.
3. Improved parenchymal filling of liver, gallbladder and intestinal wall.
4. Enhanced visualization of portal vein.

Conclusions: In special cases, vasoactive substances are undoubtedly helpful in clarifying visceral angiograms (Fig. 14). However, vasoconstrictors by no means permit a positive differentiation of neoplastic and inflammatory changes (DOPPMAN et al., 1969; KAHN and WISE, 1967; ROCKOFF, 1966).

Further, the effect of drugs on the diagnostic yield in cases of gastrointestinal bleeding has by no means been fully elucidated. Injection of epinephrine as well as of vasodilators has in individual cases helped pinpoint gastrointestinal sources of bleeding where no extravasation had previously been visible (STECKEL et al., 1971). The use of vasodilators evidently improves the visualization of hollow organ walls.

On the other hand, when drugs are to be used in visceral angiography, one must always take into account possible side effects. Thus, bradykinin causes a blood pressure rise and possibly cardiac arrhythmia, while isoproterenol can provoke cardiovascular reactions, glucagon nausea and vomiting, and tolazoline can cause hypotension, dizziness, and fainting spells.

The therapeutic potential of pharmacoangiography is described in the chapter on gastrointestinal bleeding (p. 34).

According to our own experience and the literature, the outlook for pharmacoangiography does not appear very bright at the moment. In our opinion, the subject is still very much in a state of flux – none of the findings to date are conclusive. We shall have to await the outcome of further experimental and clinical studies.

9 Magnification

Among advances in the field of abdominal angiography we should also mention the development of magnification techniques, spurred on by the desire for a higher data yield and for visualizing smaller structures.

According to BOOKSTEIN (1971), the primary twofold enlargement of the roentgenogram with an 0.3 mm focus and curtailment of radiation scatter by increased lens-to-film distance more than double the resolution of paired lines as compared to the conventional filming technique with a 1 mm focus. The decisive factors for the quality of the film are a small focus and the elimination of screen lines.

The better the resolution of the film/screen combination the smaller the benefits to be derived by the magnification technique. However, modern equipment can either eliminate or minimize the disadvantages associated with magnifying techniques, such as increased radiation exposure for the patient, reduced frame size, and greater geometric blurring.

The use of a small focus necessarily leads to longer exposure times with the risk of blurring due to motion; on the other hand, increased tube voltage entails reduced contrast. The 0.3 mm focus can be used with currents of low amperage only; at 100 ma the size of the focus increases (MATTSON, 1968).

Magnification has initially been used in renal angiography. Conceivably, the technique is suitable for early detection of tumors, notably for the differentiation of malignant neovascularity. Despite superior definition of individual vessels, "even the modern magnification techniques do not permit differentiation of vessels with a diameter below 300 microns" (VOEGELI, 1971).

10 Abdominal Stereoangiography

Stereoradiography has lost much of its clinical usefulness as a diagnostic tool and little has been said about it in recent years. On the other hand, the angiogram affords optimal conditions for imparting to the viewer a three-dimensional impression.

To our knowledge, it was HETTLER (1961) who first dealt with a stereoscopic procedure, documenting its diagnostic potential in abdominal angiography with appropriate pictorial examples. His method is based on use of a conventional serial filming apparatus, alternately covering one of two opposing tubes firing simultaneously.

The idea of preparing stereoscopic serial angiograms without the need for a second tube was fathered by the usual difficulty of clearly visualizing the vascular architecture, even when viewed in two planes, in examinations of pancreatic vessels.

GAJEWSKI et al. described in 1971 a technically simple stereoradiographic system in which the x-ray tube remains stationary and the parallax effect needed for three-dimensional perception of the pair of stereo pictures is produced by rotating the patient by a certain number of degrees. If the rotation is continued at a predetermined speed within a suitable range of angles, it is possible to produce with a large film changer or a 70 mm video amplifier, without much technical effort, an automatic sequence of paired stereo pictures of considerable diagnostic value (Figs. 35, 38b).

The diagnostic value of the procedure is not yet firmly established. However, the stereoangiograms so far obtained, notably of stenoses of the major aortic branches near the trunk or at the origin, and also for the interpretation of celiac studies and superselective angiograms have proved at times striking, largely obviating the need for two-plane roentgenography.

The angiograms, whether in the 70 × 70 mm format or enlarged to 35 × 35 cm, are displayed as usual side by side on the viewing box or a simple frame specially fitted for the 70 mm film, for evaluation with the aid of a stereoscopic viewer.

Recently, GEORGI (1970) studied the stereoscopic evaluation of angiograms in oncologic gynecology and suggested a procedure for determination of ventral and dorsal tumor extension from angiograms in the sagittal path of the x-ray beam.

11 Electronic Improvement of Angiograms: Subtraction and Color Subtraction

Poor contrast in vascular regions and organs can considerably hamper the assessment of abdominal angiograms. The poor picture quality may be due to obesity; improper positioning of the catheter; insufficient amount of contrast medium or insufficient flow of contrast medium per second; absorption of radiopaque agent in the capillary bed of enlarged organs; dilution of the medium in dilated veins, and other causes. To this must be added the disturbing superimposition of the spinal column, ribs, or the pelvic bones.

In 1935, ZIEDSES DES PLANTES published a method for the photographic subtraction of x-ray pictures that permitted elimination of interfering overshadows of bones with increase in the contrast of relevant image portions.

The most important application of this procedure, because of its very nature, is in cerebral angiography (DECKER and BACKMUND, 1968, and others).

The photographic subtraction process is costly and time-consuming, so much so that it did not become a routine diagnostic tool until the advent of electronic subtraction systems.

Little is known about the value of image subtraction in visceral angiography (WISE and GASON, 1966; CHÉRIGIÉ et al., 1967; ROTH et al., 1969). In a series of 325 selective visceral angiograms, we found 104 (33%) in which subtraction facilitated and improved, or actually made possible, examination of the veins. Out of 183 celiac angiograms, we found complete or partial visualization of the pancreatic parenchyma in 44 cases (27%). Eleven out of 142 mesenteric angiograms gave us a partial outline of the pancreas. On the whole, the method made is easier to differentiate poorly filled vessels and small arteries and veins (Fig. 147) (ERNST, 1971).

A further refinement in the evaluation of x-ray pictures is the production of color roentgenograms from black-and-white subtracted negatives. The image subtraction is done electronically; a color filter is superimposed on the arterial picture and photographed with a camera. Next, a filter of a different color is superimposed for double exposure of the venous or capillary phase (electronic photography by the method of GROH and HAENDLE, 1968). Thus, additive mixing of colors indirectly produces a color radiograph of undisputed didactic value as compared to the conventional black-and-white picture in that it emphasizes the key diagnostic features by color. The fully electronic process was first employed by FISCHER and GERSHON-COHEN (1958) as well as OOSTERKAMP et al. (1966).

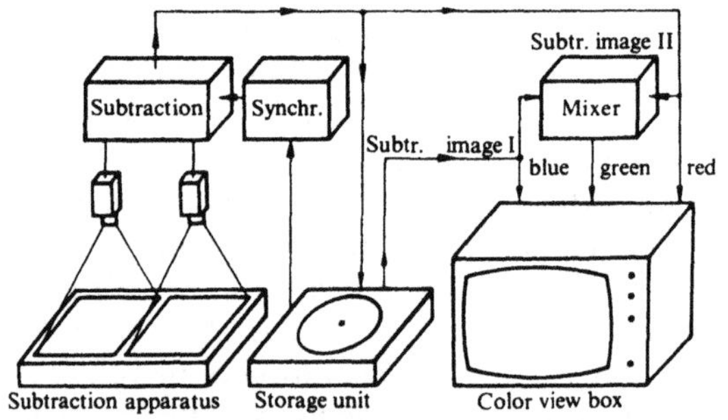

Principle of electronic color subtraction

For evaluation of the angiogram, this method speeds the topographic correlation and classification of vascular systems as the arterial and the venous phase can be displayed side by side in a color image. Evaluation of the venous phase is facilitated, the definition of organ and tumor masses is enhanced, and overall appraisal of blood flow through an organ is simplified in a color subtraction picture.

The definitive role of color radiograms remains to be established, but the physiology and psychology of vision alike indicate that color vision is superior to black-and-white vision, because of greater depth impact and the better visualization of details resulting.

Both methods, image subtraction and indirectly produced color radiography, are subject to the following limitation: *An "improved" picture modified electronically or by color never contains more information than the original.* Still, it provides faster and more reliable information that is decisive for diagnostic purposes (for a comprehensive literature review see ROTH et al., 1971).

12 Hemodynamic Changes Associated with Angiography

With the widespread use of abdominal angiography, the question arises whether the injection of contrast media may put the patient in added jeopardy. Apart from infrequent allergic reactions, as long as one observes the dose limits, the contrast medium is unlikely to cause toxic injury; however, hemodynamic changes such as have been observed after the injection of contrast media in the cardiac atria and ventricles must be expected (FODA, 1965; CASTILLO et al., 1965; FELIX et al., 1969).

Their effect on the blood circulation is determined by two factors:

1. Increase of volume at the site of the injection, and
2. change in osmolarity caused by the highly viscous and hypertonic contrast medium.

Depending on the quantity of contrast medium injected and the speed of injection, the increased volume entails a transient, initial pressure rise followed in short order by a pressure drop, attributed by LÖHR and associates (1968) to the peripheral effect of the contrast medium, viz. dilatation of the capillary bed, hence decrease of peripheral resistance.

Furthermore, the hypertonic, highly viscous contrast medium causes fluids from interstitial spaces to enter the circulatory system (FISCHER, 1965). As a result, the isotonic balance of the blood, disturbed by the high osmolarity of the contrast medium, is restored.

Investigations by EFSEN and MUNKNER (1968) demonstrated the effects of the osmolarity of the contrast medium by a measurable increase of cardiac output. This circulatory reaction is attributable solely to the hypertonic properties of the contrast medium. This is shown by the fact that injections of physiologic saline will cause a comparable, mechanically induced initial blood pressure rise without the subsequent hypotensive reaction or increase of cardiac output.

In a series of 102 successive angiograms, we made direct pressure recordings before, during, and after injection of the contrast medium, utilizing Urografin 76% (SCHERING, Berlin). These arteriographic examinations included:

1. Thoracic aortography }
2. Abdominal aortography } (catheter examination)
3. Selective arteriography }
4. Translumbar aortography (direct puncture)

For the catheter examination, we used open-end Oedman catheters with side holes and pressure syringes. The injection rates varied between 6.0 and 15.0 ml/sec. For selective arteriography, we used catheters with only an end hole. Injections were manual in these examinations as well as in translumbar aortography. The contrast medium volumes ranged from 10 to 50 ml and, for survey aortographies, between 35 and 60 ml. Blood pressure was measured within the vessel with a Statham gauge and recorded on a Hellige four-channel recorder.

A characteristic blood pressure curve with the corresponding roentgenogram is shown in Fig. 36.

Here, two needles were introduced separately for injection of contrast medium and for measurement of blood pressure. A transient blood pressure increase occurred during the injection, followed by a hypotensive reaction lasting only about 20 seconds.

The normal initial pressure level was restored after about 40 seconds.

In selective arteriography, the initial pressure rise is barely noticeable and the subsequent blood pressure drop is also minimal. These small pressure swings can be explained by the slower injection (manual) and the smaller quantities of contrast medium used.

In contrast to the examination techniques mentioned so far, translumbar aortography may be performed under general anesthesia. In these cases, blood pressure measurements were not initiated until after the induction of anesthesia, with the patient shifted to a prone position, when the pressure levels were stabilized.

Blood pressure readings after injection of Urografin 76%

	Average BP in mm Hg $\left(=\frac{\text{syst.}+\text{diast.}}{2}\right)$		
	Before injection	During injection	After injection
Thoracic aortography (n = 15)	125	135	89
Translumbar aortography (n = 15)	129	141	104
Catheter aortography (n = 13)	143	152	106
Selective visceral arteriography (n = 42)	108	112	98
Injection of physiologic saline	124	132	119

This tabulation gives an idea of average blood pressure changes before, during and after injection of the contrast medium. Peak increases of 12 mm are seen in translumbar aortography, while in selective arteriography the changes do not exceed 4 mm Hg. The subsequent hypotensive reaction is very pronounced in thoracic and abdominal aortography (36 and 37 mm Hg, respectively), but in selective arteriography, too, it reaches 14 mm Hg.

For control purposes, six patients received an injection of normal saline solution; here the increase was limited to 8 mm Hg and the drop to 13 mm Hg, reflecting the mechanical effect of the pressure wave. The individual values are a function of the rate of injection, the lowest being recorded in selective arteriography with manual injection. In this group, there was no evidence of the blood pressure changes otherwise observed after injection of the contrast medium; what modest variations did occur were within the margin of error of the test method.

To recapitulate, these investigations warrant the conclusion that the injection of concentrated, highly viscous contrast media in aorto-arteriography results in measurable hemodynamic changes. Thus, there is an initial transitory blood pressure increase due to local volume expansion (averaging 12 mm Hg in translumbar aortography), followed by a pressure drop averaging 27 mm Hg 20 to 40 seconds later. We consider this drop to be a reaction of the peripheral vascular system to the increased osmolarity of the contrast medium.

We found no clearcut difference in this respect between patients with and without arteriosclerosis. Our findings warrant the conclusion that patients with stable circulation run no hemodynamic risk in aorto-arteriography, but that complications cannot be ruled out in cases with preexisting cardiocirculatory insufficiency and pronounced hypovolemia when arteriographic studies are carried out with sizable amounts of contrast medium (WENZ et al., 1970; HALL, 1970).

Blood pressure changes in mm Hg after injection of Urografin 76% as compared with different initial pressure levels

Systolic BP before injection	Average pressure drop after injection	
	Systolic	Diastolic
Up to 150 mm Hg	13.7	7.5
155 to 200 mm Hg	38.1	20.0
Above 205 mm Hg	54.4	28.1

If the findings are viewed in relation to groups of different baseline values of blood pressure, it becomes clear that hypertensive individuals with systolic values in excess of 200 mm Hg exhibited the greatest blood pressure drop, averaging 54.4 mm Hg systolically and 28.1 diastolically, and should therefore be watched with special care.

13 Complications of Abdominal Angiography

If abdominal angiography is to be performed, certain conditions have to be met (see p. 8). An absolutely aseptic procedure is a requirement. The needles and catheters must be thoroughly cleaned and perfectly sterilized. All patients should remain under clinical observation for at least 24 hours after angiography. Translumbar aortography and catheter examinations should be carried out on an in-patient basis.

Visceral angiography applied directly by the "cannula-method" as well as indirectly by catheter may be followed by complications, but these are fortunately rare. The table below summarizes a number of papers reporting experience in more than 1 000 examinations, some of them published in the form of statistical surveys (McAFEE, 1957; LANG, 1963; BEALL et al., 1964; CORMIER et al., 1966).

Mortality and complications after angiography

	Number	Mortality %	Major complications %
LANG (1963)	11 402	0.06	0.71
SAUR (1964)	6 155	0.05	1.7
HALPERN (1964)	1 000	—	2.4
SEIDENBERG (1966)	1 500	—	1.8
BAUM (1966)	1 600	—	0.6
CORMIER (1966)	5 387	0.15	2.0
FOLIN (1968)	1 319	—	1.2
HEGER (1969)	1 455	—	0.9
Total	29 818	0.03	1.41

When we look into the question how such surveys are produced, the initial, relatively favorable impression is somewhat dimmed. Once the radiologist has made certain that there is no more bleeding from the puncture site and the foot or radial pulse is readily palpable, he generally loses sight of the angiographed patient very quickly. The patient is provided with a compression dressing and sand bag and returned to his ward or to the referring hospital; only if something out of the ordinary happens then is the radiologist notified of the complications, such as afterbleeding, thrombosis, embolism, or the development of aneurysms at the puncture site (Fig. 41).

Since follow-up examinations by the radiologist are exceptional, some of the above-mentioned surveys of postangiographic incidents may not be too reliable, for in the absence of specific follow-up examinations only those complications will be reported that require surgical intervention or that lead to permanent injuries. PAULIN and associates studied this problem in 1968 and tried to record objectively cases of thromboembolism that did not attract clinical attention. By applying these stricter and more objective diagnostic criteria they discovered thromboembolic episodes in as many as 25% of cases.

In 1968 PAULIN et al. drew certain conclusions from their observations in a total of 880 oscillographically monitored angiographic studies: The incidence of complications was highest after serial-film coronary angiography, followed by transthoracic aortography and celiac angiography. No incidents occurred in abdominal aortography. The complications were unrelated to age or sex and to pre-existing coronary disease or malignant tumors. A marked difference was found, however, when different catheter lengths and calibers were compared in that thromboembolic complications were more frequent after the use of long and large-caliber catheters.

JACOBSSON (1968) was able to show that platelets tend to deposit on the catheter in the form of reversible aggregations in much the same way as they do on a damaged vessel wall. Under the action of locally formed thrombin this structureless aggregation may change into an irreversible platelet thrombus. This mechanism—in contrast to development of the so-called red thrombus—is refractory to anticoagulants. As the catheter is withdrawn, the platelet deposits on the arterial wall opening are stripped off like a collar and so become the nucleus for local thrombosis.

In the light of these observations we carried out a follow-up oscillometric study of a random series of catheter angiographies performed among our own patients. According to measurements in 100 patients, there was an increased incidence of complications with the wider-caliber yellow Oedman catheter and an increase in pathologic findings with increasing catheter length. No correlation was found with the retention time of the catheter in the vascular lumen (SPÄH, 1971). A temporarily pathological oscillogram was obtained in 21% of the cases. Figure 37 depicts one case of thromboembolic complication.

Although the incidence of complications relative to the total patient population represents an acceptable risk when weighed against the advantages of this diagnostic method, we should endeavor to create conditions under which such incidents will be avoided.

Thromboembolic complications following catheter angiography

Author	No. of cases	Technique	Incidence %	Method of investigation
LUKE and McGRAW (1963)	271	abdominal	0.4	?
	93	thoracic	4.3	?
KOTTKE et al. (1964)	195	abdominal	5.7	Palpation of pulse
	44	thoracic	25.0	Palpation of pulse
PAULIN et al. (1968)	88	abdominal	3.5	Oscillometry
	32	thoracic	12.0	Oscillometry
JACOBSSON (1968)	76	thoracic	8.0	Oscillometry

The complications of lumbar aortography include para-aortic injections with dissecting aneurysms, hemorrhages, intestinal gangrene, anesthesia incidents, spinal cord lesions, renal damage, and less common sequelae.

Catheter examinations are occasionally complicated by local thrombosis, detachment of intimal plaques causing peripheral embolism, perforation of the vessel wall with dissection, and arteriovenous fistulas. In exceptional cases the flexible tip of the guide wire can break off, necessitating surgical removal. In very rare cases a large hematoma forms at the catheter entry site, requiring surgical intervention.

Bleeding, thrombosis and embolism are by far the most commonly encountered angiographic complications and certain factors favoring their development ought to be mentioned: Pre-existing vascular diseases; large-caliber catheters; repeated traumatizing punctures; long duration of examination (LUKE and MCGRAW, 1963); forced or neglected compression of puncture site; hemorrhagic diathesis or treatment with anticoagulants (Marcoumar) (DIEMEL and SCHMITZ-DRAEGER, 1969).

One of the most serious aortographic incidents is temporary or permanent damage to the spinal cord, which according to estimates by HORNYKIEWITSCH and BARGON (1962) as well as by SCHOEN (1962), based on extensive American surveys, occur in 0.2% of all aortographic examinations. It is all the more surprising that there are no detailed case histories in the German-language literature of recent years. Lately, BROY (1971) has called attention to neurologic incidents of this kind. He reports the case of a patient of his, a woman of 39, in whom renal arteriography was performed because of painless gross hematuria. In the course of the examination the tip of a red Oedman catheter slipped into the ostium of the first lumbar artery a few millimeters below the renal artery. Following manual injection of 8 ml of Angiografin in about 2 to 3 seconds, the patient reported that her legs felt completely numb and weak. She had a transverse myelitis which proved refractory to therapy and progressed on the following day as far as the 11th thoracic vertebra, causing anesthesia, analgesia, and flaccid paraplegia including bladder and bowel incontinence. Her paraplegia is probably irreversible.

Examination of the films revealed that the greater radicular artery was filled with contrast medium from the first lumbar artery. The muscular branches of the first lumbar artery were flooded with contrast medium, as manifested by a dense, cloudy paravertebral extravasation. The toxic postangiographic myelitis described here is a relatively rare complication of this technique which can still not be fully explained. Such a spinal incident may be expected to result from a combination of unforeseeable circumstances including flooding of the greater radicular artery with contrast medium, a poorly developed anterior spinal artery, anomalies in the arterial supply of the spinal cord, and possible individual differences in neuronal sensitivity to the contrast medium.

The rare *deaths*—reported mostly in older surveys—are in large part attributable to toxicity of the contrast medium but have also been caused in some cases by hemorrhages, thrombosis, spinal cord lesions, renal failure, or nervous system disorders. Today, fatalities could occur only through the coincidence of a number of complicating associated diseases. An illustration is provided by one of our own cases:

A four-year-old girl with severe hydrocephalus, myelomeningocele, and excessive thoracic and lumbar scoliosis was to undergo surgery to straighten the spine. The child had transverse paralysis and had to be attended to and fed in prone position. It was planned to remove several vertebrae to enable the child to sit up straight. For exploration of the vascular topography at the level of the proposed operation, the child was referred to us for catheter aortography, which was carried out without difficulty (see Fig. 100).

However, the child never awakened from anesthesia. The actual cause of death could not be established at autopsy. We assume that her organism was too severely damaged to withstand the strain of contrast medium and anesthesia.

The vitally indicated diagnostic workup comprised preoperative abdominal angiography in this gravely ill child. Its risks were dicussed at length beforehand, but in this desperate situation no other diagnostic method was at hand.

Among a total of 1932 lumbar aortographies for visualization of the lower extremity vessels because of arterial occlusion, we have seen a total of two fatalities, both involving patients with a history of serious disorders: (1) Emergency aortography for acute occlusion of the iliac artery secondary to a bifurcation bypass. Cardiac failure at the end of anesthesia, with no technical difficulties arising in the angiography. Autopsy disclosed a recent thrombosis of coronary and renal arteries. (2) Severe general arterial occlusive disease with bilateral stenosis of iliac arteries. Bleeding from the translumbar puncture requiring surgical repair. On the day after the operation the patient died of postoperative consumption coagulopathy.

Apart from some clinically uneventful extravasations during aortography and innocuous hematomas at the catheter entry site in the inguinal region, we witnessed the following more serious incidents:

Age and sex	Exploratory technique and Indication	Concomitant aggravating condition	Complication
41, ♂	Catheter aortography, small kidney	Hypertension	Local hematoma (operated)
34, ♀	Catheter aortography, pheochromocytoma	Hypertension	Local hematoma (conservative therapy)
20, ♀	Celiac angiography, suspected liver tumor	Got up too soon	Thrombotic occlusion of femoral artery (operated)
54, ♂	Retrograde arteriography, rejection reaction	Hypertension, kidney transplant	Local hematoma (operated)
64, ♂	Celiac angiography, suspected liver abscess	Arteriosclerosis	Embolic popliteal occlusion (operated)

The role of hypertension is readily apparent from this tabulation. However, sizable injury to the artery from introduction of the catheter in previous angiographic examinations and incomplete bed rest by the patients after the examination must also be incriminated.

While the five thromboembolic complications among our patients were also related to thoracic angiography, the following serious incidents were associated with *abdominal angiography* carried out at the Radiological Division of the Heidelberg Surgical University Clinic:

1 fatality (0.04%)

4 extensive hematomas (surgery in 3 cases!), and

2 cases of thromboembolism (0.3%).

The frequency of adverse reactions to angiography can be minimized if the following rules are strictly observed:

Retrospective summary of iatrogenic vascular injuries at the Surgical Clinic, University of Heidelberg (according to TREDE et al., 1972).

Period of observation 1960 to 1971. N = 26	
Non-angiographic vascular lesion (ligature of femoral artery, radiation ulcer with vascular erosion, etc.)	7
Thromboembolic sequelae of angiography performed elsewhere	14
Thromboembolic sequelae of angiography performed at the Radiologic Division, Surgical Clinic, University of Heidelberg. (Indications: 1. Suspected liver tumor; 2. occlusion of common carotid and stenosis of vertebral artery; 3. suspected liver abscess; 4. stenosis of subclavian artery; 5. obstruction of subclavian artery.)	5

— Performance of examination in hospitalized patients
— Compelling need for examination
— Acceptable patient risk
— Therapeutic consequences considered
— General clinical examination beforehand
— ECG, blood count, coagulation status, urinalysis.

To reduce the risk of thrombosis, we add heparin in a ratio of 1:1000 to the normal saline solution for rinsing of the catheter.

Owing to the hazard of bleeding from the puncture site this should be compressed for about 10 minutes, and in hypertensive patients for about 30 minutes. In addition, we place a sand bag on the corresponding lumbar region for six hours. After the angiographic examination each patient is seen by the radiologist himself at least once. He examines the puncture site as well as the patient's pulse.

13.1 Diagnosis and Therapy of Angiographic Complications

Incidents following direct aortic puncture are generally easy to detect. The angiogram itself will reveal extravasations (Fig. 40), a faulty injection site (Fig. 42), and dissections (Figs. 43, 44). Larger hematomas, which usually spread retroperitoneally, cause severe pains and lumbar bulging at the level of the puncture site. Not infrequently, subileus or ileus develops within a few hours as a reaction to the hematoma. In such cases immediate arrangements should be made to check the blood count and provide continuous monitoring of hemoglobin and hematocrit, pulse rate and blood pressure, and to observe the patient in an intensive care unit. If the bleeding does not stop or progressive clinical signs of dissection occur, surgical repair is indicated.

The detection of thrombotic or embolic changes following direct aorto-arteriography or catheter examination may prove more difficult. As a rule, such episodes involve an acute arterial occlusion that may be expected to produce marked objective and subjective signs. However, a number of such incidents may at first escape the radiologist's attention because the patient remains in bed after the angiographic examination, so that straining of the extremity, as an important causative factor of painful hypoxia, is avoided. The symptoms of inadequate blood supply may be slow to develop, and when they do appear, they may no longer be attributed to the radiologic study.

In typical cases the patient will complain of pains in the leg or in the arm and report a distinct sensation of chill. This should be the signal for an immediate check on the pulse. Subsequent oscillometry will usually reveal the occlusion. Conservative treatment with low positioning of the extremity, application of cotton dressings, and administration of vasodilators is permissible during the first one or two hours. We have never observed the repeatedly reported episodes of arterial spasms and therefore have little faith in the effectiveness of antispasmodics.

Management of postangiographic thromboembolism (KAPPERT, 1969)

Signs	Patient complains of pain and sensation of cold
Diagnosis	Pulse status, skin temperature, oscillometry (renewed angiography!)
Therapy in first 2 hours	*Cotton dressing* *Leg positioned low* *Analgesics* (in severe cases morphine, otherwise methampyrone + tranquilizers *Vasodilators* (Complamin or Ronicol intraarterially plus 0.5 mg Hydergine in 500 ml fructose 5% i.v.)
After 2 hours	*Surgical treatment* (Fogarty catheter) absolutely indicated in case of main extremity arteries. *Fibrinolytics* to be given in peripheral occlusions only

The 1970 "Symposium on Vascular Thrombosis After Catheter Angiography" did not reach a clear consensus on the management of acute iatrogenic occlusions occurring on the x-ray examination table. Some favored immediate surgical intervention after 1–2 hours (HASSE et al., 1970), while others advocated the use of fibrinolytic agents (JÜRGENS et al., 1970).

We ourselves have had so little experience with thromboembolic complications that we are hardly in a position to express an opinion. We referred our patients immediately to a vascular surgeon, who immediately performed a successful thrombectomy in cases of unmistakable total occlusion.

Whichever the choice, fibrinolysis or surgery, the postangiographic occlusion has to be diagnosed by the radiologist himself, who should attend to it immediately in cooperation with the internist and the surgeon.

IV The Abdominal Syndrome and Angiography

1 Disorders of Visceral Blood Circulation

Pathologic changes of the visceral arteries can lead to clinically demonstrable disorders of the gastrointestinal tract and the parenchymatous organs. In the days before angiography, antemortem diagnosis of acute occlusions was mostly made during exploratory laparotomy, while chronic obliterative processes generally escaped notice until autopsy. This inability to arrive at a timely and exact diagnosis and institute effective therapy accounts for the lack of interest in abdominal blood flow disturbances that persisted for a long time.

1.1 History

At first, a few pathologists made studies of occlusive diseases of visceral arteries (CRUVEILHIER, 1830), without paying any attention to the decisive criterion, a functional collateral system.

One praiseworthy exception was the Heidelberg anatomist FRIEDRICH TIEDEMANN whose 1843 monograph on the "Constriction and Occlusion of the Arteries" described a chronic occlusion of the superior mesenteric artery in a 60-year-old beggar. With the aid of dye injections Tiedemann was able to show that the blood reached the superior mesenteric artery by way of collateral vessels: from the celiac artery via the dilated superior pancreaticoduodenal artery and from the inferior mesenteric via the ramus anastomoticus magnus of the left colic artery.

His work is rightly considered fundamental to all the functional and anatomic knowledge contributed by subsequent generations, notably through the employment of angiography.

The collateral link between the inferior and the superior mesenteric arteries mentioned by TIEDEMANN bears the name of the Parisian anatomist JEAN RIOLAN (1580–1657). However, according to DIEMEL et al. (1964), RIOLAN merely saw the vascular arch located at the inner margin of the large intestine and did not recognize its functional role.

In 1969, CHIENE reported a case of total obstruction of all three visceral arteries, yet the cause of death was not attributable to this occlusion (cf. also CEN et al., 1972). Similarly, ROB reported in 1970 on a total of 6 patients with celiac and superior mesenteric occlusion, not accompanied by clinical manifestations of pathologic deficiency.

Clinical manifestations of visceral vascular occlusion depend above all on the functional efficiency of the collateral system. Since this is by no means always sufficient to sustain functional blood flow, the condition gives rise to a clinical syndrome variously known as abdominal angina, intestinal angina, mesenteric angina, visceral angina, abdominal angina syndrome, abdominal intermittent syndrome, abdominal claudication, intestinal claudication, intermittent intestinal dysbasia, intermittent angiosclerotic intestinal dyspepsia, intermittent anemic dysperistalsis, intermittent mesenteric ischemia, mesenteric arterial insufficiency, Orthner's disease, Orthner's claudication, Pal's syndrome and Pal's crisis.

VOLLMAR (1968) distinguishes between an acute and a chronic occlusive syndrome of visceral arteries.

1.2 Acute Occlusion of Visceral Arteries

According to VOLLMAR (1968) the acute obstruction of one or more visceral arteries may be caused by:

1. Arterial embolism.
2. Arterial thrombosis.
3. Aneurysm of the abdominal aorta and the mesenteric vessels.
4. External compression of the artery (strangulation, tumors, etc.).
5. Trauma (arterial avulsion, arterial thrombosis).

Among these factors, arterial *embolism* and *thrombosis* are about equally common, while the other causes are rare events (ZAHN and GOERTTLER, 1971). One possible exception is *vascular injury* due to abdominal trauma; at any rate, we have seen an increasing number of such alterations on our angiograms, notably in cases of ruptured spleen (cf. chapter "Abdominal Trauma" p. 43).

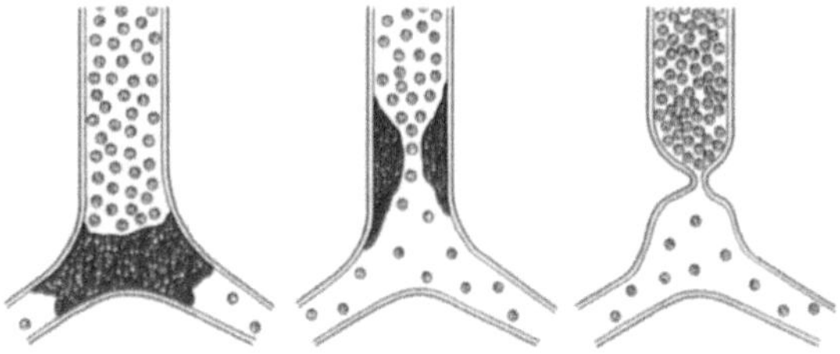

Causes of chronic occlusion of visceral arteries

Acute vascular occlusion is followed by ischemia, which is in turn determined by the location and extent of the block. Contributing factors are (1) lack of an adequate, immediately available collateral circulation, (2) the fact that visceral arteries are functional end-arteries, and (3) that the so-called ischemic tolerance of the gastrointestinal tract and the abdominal organs being supplied is limited to a period of 120–180 minutes.

Not infrequently, an arterial occlusion is followed by a secondary thrombosis of mesenteric veins due to the blood stagnating in the venous draining system. Fig. 45 shows such a stationary column of contrast medium recorded serially in the mesenteric veins more than 30 seconds after the injection. The cause of this surgically verified thrombosis at the confluence with the portal artery was a recent embolus in the distal leg of the superior mesenteric artery.

According to GOERTTLER (1968), embolism of visceral arteries affects the superior mesenteric artery and its ramifications in over 90% of cases. In large part this seems to be due to the fact that, in probing the branches of the abdominal aorta, the tip of the catheter time and again literally "drops" into the very wide drainage funnel and also to the position at the apex of the ventroconvex lumbar curvature of the abdominal aorta. In our own patient population we were able to demonstrate celiac occlusion in a single case among acute occlusions of visceral arteries.

For specific and *timely therapy* rapid localization of the occlusion is essential. Angiography is the only method that can quickly provide this anatomic diagnosis before laparotomy. A radiologist who wants to be more than just a technical assistant to the clinician must be familiar with the clinical picture and, above all, the proper timing of his procedure, on which the health and the life of his patient may depend.

An acute occlusion of the celiac trunk is an exceedingly rare occurrence. Sudden crushing pain in the epigastric region, nausea, blood-tinged vomitus, suggest diagnoses such as myocardial infarction, gastric perforation, acute pancreatitis, incarcerated diaphragmatic hernia, cholelithiasis, etc. Even in the acute phase, the radiologist plays a major role in the establishment of an accurate diagnosis. A plain abdominal x-ray film can be decisive, particularly in advanced stages in which retention of fluid and gas in the lower ileum and the right half of the colon is accompanied by edematous thickening of the intestinal walls and signs of peritonitis (AAKHUS and BRABRAND, 1967). In earlier stages of the acute visceral artery occlusion, however, the survey film often fails to yield any abnormal findings.

According to MCCORT (1960), clinical symptoms are unlikely to be found after an acute obstruction at the level of the inferior mesenteric artery unless there are concomitant occlusions in the area of the superior mesenteric and the left internal iliac artery, or congenital anomalies of the preformed vascular bridges.

Among our patients, we saw only one acute occlusion of the inferior mesenteric artery secondary to an aortofemoral bypass with ligation of this artery, which led to clinical manifestations (mucosanguineous stools) and in which we discovered a segmental stenosis of the sigmoid colon with mucosal atrophy. In none of the cases did angiography ever disclose an acute occlusion of the inferior mesenteric artery.

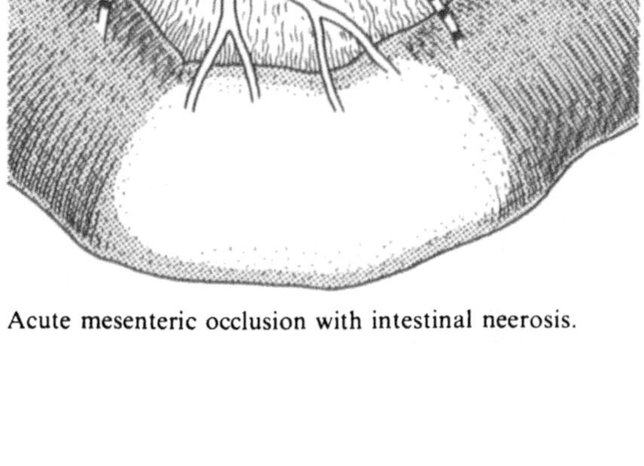

Acute mesenteric occlusion with intestinal necrosis.

The situation is quite different in sudden obstruction of the superior mesenteric artery or its branches. Intestinal necrosis is a virtually inevitable outcome, dominating the overall clinical picture:

Acute mesenteric occlusion (according to BURY, 1969)

Initial stage (1–2 hours)	Acute abdominal vascular pain; retching; hyperhidrosis; tachycardia; prostration; hyperperistalsis, bloody diarrhea; leukocytosis; discrepancy between poor general condition and scarcity of objective findings
Latent stage (2–12 hours)	Atypical complaints; poor general condition; absence of intestinal sounds; tachycardia
Irreversible stage of intestinal necrosis (past 12 hours)	Localized or diffuse peritonitis; ileus; toxic circulatory insufficiency

Most of our patients with mesenteric occlusion were studied in the latent stage. Considering the atypical nature of the clinical symptoms, it is understandable that a number of other diagnoses were first excluded. Nevertheless, we believe that while the results of treatment of acute mesenteric obstruction remain so dismal, every effort to arrive at a firm diagnosis as quickly as possible is justified.

1.2.1 Angiographic Indications and Techniques

It is essentially up to the internist or the surgeon to establish the indication for visceral angiography. The radiologist can help by watching for two signs which have often proved helpful to us, namely, severe tachycardia inconsistent with the acute abdominal picture and incipient abdominal x-ray changes pointing to peritonitis. Not infrequently, a few loops of the small intestine will overlap in this intermediate stage, signifying that some intestinal wall damage has already occurred.

In acute abdomen of unknown origin, it is of course necessary, first of all, to rule out free perforation of a hollow viscus, an obstruction in the gastrointestinal tract, acute pancreatitis, recent myocardial infarction, or acute hepatic vein obstruction. The radiologist bears a heavy responsibility in most of these diagnoses by exclusion. The decision to proceed with early angiography will be facilitated if possible sources of dissemination of emboli are known or detected in the course of the clinical examination (atrial fibrillation, mitral stenosis, complete arrhythmia, aortic aneurysm).

Inasmuch as there is very rarely clinical evidence of the anatomic localization of the vascular occlusion, the idea that flush aortography should first be done for purposes of orientation is not far-fetched. It has been our experience, however, that better results can be obtained by immediate selective arteriography unless a lateral-view aortogram discloses an occlusion (Fig. 46).

The reasons are that acute occlusions tend to occur unilaterally in the superior mesenteric artery, while on the other hand selective arteriography makes possible a far more exact diagnosis since it visualizes circumscribed vascular regions without overshadows, so that even small peripheral emboli become detectable (Fig. 47).

Last but not least, selective arteriography makes it possible to visualize the return of venous blood and detect any coexisting venous obstruction.

The objection that selective arteriography is more time-consuming than aortography in defining the superior mesenteric artery is valid only in the presence of severe vascular arterio-

Treatment and results in 45 patients with acute occlusion of mesenteric arteries and veins at the Surgical Clinic of the University of Heidelberg, 1964 to 1970 (from LAUBACH, 1971)

	Number of Patients	Operated on	Not Operated on	Surviving
Embolism	16	13	3	–
Thrombosis	15	13	2	1
Venous occlusion	9	8	1	2
Combined occlusion	4	4	–	1
Undetermined	1	1	–	–
	45	39	6	4 (9%)

sclerotic changes. In individuals of advanced age, a survey aortography is the first step; if there are obstructions in the course of the pelvic arteries, immediate preference would be given to high translumbar aortography. Since this procedure requires general anesthesia, it should be followed directly by surgical intervention if a vascular occlusion is demonstrated.

If it turns out that the arterial and venous trunks of the superior mesenteric vessel are unobstructed, we follow up with celiac angiography and only then perform flush aortography if the clinical findings are suggestive of vascular occlusion.

BONAKDARPOUR (1970) experimentally investigated the angiographic findings of a mesenteric occlusion in 18 dogs. After ligating the afferent branches of the artery at various distances from the origin of the aorta, he found the following changes:

1. Stagnation of the contrast medium in the ligated vessels (stagnation sign).
2. Visualization of the vascular stump (stump sign).
3. Delayed filling of the arteries in the ischemic area.
4. Reduced vascularization of the affected intestinal regions.

So far, the results of surgical treatment have been disappointing. In 1965, SCHRÖDER reported that a review of the literature yielded only 45 successful operations for occlusion of visceral arteries. No doubt, the reason for this disheartening statistic is the tardiness in performing laparotomy, that is, the fact that the vascular disease was detected too late or not at all. This state of affairs is not likely to change unless the clinician recognizes the possibility of a visceral artery occlusion sooner and orders an angiographic examination at the earliest possible moment. This in turn presupposes active collaboration with the radiologist, who must of course provide round-the-clock angiographic services for prompt examination of the many patients that are brought in late at night (WENZ, 1969).

1.3 Chronic Occlusion of Visceral Arteries

1.3.1 Etiology

Congenital stenosis of visceral arteries is rare. It is marked by a symmetrical constriction of the vascular lumen (*1*). The rare fibromuscular wall hyperplasia (*2*) can occur not only in the renal arteries but also in visceral arteries, as has been described by PALUBINSKAS and RIPLEY (1964) and RIPLEY and LEVIN (1966). External arterial compression (*3*) is also conceivable in the presence of suggestive clinical symptoms, e.g. in cases of malignancy (carcinoma of the pancreas; WEISSLEDER et al, 1966).

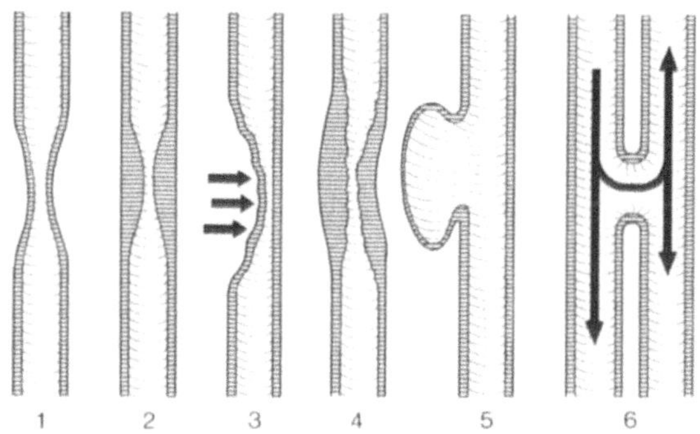

Causes of chronic visceral artery occlusion

A rarity is the so-called *median arcuate ligament compression syndrome*. Such compression is usually associated with a constant epigastric bruit which may vary in intensity during respiration and is most often seen in young females. The lateral aortogram shows a characteristic concave impression on the cranial surface of the celiac artery just beyond its origin (Fig. 51). If the aortogram is performed in both full inspiration and full expiration, the degree of stenosis usually changes. In the case of selective arteriography it is often possible to catheterize the celiac artery. Since the catheter tip lies beyond the stenosis, no abnormalities may be seen on such an angiographic series (REUTER and REDMAN, 1972). Injection of the superior mesenteric artery, however, generally shows filling of some or all of the celiac distribution through dilated, elongated pancreaticoduodenal arcades.

Among chronic stenosing vascular diseases, arteriosclerosis (*4*) of degenerative or mixed degenerative-inflammatory origin occurs most frequently, at a 90% incidence as compared with about 10% for arteritis. *Polyarteritis nodosa* as a special form is characterized by progressive necrotizing arteritis of the medium and small arteries. The symptom complex of an individual patient depends on the organs involved: the gastrointestinal tract in 51%, the liver in 66% and the kidneys in more than 80%. Angiographic findings in polyarteritis nodosa include multiple fusiform or saccular aneurysms associated with irregular caliber of the medium and small arteries (Fig. 52). The aneurysms may rupture, causing hemorrhage into the perirenal, retroperitoneal or intraperitoneal spaces. Hemorrhage may be a terminal event in this disease. Angiography is a diagnostic test for assessment of the extent of pathologic involvement, or to locate the site of acute bleeding. No other disease process produces a similar angiographic appearance of extensive small aneurysm formation with associated vascular irregularity. Recently, CITRON et al. (1970) reported necrotizing angiitis in young people following multiple *drug abuse*. The pathologic and angiographic appearance is the same as in polyarteritis nodosa. Calcifications and mural thrombi predominate, followed at some distance by aneurysms (*5*) and arteriovenous shunts (*6*) (GOERTTLER, 1969).

Besides the abovee-mentioned chronic stenosing vascular lesions, the following vascular abnormalities are very rarely observed: *Ergotism* as a form of *drug toxicity* can cause irregular narrowing of the mesenteric and hepatic arteries, which have areas of marked narrowing alternating with areas of normal caliber much more common in the peripheral circulation. These vascular changes will revert to normal as the drug toxicity regresses. *Intraarterial barbiturates* will cause severe vascular spasm (REUTER and REDMAN, 1972). Peripheral vascular occlusions due to intimal proliferation and gastrointestinal hemorrhage are observed in a hereditary disease, *Pseudoxanthoma elasticum*, causing widespread degeneration of elastic fibers and early calicification of the arterial intima and media. Angiography has demonstrated angiomatous malformations, aneurysms of small arteries and irregular arterial narrowings (BARDSLEY et al., 1969). The superior mesenteric artery is involved in some rare cases of *Takayashu's arteritis*. The disease is a primary arteritis of unknown etiology more frequently seen in women. The course is progressive for a period of years with more stenosis than dilatation and prominent collateral circulation. Symptoms similar to abdominal angina have been described in one patient with celiac involvement (KATER, 1967).

1.3.2. Collateral Circulation

The visceral arteries—celiac, superior mesenteric and inferior mesenteric—are arranged in three tiers and are linked by preformed natural vascular bridges. Normally, these anastomoses are of small caliber and serve only to supply blood to the area in which they are distributed. Under certain pathologic conditions, however, these insignificant vessels form large collateral systems, which often possess a surprisingly large capacity. It is this compensatory power of the collateral vessels that explains the generally marked discrepancy between the magnitude of the blood flow disorder and the frequent absence of clinical manifestations (KRIESSMANN, 1967).

A distinction must be made between collateral vessels between the above-mentioned three-tiered visceral system and those vascular bridges that encompass other arteries alien to the system, such as the intercostal or iliolumbar arteries. In a craniocaudal direction, the most important intervisceral connecting vessels (Fig. 54) are the following:

1. The anterior and posterior pancreaticoduodenal arcade linking the celiac and superior mesenteric arteries. It can go into action when either the celiac or the superior mesenteric artery is occluded (Fig. 55).

2. Connecting vessels between the medial and the left colic arteries, constituting Riolan's anastomosis, which shunts the inferior and the superior mesenteric in both flow directions (Fig. 4, 59). The collateral vessel is the bypass for occlusions of the superior or inferior mesenteric artery. Normally, the vessel can barely be seen in the angiogram but under these conditions its caliber may approach the width of the superior mesenteric.

3. The link between the inferior mesenteric and the left internal iliac artery by way of the superior hemorrhoidal artery (Fig. 58). With a well-developed collateral system, the pelvic arteries may draw so much blood from the mesenteric system as to cause a relative circulatory insufficiency of the intesine, even if the visceral arteries are unobstructed (the so-called mesenteric steal syndrome, VOLLMAR et al., 1964; iliofemoral steal syndrome, VOLLMAR, 1971).

While the many anastomoses existing within the arcades of the small intestine play a secondary role in the maintenance of collateral circulation, other collateral vessels between the common or left hepatic artery and the left gastric artery, between the gastroepiploic and the splenic artery, etc. have been described (cf. DÜX et al., 1966).

Collateral vessels not belonging to the visceral system include (Fig. 56):

1. Intercostal arteries
2. Diaphragmatic arteries
3. Epigastric arteries
4. Lumbar arteries
5. Iliolumbar arteries communicating with the inferior mesenteric via the internal iliac artery.

very slowly and the other vascular segments fill the breach through the intermediary of fully functional collaterals (CEN et al., 1972).

Such a situation is shown in Fig. 4, where the only open passages are the afferent artery of a residual kidney and the stenosed inferior mesenteric. The patient was a 42-year-old man with hypertension and peripheral circulatory disorders who weighed 82 kg and had no digestive complaints of any kind.

This case shows that it is impossible to draw inferences regarding the clinical picture from the arteriogram. We therefore reviewed our patient records with respect to stenoses and occlusions of visceral arteries.

Localization and distribution of obliterating visceral vascular diseases with clinical symptoms in 769 consecutive aortographies (Radiology Department, Surgical Clinic, University of Heidelberg, 1961–1969). (WENZ et al., 1971). Most of the patients presented with arterial obstructions in the lower extremities.

	Occlusions	Proximal stenosis	Peripheral stenosis	Total
Celiac artery	5	5	–	9
Common hepatic artery	–	2	–	2
Gastroduodenal artery	4	3	–	7
Splenic artery	1	1	–	2
Superior mesenteric artery	6	7	6	19
Middle colic artery	–	1	–	1
Ileal and jejunal arteries	1	–	1	2
Inferior mesenteric artery	8	3	2	13
	25	21	9	55

Among the 769 patients so evaluated, there were 167 with stenoses and occlusions of visceral arteries, of whom only the 55 (7%) listed in the table reported abdominal complaints. In the same period only six patients required surgery for so-called abdominal angina.

The controlling factor in the development of a functionally efficient collateral system is the pressure drop in the particular vascular segment, with a pressure gradient between the "throttled" vascular area and the adjoining artery. The blood invariably flows toward the vascular region with the lower pressure.

Other important aspects are the span of time available for adaptation of the collateral system and the integrity of the affected vessels as well as the global cardiocirculatory status.

According to VOLLMAR (1968), the functional efficiency of the collateral bridges between the three tiers of visceral vessels declines in caudocranial direction. Even combined stenoses and segmental occlusions of two or even three visceral arteries, e. g. the celiac trunk and the superior mesenteric artery, can be tolerated provided the occlusive processes develop

By comparison, MÜNSTER and MÜLLER (1967) found among 1200 unselected aortographies a 4% incidence of celiac and superior mesenteric artery obliterations. Four-fifths of them occurred past the age of 40, primarily in patients with obstructive diseases of limb arteries. In the opinion of these authors, 85% of the occlusions were discovered by chance. Among a total of 50 patients with obliterative diseases there was a single woman exhibiting symptoms of an abdominal circulatory disorder.

The probability of clinical manifestations of insufficiency in occlusion of one or more of the visceral arteries (Fig. 3) increases in the presence of other factors affecting the collateral system, such as tumors (Fig. 61), inflammations, and scarring. For example, after gastric resection involving primary or secondary obstruction of the gastroduodenal artery, the pancreatic arcades can no longer serve as a bypass for a celiac, hepatic or mesenteric occlusion. Of special importance, too, is the localization of the occlusion in relation to the terminal artery; the more peripheral the occlusion, the smaller the chance for collateral compensation.

Nor should the relation between advancing age and the consequent decline in "circulatory reserve" (ZAHN and GOERTTLER, 1971) be disregarded. Arteriosclerotic changes of old age impose varied limitations on the intestinal network of arteries. This leads to a reduced increase in flow rate in response to increased peripheral demand, which arises in the abdominal organs after meals (after intake of food the volume of blood circulating in the visceral arteries increases by about 30%).

Therefore, elderly individuals should beware of overburdening their intestinal arterial system and avoid heavy meals necessitating a considerable increase in blood flow (ZAHN and GOERTTLER, 1971).

Another danger due to visceral arteriosclerosis is posed by hemodynamic disturbances, which may culminate in poststenotic thromboses. Similarly, calcium salt deposits spreading to the vascular lumen may act as "platelet traps" and form the head of a thrombus (Fig. 5).

In this connection we may touch upon a problem that to us seems far from settled. Following studies by MIKKELSEN (1957 and 1959) this author's view that only an occlusion or stenosis of two major visceral arteries can cause a clinically detectable circulatory deficiency gained wide currency. This opinion has been repeated in the great majority of English-language papers published on the subject. Recently, doubts have been voiced by WARTER and associates (1970) who evaluated no fewer than 60 cases of isolated celiac stenosis, some of which were associated with severe clinical symptoms.

Other individual reports also indicate that a circumscribed occlusion of a single visceral artery can lead to serious symptoms (Fig. 48). Thus, LÉGER et al. (1967) report the case of a 52-year-old woman presenting with postprandial epigastric pain and diarrhea in whom angiography revealed a filiform stenosis at the origin of the hepatic artery. A fibrous ring (stenosing periarterial fibrosis) was severed during surgery, and this instantaneously relieved the symptoms.

No doubt, isolated observations of this kind do not by themselves constitute proof. However, SCHIMANSKI and SCHMIDT (1971) carried out a very critical review of the literature on occlusion or stenosis of a single visceral artery associated with clinical symptoms, and were able to cite a number of relevant papers (op. cit.). They themselves found among 16 cases of visceral circulatory insufficiency 9 patients with isolated stenosis or occlusion of the main trunk of a visceral artery. In seven cases, 2 or 3 arteries were stenosed. In addition, 8 patients suffered from recurring peptic ulcer in conjunction with stenosis of the celiac artery.

It seems to have been established that the onset of clinical symptoms is related to the degree of ischemia rather than to the number of arteries that are occluded.

1.3.3 Angiographic Indications and Findings

Even though the majority of visceral stenoses and occlusions are clinically asymptomatic, there can be no doubt that the underlying visceral circulation disorder is reflected in clinical pathology. The triad of

postprandial pain
malabsorption syndrome
epigastric vascular sounds

points to the so-called abdominal angina. In typical cases the diagnosis may be established on purely clinical grounds; nevertheless, most patients undergo a number of fruitless examinations until they are eventually referred for angiography, which usually clarifies the situation at once.

The procedure consists in preparing a flush aortogram either by way of a catheter or, in generalized occlusive disease, by way of translumbar aortography (Fig. 6).

The direction of the blood flow in collateral vessels is usually determined by selective arteriography, and we therefore try a selective approach from the start in the majority of cases.

Typically, the vascular segment distal to an extensive stenotic process or total occlusion fails to fill. Filling occurs with variously long delays by way of the collateral vessels.

In contrast to the aortogram of healthy individuals, these collateral pathways—mostly pancreatic arcades or Riolan's anastomoses—are usually so strongly developed as to be immediately visible. Indeed, their caliber may match that of a visceral artery trunk.

While in anteroposterior projection the delayed filling is an important angiographic characteristic of occluded visceral arteries or advanced stenosis, only a lateral view positively demonstrates a stenosis at the origin or total occlusion of the unpaired visceral arteries owing to their ventrally directed origin. It should be noted, however, that in obese patients the quality of lateral angiograms is generally poor.

2 Gastrointestinal Bleeding

Clinical statistics and autopsies alike show peptic ulcers and esophageal varices to be far and away the leading causes of gastrointestinal bleeding (Dalichau et al., 1968). In our own case records from the years 1963 through 1968, peptic ulcers predominated. The proportion of unexplained bleeding was 11.7%; included were 13 patients with hematemesis and melena, who became symptom-free within a very short time and in whom x-ray studies and endoscopy failed to detect the source of bleeding. In all likelihood, most of these patients suffered from acute erosions that escaped notice at the time. Four patients died before a thorough diagnostic workup could be done, and no autopsy was performed; in another three, even laparotomy failed to determine the cause.

Conventional methods of x-ray examination, including aortic flush angiograms, upper G.I. series, and barium enemas, err in 10 to 50% of attempts to localize the source of intestinal bleeding (Berkowitz, 1954; Birke and Engsted, 1956; Jones et al., 1959; Prévôt and Lassrich, 1959; Wenz, 1967 and 1969).

Even exploratory laparotomy fails to discover the source of bleeding in 6 to 8% of cases (Kelley et al., 1963; Spencer, 1964; Brick and Palmer, 1964), and pathologists, too, are at times hard put to find it.

No doubt it is due to endoscopy that erosive gastritis is today more frequently being recognized as the cause of bleeding (see tabulation below).

Etiology of Gastrointestinal Bleeding (Katz et al., 1964)

Author	Endoscopy	Year	No. of cases	% Erosive gastritis
Brown et al.	No	1950	324	—
Marthin et al.	No	1953	246	5
Atik and Simeone	No	1954	293	2
Berkowitz et al.	No	1956	500	1
Zimmermann et al.	No	1956	200	—
Palmer	Yes	1952	121	22
Jones	Yes	1956	1910	30
Palmer	Yes	1962	650	15
Katz et al.	Yes	1963	150	26
Hirschowitz et al.	Yes	1963	216	22

Angiography provides fundamentally new approaches to the diagnosis of gastrointestinal bleeding: (1) Direct-contrast visualization of the source of bleeding (tumor, ulcer); and (2) delineation of the bleeding site by the contrast medium extravasated into the intestine.

2.1 Experimental Groundwork for Angiography

The application of angiographic techniques for the localization of occult gastrointestinal bleeding is based on a report by Rastelli and associates (1959). The authors tried to locate the source of bleeding postmortem by filling the aorta with contrast medium and visualizing the escape of the medium into the intestinal lumen in a case of duodenal ulcer and arterial erosion. They made a similar experimental study in dogs.

Initial quantitative investigations aimed at setting a lower limit for angiographically detectable bleeding were done by Jaffé and associates (1964). They applied a throttle clamp to a mesenteric twig implanted into the patent intestinal lumen, which enabled them to vary the intensity of bleeding and determine by serial arteriography the minimum intensity of intestinal bleeding demonstrable by contrast medium. In these experiments it was possible to detect bleedings at a rate in excess of 6.0 ml/min by flush techniques, whereas bleeding rates below 3.0 ml/min never led to a recognizable intraluminal escape of contrast medium.

Frey and associates (1967) succeeded in recording less copious intestinal bleeding at rates as low as 0.6 ml/min. They accomplished this by selective filling of individual visceral arteries, a procedure the authors had used for that purpose for the first time.

In 1969, WENZ et al. conducted 62 experiments in 8 dogs and obtained the following threshold values for artificially induced bleeding from the superior mesenteric artery: the minimum bleeding rate demonstrable by selective arteriography was 1.3 ml/min using 2.0 ml Urografin 76% per kg of body weight (Fig. 69). At a blood flow of more than 3.0 ml/min, 1 ml Urografin per kg of body weight proved sufficient. The optimal injection pressure proved to be 0.25 kiloponds/cm^2, which is equivalent to an injection rate of 1 ml/sec (Fig. 70). The viscosity of the contrast medium is of secondary importance in the diagnosis of occult intestinal bleeding. The following diagram shows the relation between the detection of bleeding by serial angiography and the dose of contrast medium as well as the injection pressure in experimental gastrointestinal bleeding of varying intensity in animals. At a bleeding rate of 3 ml/min, 1 ml/kg of Urografin is sufficient; at a bleeding rate of 3 ml/min or less, 2 ml/kg of Urografin is required.

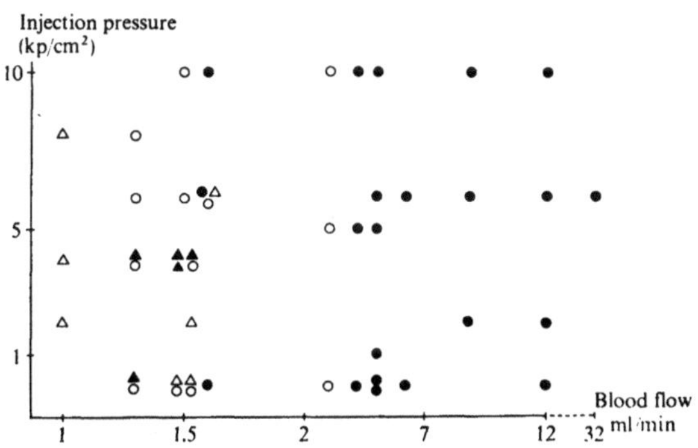

- ● 1 ml/kg Urografin—positive result
- ▲ 2 ml/kg Urografin—positive result
- ○ 1 ml/kg Urografin—negative result
- △ 2 ml/kg Urografin—negative result

Serial angiographic demonstration of bleeding as dependent on dose of contrast medium and injection pressure

2.2 Clinical Observations

Experimental experience is the basis for the angiographic localization of bleeding in patients. Most publications on the subject are of very recent date:

In 1960, MARGULIS et al. injected intraoperatively contrast medium into the mesenteric branches of two patients to localize bleeding from the colon. The exact bleeding site was identified through the escape of contrast medium into the intestinal lumen.

In 1963, NUSBAUM and BAUM tried angiography in looking for the cause of intraabdominal hemorrhages. Coincidentally, they discovered a vascular malformation in the duodenal wall. The same group (NUSBAUM et al.) reported in 1965 on angiographic diagnosis of acute gastrointestinal hemorrhages. In two out of eight patients they diagnosed gastric ulcer; in one, esophageal varices, and in another, a Mallory-Weiss syndrome. Three cases defied diagnosis even after laparotomy, and one patient was not operated on. In 1967, BAUM et al. mentioned 21 angiographed patients with unexplained gastrointestinal bleeding; by 1969, according to a report of NUSBAUM et al., the number had already increased to 100 examinations for acute and chronic gastrointestinal bleeding. Included in these cases were hemorrhages in the gastroesophageal passage, gastroduodenal ulcers, erosions, tumors, bleeding from colon diverticuli, postoperative stress ulcers, and arteriovenous malformations.

With the aid of a small focal spot tube the authors were able to differentiate vessels down to a diameter of 50–90 microns. They thus succeeded in identifying the causes of 45 out of 60 cases of acute gastrointestinal bleeding. Among 40 other patients with a history of severe gastrointestinal hemorrhage or occult bleeding, 12 were shown to have dilated vessels or arteriovenous malformations. In 15 cases, mesenteric angiograms provided indirect evidence of the source of bleeding. The authors found it possible to define the cause of bleeding in 72 out of a total of 100 cases.

In 1967, FREY et al. angiographed 8 patients because of gastrointestinal bleeding and found small-intestine tumors in several of them. The following authors published individual case reports with sometimes dramatic angiographic findings capping prolonged but fruitless diagnostic efforts: BERCHTOLD and FUCHS (1966)—telangiectatic leiomyoma of the small intestine ulcerating into the intestinal lumen; BREHM et al. (1967)—eroded cavernous hemangioma of the jejunum; WENZ and KREBS (1967)—bleeding small-bowel neurinoma.

As early as 1964, French authors (DEBRAY at al.) called attention to the possibility of angiographic diagnosis of bleeding small bowel tumors, and also to the usefulness of the method in bleeding gastroduodenal ulcers (WEILL et al., 1970). With the aid of selective angiography, KATNER et al. (1968) uncovered decidedly rare causes of bleeding, such as arteriovenous malformations of the jejunum, ulcerative enterocolitis, duodenal leiomyoma, Kaposi sarcoma of the jejunum, and 3 cases of bleeding colon diverticula. BAUM et al. (1970) have reported success in angiographic localization of bleeding in the medial portion of the duodenum.

Other authors who have helped to perfect this angiographic method of localizing intestinal bleeding may be found in the English-language literature (ANNES et al., 1967; BOIJSEN and REUTER, 1967; KOEHLER and SALOMON, 1967; HALPERN et al., 1968; REUTER and BOOKSTEIN, 1968).

Whether and when to make the radiologic examination is decided on the basis of a thorough clinical workup in collaboration with the radiologist. Once the hemorrhagic shock or collapse has been brought under control, x-ray localization of the source of bleeding should be attempted as quickly as possible. At our clinic, we have had excellent results with such "early examinations."

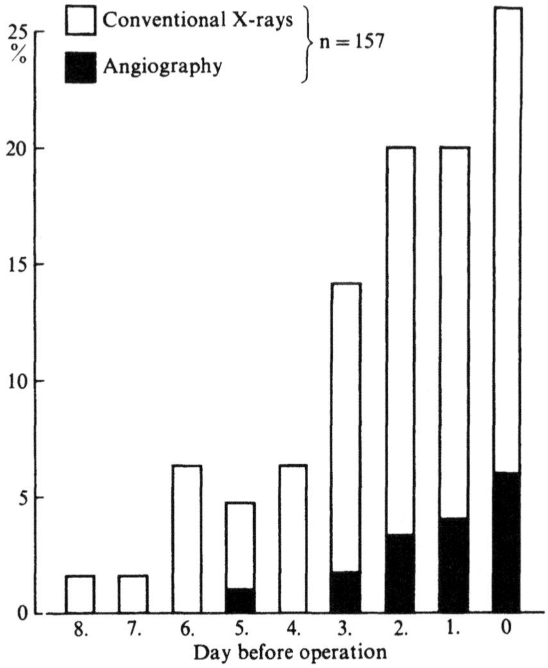

Timing of x-ray examination in gastrointestinal bleeding (WENZ, 1969)

The superior surgical results obtained by early treatment of the most common cause of bleeding, peptic ulcer (SCHREIBER et al., 1965; DALICHAU et al., 1968), should encourage radiologists to localize sources of bleeding as rapidly as possible (Fig. 68). Depending on the suspected site of bleeding, use is made of a plain x-ray, a GI series, or barium enema. It should be borne in mind that the administration of barium precludes angiography immediately afterwards. Therfore, immediate angiography is advisable in heavy intestinal bleeding; if the result is negative, one may always follow through with the conventional barium transit. We have no hesitation to perform angiography to localize the source of bleeding immediately before a scheduled operation, while a transfusion is being given.

Experience with our own patients, some of whom had gone through numerous radiologic and endoscopic examinations with negative results, has strengthened us in following this active course. A case in point is that of a woman with ileal hemangioma who had been subjected to a total of 25 x-ray and endoscopic examinations and no fewer than 22 blood transfusions before being referred to our clinic, where she underwent angiography immediately. In 2 other patients, arteriography was the only radiologic study between two laparotomies that were performed because of a bleeding small-bowel neurinoma and hemorrhage following a Billroth II resection, respectively (Figs. 7, 64, 66, 170).

2.3 Angiographic Technique

The procedure of choice is selective angiography on account of the clear delineation of circumscribed intestinal segments and overshadow-free visualization of visceral vascular branches. Flush aortography offers less of a chance to localize the source of bleeding because of contrast medium dilution in the nonselective technique and the superimposition of extraneous vascular regions. Nevertheless, BREHM et al. (1967) succeeded in localizing a previously obscured hemorrhage with the aid of flush aortography. Aortography can also be valuable in localizing tumors which are not supplied by visceral arteries but invade the adjoining intestinal loops, causing gastrointestinal bleeding (e.g. retroperitoneal sarcoma).

When a gastric source of bleeding is suspected—that is, in virtually every case of hematemesis—the first procedure will be celiac angiography. In the venous phase, attention will focus on opacification of the portal vein and on possible filling of varicose collaterals to the esophagus in portal hypertension.

If the history, the clinical picture, or repeated fruitless endoscopic and roentgenologic examinations point to a deeper location of the bleeding, first the superior mesenteric and then the inferior mesenteric artery will have to be visualized.

Techniques used for angiographic demonstration of bleeding

Celiac angiography	34
Mesenteric angiography	29
Splenic arteriography	1
Left gastric arteriography	1
Aortography	8
Total	73
in	47 patients

The quantity of contrast medium we use does not as a rule exceed 30 ml of Urografin 76% for each visceral artery. This dosage is adequate for acute severe hemorrhages, the more so as in case results are negative the injection has to be repeated into other visceral arteries or the aorta itself and then doses of 100 ml or more are needed. When an oozing hemorrhage or bleeding from a tumor is suspected, we have been injecting—so far without any complication—50 ml Urografin 76% into the superior mesenteric artery. A dose of 30 ml Urografin 76% is sufficient for the inferior mesenteric artery. The rate of injection is adjusted to the extent of the bleeding. In practice, the injection is done manually when the hemorrhage is profuse, while for minor hemorrhages or during bleeding intervals we use the automatic injector at rates up to 8 ml/sec. This procedure is most reliable for visualization of small bowel tumors, for example.

It is clear from all animal experiments that bleeding must exceed a minimal limit of severity to be detectable angiographically. All of our patients who were successfully angiographed had posthemorrhagic anemia with sharply reduced hemoglobin and hematocrit levels. The sole exception, with virtually normal hemoglobin values, was a 52-year-old patient who was angiographed immediately after the first intestinal hemorrhage. He was found to have a small polyp of the jejunum (Fig. 67). Future studies will show whether further refinements of techniques will also make the so-called microhemorrhages accessible to angiographic detection.

What can the angiogram be expected to show in gastrointestinal bleeding?

1. The *hemorrhage* itself can be localized directly. Only in very few cases will the contrast medium escaping into the gastrointestinal tract through the perforated vessel produce a distinct opacification of mucous membranes. Far more frequently, there will be persistent minute extravasations of the contrast medium, which are not always easy to detect.

As a rule of thumb, this means that the heavier the bleeding the easier its localization (cf. experimental results).

2. The *source of bleeding* may also be demonstrated directly. A bleeding tumor (small-bowel neurinoma or the like) or the inflammatory marginal reaction of an ulcer crater can betray its presence by increased vascularization or, in the case of a malignant tumor, by pathologic neovascularity. In the presence of such symptoms, angiography can prove diagnostic even in cases in which laparotomy or endoscopy fails.

The table below presents results of selective angiography for localization of causes of bleeding in our patients.

Angiographic localization of gastrointestinal hemorrhages

Positive	19	(gastric erosion, 6; peptic ulcer, 5; tumor, 4; other, 4)
Doubtful	11	
False	4	(duodenal ulcer, 3; tumor, 1)
Negative	15	(duodenal ulcer, 3; peptic ulcer of jejunum, 1; hemangiomatosis, 1; erosion, 1. Surgery was also unsuccessful, 1; no operation, 8)

2.4 Use of Vasoactive Agents for the Treatment of Gastrointestinal Hemorrhages

The idea of utilizing the catheter inserted in the bleeding visceral vessel for therapeutic purposes suggests itself. The first references to specific administration of hemostatic agents for the therapy of gastrointestinal hemorrhages were made by NUSBAUM et al. (1968) and STECKEL et al. (1968), who studied the vasoconstrictive effect of different substances upon the mesenteric vessels and who first demonstrated a definite therapeutic effect in hemorrhages due to portal hypertension.

American workers use almost exclusively vasopressin, a synthetic polypeptide already used by BAUM and NUSBAUM (1971) in 48 cases of gastrointestinal bleeding. In 28 cases of portal hypertension and bleeding esophageal varices, the catheter was threaded into the superior mesenteric artery and vasopressin was injected with a motor-driven pump at a rate of 0.2 pressor units per ml a minute. After 10 minutes of continuous vasopressin infusion, a control arteriogram revealed considerable vasoconstriction. In 27 cases the acute hemorrhage was stopped; 24 patients subsequently underwent surgery (portocaval shunt).

Similar favorable results were achieved with vasopressin injections in 6 cases of arterial bleeding (Mallory-Weiss syndrome, gastric erosion, etc.). In two patients the dosage had to be raised to 0.3 pressor units/ml/min and the infusion time extended to 5 days.

The anticipated cardiac complications of intravenous vasopressin injections did not occur in selective arteriography. However, because of the potential antidiuretic effect of this substance, we used Oxypressin (Sandoz), which reportedly does not have this side effect, in cases of severe gastrointestinal bleeding. As of now, our experience has been fairly limited. Still, when faced with a life-threatening gastrointestinal hemorrhage, particularly in a patient whose poor general condition precludes surgery, one should consider this effective "arterial pharmacotherapy". Somewhat comparable to the therapeutic use of catheter angiography are efforts to arrest hemorrhage with the aid of a balloon catheter (WHOLEY et al., 1970).

2.5 Visceral Angiography and Hemorrhagic Shock

In discussing acute gastrointestinal hemorrhage as an indication for visceral arteriography, we have repeatedly mentioned that the patients are frequently in hemorrhagic shock, a condition with which the radiologist is rarely, if ever, confronted under normal circumstances.

Since it has been shown that the exact angiographic localization of the source of bleeding is, among other things, dependent on the intensity of the hemorrhage, visceral angiography will occasionally have to be performed at times when shock is imminent or has just been overcome (WENZ et al., 1969). The problem then is not only to establish the clinical symptoms and the pathogenesis of the shock but to evaluate the changes detected by radiography. Peripheral vasoconstriction and diminution of blood flow in tissues and organs are detectable, as we know, by (1) dye dilution, (2) plethysmography, and (3) isotopes. In contrast to these indirect procedures, hemodynamic changes have so far hardly been investigated by optical and/or roentgenologic methods. Microscopic studies of intravital capillary preparations under incident light have been described. The shock-constricted capillaries can be visualized directly.

Serial angiography is another method for direct visualization of the vascular and fluid mechanics of shock. In animal experiments on six dogs in hemorrhagic shock, we prepared serial angiograms of the superior mesenteric artery in order to explore the nature of the changes due to shock (for details of method see CZEMBIREK et al., 1971).

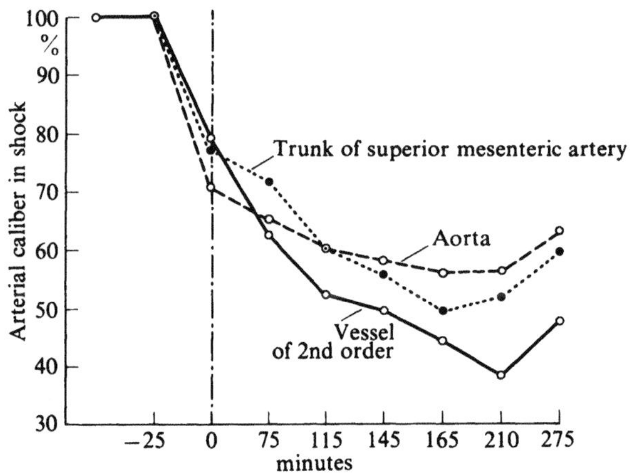

Change in caliber of visceral arteries in shock

These studies on the superior mesenteric artery revealed changes of caliber affecting not only the minor vessels but also the aorta and the trunk of the superior mesenteric artery (Fig. 65). In addition, the number of perfused arteries is distinctly reduced in shock. While about 80% of the vessels can be visualized in the early stages of shock, the number drops to 60% in compensated shock. There is no evidence of an increase in the number of demonstrable vessels in the late oligemic phase or after reinfusion.

The steady film sequence in serial angiography makes it possible to determine exactly the flow time of the contrast medium. During the hemorrhagic shock, the arterial phase is prolonged by comparison with the control angiogram, the contrast medium remaining visible in the arterial system an average of 3 seconds longer. Similarly to the arterial changes, the venous system also shows a constriction of the vascular lumen down to about 40% of the baseline caliber of the greater veins, depending on the stage of shock. In shock, the venous system is filled an average 2 seconds sooner. This may be considered an established fact since a premature venous phase is seen despite the reflux of contrast medium into the aorta and the constriction of the arteries.

Inasmuch as the changes involve both the arterial and the venous phase, they may be taken as evidence that the measured caliber changes reflect active vasoconstriction. According to several authors, the site of the active vasoconstriction is at the level of the muscular elements of the vessel wall (FINE et al., 1962). This active vasoconstriction is attributable to humoral factors, among which acetylcholine, histamine, and epinephrine in particular (KATZ and STRENGE, 1938) have been studied.

The greater constriction of the veins which we found is consistent with findings by FOLKOW (1961). They indicate that the venoconstrictive mechanism is stronger and less responsive to the vasodilating action of metabolites.

So far there has been no optical evidence of the "arteriovenous shunt" proposed in the literature (CLARA, 1939; STAUBESAND, 1968; and WATZKA, 1936). This is understandable if we compare the resolving power of x-ray machines with the caliber of the assumed shunt. According to STAUBESAND (1968) the diameters of these shunts are less than 300 microns, that is to say, below the present radiologic detection limit in serial angiography. However, the early venous filling is indirect evidence of the existence of mechanisms which enable the arterial blood to reach the venous system more rapidly.

For the reasons stated we are unable to draw any angiographic conclusions as to the nature of the shunts. However, there is angiographic evidence of distinct vasoconstriction during and immediately after severe acute gastrointestinal hemorrhage. We had noted on several previous occasions a premature filling of the portal vein system in these angiograms. This was particularly conspicuous in a patient with a ruptured spleen due to non-lacerating abdominal trauma, though rupture of the splenic sinus and the possible traumatic formation of an arteriovenous shunt would be a plausible explanation in this case (cf., also chapter on splenic rupture, p. 75).

To sum up, it may be said that visceral angiography lends itself to experimental investigations of hemorrhagic shock as well, permitting verification of previous findings. The experience acquired in this field assumes clinical importance when angiography must be performed in cases in which hemorrhagic shock is imminent or has just been overcome. These are the angiographic signs of hemorrhagic shock:

1. Constriction of arteries and veins
2. Reduced capillary area
3. Premature venous filling

These changes should be taken into account in the angiographic diagnosis.

3 Portal Hypertension

3.1 Pathophysiology

A great many ailments in the region of the portal vein are associated with congestive manifestations; those occurring in cirrhosis of the liver were already correctly observed by VESAL (1514–1564). On the basis of exact pressure measurements, WHIPPLE (1945) introduced the concept of portal hypertension as the dominant symptom common to a variety of pathologic conditions.

Flow obstruction is reflected morphologically in visualization of the collateral circulatory pathways. Such anastomoses are as well known in the retroperitoneal region, in the hemorrhoidal plexus, and in the ligamentum teres along the obliterated umbilical vein as are collaterals on the lesser curvature of the stomach. The venous plexus of the lower third of the esophagus communicating with the superior vena cava by way of the azygos vein drains into the superior gastric veins, which course along the greater curvature of the stomach—as short gastric veins—into the splenic vein and converge to the vena coronaria ventriculi along the lesser curvature.

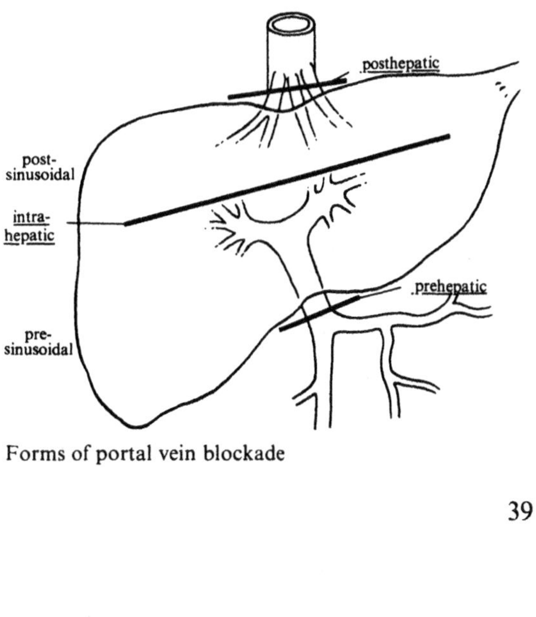

Forms of portal vein blockade

The valveless portal circulation receives its flow impulses essentially from the intestinal peristalsis, from arterial pressure pulses imparted via the arteriovenous anastomoses in the villi of the intestine, and from rhythmic contractions of the spleen. The interplay of these forces with variable resistances in the drainage area determine the pressure in the portal venous system, which averages between 100 and 150 mm of water column (BÖRGER, quoted by HELLNER et al., 1957).

The diagnostic task of radiology is to localize the obstruction in the portal circulation. The block may be prehepatic, intrahepatic or posthepatic.

3.2 Prehepatic Block

Prehepatic obstructions can develop outside or inside the vessel. Tumors and inflammatory changes along the course of the splenic and portal veins, notably at the level of the pancreas, the stomach or the duodenum, as well as enlarged lymph nodes in the area of the hilus of the liver, can cause stenosis or complete blockage of the extrahepatic portion of the portal vein.

Intravascular obstructions are caused by thrombosis or thrombophlebitis making the portal vein or the splenic vein alone (thrombosis of splenic vein) impassable. Thrombi can be angiographically visualized if the contrast medium flows around the obstruction or bypasses it via collaterals. Extrahepatic stenosis of the portal vein and, less frequently, of the splenic vein has also been ascribed to traumata.

In children, prehepatic portal hypertension can be caused especially by umbilical vein sepsis in the newborn (Fig. 74) and also by pyelophlebitis secondary to appendicitis, but there may be more distant primary foci such as osteomyelitis, otitis and the like.

3.3 Intrahepatic Block

The intrahepatic block is far less important in childhood than in adults, being by and large limited to rare cases of congenital fibrosis of the liver and congenital dilatation of intrahepatic portal vein branches. In the adult, cirrhosis of the liver of varied origin is the most common cause of intrahepatic blockage (Fig. 72).

Cirrhosis of the liver. The conventional upper GI series is sufficient to demonstrate cardial and esophageal varices related to the cirrhotic condition, but the portal vein itself must be visualized for a closer look at portal circulation. A characteristic of portal hypertension is the retrograde filling of the coronary vein. The development of collateral circulation, however, is by no means always commensurate to the extent of parenchymal liver damage.

As a general rule, the intrahepatic ramifications of the portal vein show a greatly variable course. Owing to the proliferation of connective tissue, peripheral areas are more poorly vascularized, so much so that in advanced stages of atrophic liver cirrhosis the portogram resembles a "defoliated autumn tree" (Fig. 72).

Incipient cirrhotic changes cannot be demonstrated on the portogram. There is no doubt that angiography is of very limited value as compared to liver biopsy for the early diagnosis of cirrhosis or for differentiating the stages of hepatitis. Nevertheless, much has been published on the subject and a number of authors have dealt with hepatic vascular changes in cirrhosis of the liver (BOIJSEN, 1965; HABIGHORST et al., 1964; POLLARD et al., 1966; SERVELLO, 1960; GEINDRE et al., 1967; HALES et al., 1959; POPER, 1952; RUZIKA et al., 1959; TAMAO, 1966; ROSCH, 1959). The picture is dominated by the changes of the first *venous* and *portal* branches to be affected, which range from tenuous modifications of vascular gauge to kinking and, ultimately, rarefaction and the full-blown picture of "autumnal defoliation".

By contrast, arterial alterations appear much later. Dilatation of the arteries supplying the liver does not develop until the late stages of cirrhosis, when the portal blood supply has been reduced (NEY, 1958; VIAMONTE, 1968). If the angiogram shows persistent narrowing of the lumen of the hepatic artery, the prospects for portocaval anastomosis are poor.

SAMMONS and associates (1967) found that arteriograms taken in early stages of cirrhosis or in the stage of fatty liver degeneration revealed elongated or constricted arterial branches, while the late, fibrotic stage was marked by increasing vascular tortuosity, spotty filling of capillaries and dilatation of the splenic artery. In the cirrhotic stage, one may occasionally encounter arterioportal shunts, major portal vein segments filling with contrast medium even in the early arterial phase. This makes possible the functional demonstration of the arterioportal fistulas which have long been familiar to pathologists from the work of V. BECKER.

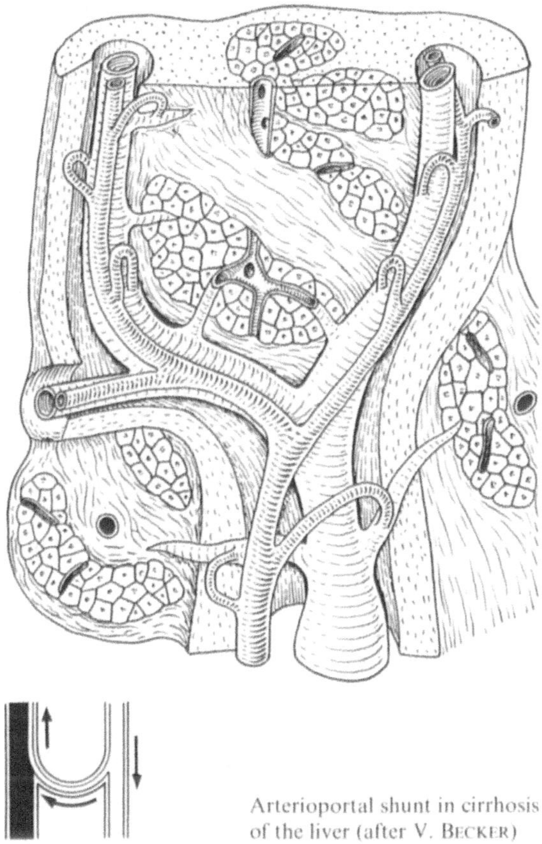

Arterioportal shunt in cirrhosis of the liver (after V. BECKER)

BOIJSEN and associates (1968) actually succeeded in demonstrating a *portal vein thrombosis* by selective arteriography of the liver: By way of the arterioportal fistula and through hepatofugal flow of the contrast medium a thrombus was visualized at the junction of the splenic vein.

The "conventional" method of visualizing the portal vein, via splenic puncture or the umbilical vein and indirectly via the splenic artery, has been described in the chapter on the technique of arterioportography. We should also mention the possibility of visualizing the portal vein in so-called *postsplenectomy bleeders;* obviously, once the spleen is removed, there can be neither splenoportography nor arterioportography by way of the celiac artery. In such cases about 50 ml of a highly concentrated contrast medium may be injected into the superior or inferior mesenteric artery in order to outline the trunk of the portal vein, which is of course very important if a shunt operation is planned.

For better opacification of the portal venous system in splenectomized patients, BOIJSEN et al. (1968) recommend adding a few micrograms of bradykinin to the contrast medium. This is useful not only in visualizing an unobstructed portal vein but also in angiograms of tumors in postsplenectomy cirrhosis of the liver, in thrombosis of the portal vein, and in exploring surgical shunts. The findings thus obtainable have been described in detail by BUCHELER et al. (1971).

Even though morphological information provided by the angiogram alone is of limited value in cirrhosis of the liver, serial angiography can be of considerable assistance to the surgeon. Thus, FUCHS et al. (1971) were able to demonstrate in a prospective study of 45 cases that shunts between the portal vein and the vena cava reduce total hepatic blood flow by 30–60%. If liver function has been reduced before the operation, however, the resultant circulatory deficit jeopardizes the outcome of the operation and leads to hepatic insufficiency. On the other hand, a shunt operation should be performed in patients with increased arterial flow volume as evidenced by a dilated artery in the presence of a narrowed lumen of the portal vein.

In many cases liver function tests suffice to differentiate between an intrahepatic portal block—mostly caused by cirrhosis of the liver in our latitudes—and a prehepatic obstruction due to thrombi and stenoses. Verification is secured by portography, notably so in patients in whom morphologically demonstrable liver alterations have led to portal hypertension but are not yet reflected in detectable functional disorders of consequence (SCHRIEFERS, 1968). For surgery, it is essential to differentiate between a peripheral splenic vein occlusion, calling for splenectomy, and a central or intrahepatic occlusion necessitating a portocaval anastomosis. Occasionally, particularly marked dilatations of the splenic vein with less dilatation of the portal vein trunk make it advisable to establish a spleno-renal anastomosis in the cirrhotic patient. Similarly significant is the finding of flat mural thrombi in the portal vein.

The differentiation of mural thrombi from functional filling defects in the splenoportogram may present serious difficulties. The number of diagnostic errors can be reduced by tracing the junctions of the superior and inferior mesenteric veins and considering laminar flow effects.

When there is a dense network of vessels in the immediate vicinity of the porta hepatis and a recognizable opacification of intrahepatic branches of the portal vein is produced, one speaks of a *cavernous transformation* of the portal vein. In such cases it is the trunk of the portal vein which is obstructed. The intrahepatic branches of the portal vein are then supplied through an angioma-like convolution of collateral vessels.

WENZ et al. (1971) have called attention to congenital intrahepatic stenoses of the portal vein with poststenotic dilatation (Fig. 73) but also to aneurysmal dilatation of the portal vein with retardation of blood flow and consequent secondary hypertension (LÉGER's portomegaly) (Fig. 71). Neither case showed signs of an antecedent inflammation or cirrhosis of the liver parenchyma.

The most important venous collaterals in portal vein occlusion are the coronary vein (1); the umbilical vein (2); links between mesenteric and systemic veins (3); and splenorenal and splenogastric anastomoses (4).

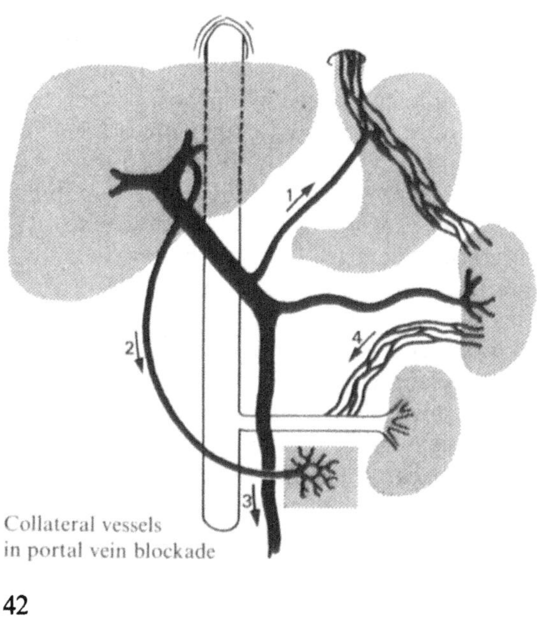

Collateral vessels
in portal vein blockade

3.4 Suprahepatic Block

As compared with intrahepatic block, the suprahepatic block is an exceedingly rare cause of portal hypertension. Reported cases in children have included congenital insufficiency of the tricuspid valve, adherent pericardium, and congenital stenosis of the hepatic vein and the vena cava.

In the adult, posttraumatic stenoses of the hepatic vein and the inferior vena cava have occurred but are extremely rare. They are caused on occasion by constrictive pericarditis, but more often they are due to endophlebitis of the hepatic veins (the BUDD-CHIARI syndrome) (Figs. 76, 77), which can at times be simulated by tumor compression.

The clinical diagnosis is based on the finding of an enlarged, congested liver with all the signs of portal hypertension.

In the arteriogram as well as in the portogram, transit of the contrast medium may be considerably slowed, so that the opacified liver presents an ivory-like appearance (Fig. 76). Evidence of retrograde flow of intraarterially injected contrast medium through the portal vein and collateral pathways to the systemic veins has been found in severe cases.

3.5 Angiographic Techniques and Indications

If the limitations and diagnostic merits of individual techniques are known, the choice of the portographic method is not difficult. No doubt the most frequent and diagnostically most useful method is *splenoportography*, whether by percutaneous or laparoscopic injection of the contrast medium. Besides sharp visualization of the portal venous system, pressure measurement often furnishes the only other objective evidence of portal hypertension and ought not to be overlooked in evaluating vascular obstructions in the portal system.

On the basis of our experience to date, arterioportography is indicated in the following circumstances:

1. Postsplenectomy hemorrhage. Without a spleen—no splenoportography!
2. Failure of splenoportography—very small or atypically localized spleen.
3. Splenic puncture contraindicated because of inflammatory or malignant organ alterations!

4. Arteriovenous fistula. Arterioportography alone allows full exploration of both the arterial and the venous phase.

Umbilical vein portography is a simple procedure in the newborn but is also occasionally employed in adults after exposure and disobliteration of the umbilical vein (Fig. 32b). The substantial surgical effort required for exposure of the umbilical vein is a hindrance to routine use of this method, which is indicated when the liver is to be subjected to prolonged selective perfusion of a chemotherapeutic agent, for example. In such cases, too, direct measurement of portal vein pressure is possible.

Hepatic venography is an essential part of the angiographic evaluation of patients with portal hypertension. An injection with the catheter tip free in a hepatic vein gives information about the degree of distortion of hepatic veins by fibrosis. The application of contrast medium through the wedged hepatic vein catheter shows the degree of sinusoidal fibrosis, the speed of emptying of the portal vein, and the direction of flow in the portal vein. The transmitted sinusoidal pressure can be obtained through the same wedged catheter.

In patients with cirrhosis, all of whom have sinusoidal or postsinusoidal obstruction, this pressure represents the pressure transmitted through a static column of blood extending from the portal vein through the sinusoids and hepatic venules to the catheter. It is the same as the splenic pulp pressure measured at splenoportography and both measurements accurately reflect total portal pressure. Normal pressures range from 40 to 150 mm of saline. If the pressure is above 150 mm of saline, the patient has portal hypertension (Reuter and Redman, 1972).

For the wedged venogram the rate of injection should be no more than 2 cc per second; the quantity of contrast medium should not exceed 8 cc.

The angiographic appearance is that of a homogeneous blush of hundreds of sinusoids with the contrast medium draining to other hepatic veins. Too rapid an injection results in reflux of contrast medium even in normal persons. In cases of fibrosis of sinusoids and obstruction of venous outflow the pattern of sinusoidal filling becomes irregular and nonhomogeneous. The increased resistance to drainage causes contrast medium to be forced into portal vein radicles. When fibrosis becomes severe and the portal vein becomes an outflow tract from the liver, the pattern of sinusoidal filling becomes markedly nonhomogeneous and the contrast medium entering portal vein radicles drains from the liver in a retrograde direction through the portal vein to portal-systemic collateral veins.

Smith et al. (1971) staged the histologic changes in the liver by the distortion of hepatic veins seen in free hepatic venography. In mild cirrhosis there is some loss in the branching, with demonstration of only third or fourth-order branches. In moderate cirrhosis these processes progress with further loss of branching and lack of sinusoidal filling. In the end stages of the disease, there is nearly complete obliteration of hepatic veins.

In our opinion, angiographic examination is justified even by suspicion of portal hypertension, particularly if there is a risk of variceal bleeding or if gastrointestinal hemorrhage and hematemesis have already occurred. In planning the operative approach, it is essential to visualize the portal vein system, a procedure that should be coupled with the measurement of portal pressure to obtain evidence of portal hypertension. In this connection the use of portography for assessing the function of a surgical portocaval shunt (Fig. 75) should also be noted.

4 Abdominal Trauma

Penetrating wounds exposing the abdominal cavity require immediate surgical repair, so that preoperative diagnosis is superfluous in most cases. By contrast, blunt abdominal trauma does not preclude any kind of injury to intraabdominal organs, so that the decision to operate and the type of surgical approach depend on the diagnostic evidence obtained.

Over a period of six years a total of 175 cases of nonlacerating abdominal trauma were seen at the Surgical Clinic of the University of Heidelberg. Of these, 128 had retroperitoneal hematomas and kidney contusions. In 47 cases—slightly more than one-fourth—there was injury to parenchymatous organs and the digestive tract. The mortality in splenic injuries occurring alone was 26%, while the mortality of multiple-organ injuries was 85%. Among cases of liver rupture occurring alone, 33% proved fatal; when it occurred in combination with other injuries the mortality rate was 100% (Gögler, 1962).

There is no question that in the face of such grave sequelae of injuries every effort is warranted to enhance therapeutic results by an exact diagnosis at the earliest possible moment. No doubt, clinical signs are sufficient to diagnose typical ruptures of an abdominal organ; rupture of a parenchymatous organ is strongly suggested by signs of internal bleeding, as is a perforating injury to hollow organs by peritonitis.

In the majority of cases the definitive diagnosis of non-penetrating abdominal injuries is far from simple. Even though most angiographic centers have still had very little experience with posttraumatic abdominal angiography, it has become quite clear during the last few years that it is possible to determine the locus and nature of an injury by means of opacification of the abdominal vessels (Figs. 13, 14).

Angiography is requested particularly in the following situations that render differential diagnosis difficult:

1. Manifestations of shock accompanied by signs of intra-abdominal trauma.
2. Differentiation of multiple abdominal injuries.
3. Masked organ injuries entailing the danger of delayed rupture.

At centers for which angiography has become a routine tool of abdominal diagnosis, the procedure is also increasingly employed in abdominal trauma, not only in preparation for reconstructive vascular surgery but also, and above all, to verify the rupture of a parenchymatous organ. According to FREEARK (1969), Chicago clinics perform more than 100 angiographic examinations each month because of sequelae of injuries. They have apparently proved highly satisfactory from the point of view of subsequent surgical treatment.

The angiogram should be prepared as soon as possible, before other contrast examinations but not before plain abdominal x-rays or fluoroscopy.

Generally speaking, every unclarified posttraumatic abdominal condition requires angiography. There is virtually no contraindication to angiography. We have been able to carry out this procedure without harm to the patient, even if he had only just recovered from shock.

4.1 Angiographic Technique

The method of choice is percutaneous catheter angiography from the femoral artery. It should be performed in as selective a manner as possible if the clinical findings emphasize specific organs.

If the angiogram is negative, it is advisable to follow through with survey aortography to rule out injury to adjoining organs. When access via the femoral arteries is barred, the catheter may be introduced by the transaxillary route or use may be made of high translumbar aortography.

Angiographic techniques in non-lacerating abdominal trauma

General aortography (translumbar and catheter)	44
Celiac angiography	65
Mesenteric angiography	20
Selective renal arteriography	72
Selective splenic arteriography	10
Selective hepatic arteriography	2
Selective left gastric arteriography	1
Total aorto-arteriographies	214

From the Radiologic Department, Surgical Clinic of the University of Heidelberg.

4.2 Angiographic Pathomorphology and Results

The table below shows possible angiographic findings and their pathomorphologic correlates ranging from vascular injury to complete detachment of an organ. A great variety of possible posttraumatic organ injuries can easily be fitted into this breakdown. It is tacitly assumed that in most cases blunt abdominal trauma results in a number of concomitant angiographic findings (Figs. 78–81).

Splenic rupture, by way of example, yields these impressive angiographic findings: Lacerations of the splenic pulp—spotty accumulations of contrast medium (*a*). Tears in smaller splenic vessels—arteriovenous shunts (*b*). Hemorrhage, spasm, compression—filling defects (*c*). Subcapsular hematoma—oval filling defect (*d*). Penetrating rupture—wedge-shaped fragmentation of organ (*e*). Subdiaphragmatic hematoma—displacement of spleen (*f*) (from VAN KAICK et al., 1970).

Pathomorphology and Angiographic Findings in Injuries to Abdominal Organs

Damage	Findings
Vascular occlusion	Interruption of vessel Defective opacification of capillary phase
Vascular perforation	Extravasation of contrast medium
Traumatic arteriovenous shunt	Premature venous filling
Intraparenchymatous hematomas	Smooth radiolucent parenchymatous areas with spreading of vessels
Subcapsular hematomas	Blurred lateral definition of organ; vascular deviation
Pericapsular hematoma	Displacement of organ and main vessel
Gaping rupture	Fragmentation of organ
Avulsion of organ	Non-opacification of organ

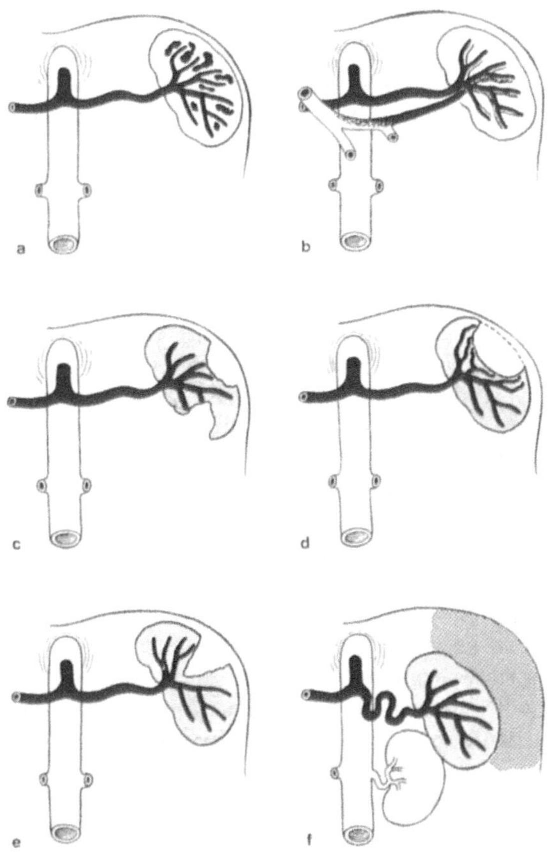

Angiographic findings in splenic rupture

Some characteristic angiograms are presented to illustrate the correlation between pathologic changes and angiographic findings. Further details on posttraumatic angiographic findings are given in the chapters dealing with individual organs.

Let us now sum up our experience to date in a few figures. We examined a total of 117 patients with an average age of 30 years. Our oldest patient was 73, the youngest 3 years old. Men outnumbered women, 99 to 18.

Among the targets of angiography in our patient population, the kidney was examined most frequently (48), followed by the spleen (20), the liver (12), blood vessels and hemorrhages (16), intestine (4), pancreas (2), and other organs (6), for a total of 97 evaluable cases, including some with multiple traumas (NIKOLAUS, 1972).

Nature of injury	Kidney	Spleen	Liver
Contusion	22	6	3
Rupture	17	13	7
Other	9	1	2

The diagnostic accuracy was high. In all those cases in which organ injury was ruled out by angiography, it was possible to dispense with exploratory laparotomy since inpatient observation in the further course confirmed the diagnosis. With the exception of two presumed injuries to the spleen, all angiographically determined organ ruptures were confirmed by surgery (see Chapter "Spleen", p. 72). One spleen and one kidney were extirpated on account of unequivocal angiographic evidence, notwithstanding unremarkable intraoperative findings. Pathologico-anatomic studies revealed a large intrasplenic hematoma and an extensive traumatic kidney infarct.

Diagnostic accuracy in organ ruptures

Angiographic findings	Surgical findings								
	Kidney			Spleen			Liver		
	+	–	?	+	–	?	+	–	?
+	16	–	–	13	2	–	4	–	–
–	1	–	–	–	–	–	4	–	–
?	–	–	–	–	–	–	–	1	–

In one case of suspected diaphragmatic rupture, the patient was in severe shock and exceedingly poor general condition, so that we could not proceed beyond flush aortography; this failed to show the splenic rupture subsequently revealed by surgery. No doubt, selective splenoarteriography would have been more successful in this case.

The high diagnostic yield of visceral angiography in blunt abdominal trauma was confirmed in 1969 by REDMAN and his coworkers. Out of 18 angiographed splenic, 7 hepatic, and 7 renal injuries, only one splenic trauma was incorrectly diagnosed by angiography.

4.3 Ruptured Diaphragm

In blunt abdominal trauma, angiography can also aid in the detection of a diaphragmatic rupture. As a rule, an injury to the diaphragm leads to prolapse of abdominal viscera. The prolapsed organs in turn may compromise pulmonary and cardiac function. Far more dangerous complications are incarceration, perforation and rupture of the prolapsed parenchymatous or hollow organs.

A clinically suspected diaphragmatic injury can be primarily diagnosed and established only by radiology. In many cases chest x-rays suffice for identification of extraneous structures belonging in the abdominal cavity. Opacification permits further clarification. An upper GI series is iseful for visualization of the stomach and the small intestine, and a barium enema for examination of the colon. Another important aid in the detection of prolapsed organs is scintiscanning, which can add a great deal to the angiographic findings.

Diagnostic difficulties can arise when the site of the rupture cannot be clearly defined, especially on the right side, or when prolapsed parenchymal or hollow organs are ruptured at the same time. The reactive pleural exudate occurring shortly afterwards or the empyema make it exceedingly difficult to differentiate rapidly the prolapsed organs and their added damage. In such cases we have found angiography useful as it has enabled us in several instances to trace the injury and identify the prolapsed organs (Figs. 83, 84).

The available literature provides little information about angiography in diaphragmatic rupture. We shall therefore cite one of our cases as an example.

A 27-year-old patient suffered a traffic accident in 1967 which caused a fracture of the third lumbar vertebra as well as blunt thoracic and abdominal trauma associated with elevated left diaphragm. After a latent period of more than 3 years he experienced an increasing sensation of fullness, eructations, epigastric pain during and after meals as well as dyspnea upon exertion and when stooped.

A chest film, which revealed gastric and colonic structures in the posterior half of the thorax besides left-sided elevation of the diaphragm, led to the diagnosis of injury to the diaphragm with intrathoracic displacement of the stomach and large intestine.

Angiography was performed to rule out or demonstrate the prolapse of other abdominal organs. A mesenteric angiogram (Fig. 83) revealed left-sided deviation and a taut course of the superior mesenteric artery, with the jejunal branches rising steeply to the left in cranial direction and being visible to the level of the middle third of the thorax on the left. A steep leftward course was also shown by the middle colic artery. A flush aortogram showed the spleen in the usual position. *Angiographic diagnosis*: Marked displacement and deviation of the mesenteric artery and its branches including the middle colic artery with intrathoracic prolapse of small bowel loops and colon and posttraumatic diaphragmatic rupture. Surgery confirmed the diagnosis.

The prolapse of viscera into the thoracic cavity following diaphragmatic rupture leads not only to displacement of the abdominal organs involved but also to changes in the position and morphology of corresponding visceral vessels. These changes constitute angiographic evidence of visceral prolapse. The arteries leading to the prolapsed organs run a craniad, mostly stretched and taut course because of the traction exerted upon them by the prolapsed organs. Other criteria of added organ injury (hemorrhage, rupture) are interruption of vessels, extravasation of contrast medium, and absence of a parenchymatous or venous phase (Fig. 84).

Angiography, preferably carried out in the form of celiac angiography with simultaneous visualization of the inferior phrenic arteries, can contribute greatly to early diagnosis and consequently to the rapid initiation of appropriate surgical therapy. Diaphragmatic injuries with visceral prolapse, representing communicating injuries at the interface between thorax and abdomen, still have a high mortality today. It amounts to 25% in acute cases, and to 75% in stages of strangulation and perforation (MILLER and HOWIE, 1968). The effects underscore the value of timely angiography in clearing up diagnostic uncertainties in case of injury to the diaphragm.

Experience in the field of posttraumatic angiography has been limited so far. However, the cases reported to date, especially concerning renal and splenic rupture (POTEMPA and WENZ, 1968; VAN KAICK et al., 1970), should encourage us to perform angiography very early in the mostly fairly young patients—in whom the examination can be completed within half an hour—in order to rule out multiple injuries or concealed organ ruptures as well as to detect previously unknown vascular injuries (Figs. 85–87). Reliable and quick posttraumatic abdominal angiography is the key to an informed choice between organ-preserving surgery and conservative therapy (WENZ, 1970).

5 Abdominal Tumors

The primacy of conventional radiographic examinations in the search for abdominal tumors has been challenged by endoscopy and angiography but also by methods of nuclear medicine. While these last are suited mainly for the visualization of liver and spleen, endoscopy permits direct inspection and biopsy in large areas of the gastrointestinal tract. The angiographic targets of choice are the vascular system, the walls of hollow organs supplied by it, and the parenchymatous organs, and their internal structure in particular.

A skillful combination of the individual techniques of conventional x-ray examinations of the abdomen, among which we may include plain x-ray, upper GI series and barium enemas, cholecystography and excretory urography, can do much to narrow down the differential diagnosis of abdominal tumors; not infrequently, however, questions regarding the specific organs involved, the true extent of the tumor, and definite evidence of malignancy and possible metastases remain unanswered.

In many of these cases angiography can be of inestimable help. The choice of vascular access routes includes the portal vein and other veins besides the aorta and its branches. On the other hand, the intestinal lymphatic vessels have not yet played any practical role in diagnosis since their visualization has not been routinely feasible until now. However, the significance of lymphography for study of the retroperitoneal space should be emphasized.

5.1 Angiographic Technique

Angiography is indicated in the search for an intra-abdominal tumor if clinical, endoscopic, or conventional x-ray examinations have failed to detect a suspected neoplasm or if there remain doubts regarding its exact localization or size. Disturbances of blood coagulation constitute the only contraindication. Further, catheter examination from the femoral artery may be hampered to such a degree by alterations of the pelvic artery that it becomes necessary to use translumbar aortography, or catheter, proceeding via the brachial artery. Pulsating tumors require caution to prevent perforations in the presence of an aneurysm.

The choice between flush aortography and selective arteriography is not always easy to make. However, we consider it unnecessary always to start with aortography and to follow this up with selective arteriography when searching for a tumor. If the tumor is clinically assignable to a specific organ (liver, spleen, stomach, etc.), selective celiac angiography should be performed immediately and only if this proves negative—or if a pancreatic neoplasm is visualized—should the next tier, that is, the superior mesenteric artery and, following this, the inferior mesenteric artery be probed and visualized.

In the great majority of cases clinical signs point at least roughly in a certain direction so that not infrequently the relatively uninormative aortography and, with it, unnecessary administration of a radiopaque agent can be dispensed with.

5.2 Angiographic Criteria for Tumors

Tissue blood flow is increased in many tumors, while in many others it is unchanged and in some reduced, usually as a result of necrosis. The following findings are made, which vary according to vascularization, localization, and size:

1. Neovascularity
2. Tumor opacification (positive contrast)
3. Arteriovenous shunts

4. Tumor radiolucency (negative contrast)
5. Signs of expansion
6. Signs of infiltration

Obviously, a tumor can betray its presence by a number of angiographic changes. Evaluation becomes difficult when there is a single sign, which may or may not be specific.

A review of critical opinions expressed in the literature shows a consensus that unequivocal evidence of neovascularity is the only reliable criterion.

5.2.1 Tumor Vessels

A tumor vessel resembles somewhat a felon on the loose: Everyone talks about him but nobody knows exactly what he looks like. A good characterization of so-called pathologic vessels was provided by STRICKLAND (1961):

> "A typical pathological vessel... is deployed seemingly without purpose, keeps to no set course and shows no progressive diminution in calibre. As it runs through the mass of the tumor, its walls may be lined by tumor cells, and... it ends its haphazard journey in amorphous spaces in the midst of areas of necrotic tumor tissue."

For a better understanding of the morphology and function of tumor vessels let us digress for a moment into ontogeny and pathology.

All the vessels in the body pass through three phases in the course of their development. In the first stage the blood is channelled through purely endothelial tubes, and to these a mesenchymal layer is added in a second stage. In the third phase, finally, different tissues arise from this mesenchymal coat so that the completed vascular wall is composed of endothelial, connective tissue with collagenous and elastic fibers, and smooth musculature. However, the arrangement of the individual elements and their relative volumes vary in different vessels (RICKENBACHER, 1971).

In the formation of granulation tissue, too, vascularization begins with the development of solid endothelial buds emanating from the capillaries, which do not provide a lumen until a later stage. It should be emphasized that these capillary buds *cannot* arise from major arteries or veins. These capillaries evolve by increases in size and through induced development of the surrounding connective tissue.

The morphological organization of tumor vessels suggests that the process of differentiation in the formation of the mural layers is disturbed: the walls of the vessels are thin in relation to their caliber; smooth muscle fibers and elastic lamellae are present in small amounts and abnormally disposed or are lacking entirely. A neural supply, too, has not been demonstrable so far. The large tumor vessels frequently show a degree of differentiation commensurate with tumor histology. In fast-growing sarcomas, for example, large vessels may consist only of an endothelial membrane and a thin layer of connective tissue (LINDGREN, 1945).

The overall arrangement of the tumor vessels is also relatively deviant. The normal vascularization of an organ generally proceeds according to rules proposed by SPALTEHOLZ (1889): In hollow organs the arteries course across the wall of the organ, which is penetrated by their branches, whereas solid organs are vascularized from a hilus, the vessels showing an arboreal ramification.

Contrary to his general rule, solid and cystic tumors are supplied from all parts of the periphery. The vessels inside the tumor are marked by irregular distribution as well as by abnormal ramification and frequently also by a tortuous, corkscrew course. Their caliber lacks the physiological taper and often shows spindle-shaped or saccular bulges.

The unphysiologic ramification, the unproportional calibers, and the pathological structure of the vessel wall not unexpectedly result also in nonphysiological circulation of the blood. The status of the tumor vessel is further complicated by the formation of thrombi, intravascular expansion of the tumor, tumor-induced compression, hemorrhage, and necrosis.

In the early stages the vessels in the foreign tissue invariably communicate with those in the surrounding tissue by way of capillaries. Thus, an artery cannot "grow" into a tumor. Preformed larger vessels are usually enclosed or destroyed by tumor tissue and are rarely taken up through linkage to the vasculature of the tumor tissue. When they are, both their course and their structure distinguish them from the actual pathological vessels (LINDGREN, 1945).

Efforts to arrive at an accurate angiographic definition of the tumor vessels on the basis of the pathologic characteristics described prove disappointing because of the unavoidable imprecision: random arrangement, erratic appearance, absence of caliber decrease, irregular margins, saccular bulges, and tortuous course (YU, 1967). It becomes evident above all that, in order to be "sure" of detection, a tumor vessel must have a substantial size, and this in turn means that the tumor itself must not be too small. Smaller neoplastic vessel are more likely to be detected by their unusual localization and disposition than by their form; however, their demarcation from hypervascularization and vascular neoformation in the context of an inflammation may present difficulties.

A proper appreciation of the efforts of pharmacoangiography to achieve improved tumor diagnosis is possible only against the background of this vascular pathomorphology. The intra-arterial injection of pharmacological substances (e.g. norepinephrine) leads to vasoconstriction of "normal" arteries but not of those tumor vessels which lack neuromuscular and humoral reactivity because of their deficient wall structure. Whereas, therefore, the sum of the vessel diameters in the area of the regular arteries will diminish by contraction, the caliber of the tumor vessels does not change, so that the flow of blood or contrast material through them will be relatively greater. This effect, of course, depends on the degree of differentiation of the tumor vessels involved; that is to say, it will not be seen or will only be faintly seen in the case of well or fairly well-differentiated vessels.

5.2.2 Tumor Opacification

Positive opacification of tumor tissue in the angiogram is possible if this tissue absorbs more radiation than the adjacent tissue. The difference must reach a certain minimum before it can become optically perceptible (Figs. 88a, 89). Both the number of vessels and their increase in diameter can increase the rate of flow of the radiopaque material. Provided there is sufficient contrast relative to the background, individual vessels can be detected at diameters as small as 300 microns. Capillaries, arterioles and venules as well as sinusoids of this order of magnitude generally fall below the limit of angiographic resolution. The homogeneous opacification of the tumor consequently requires an increase in the number of vessels within unit space at a caliber increase below 300 microns! The angiogram will not furnish any evidence regarding the nature of the vessels or the cause of the hyperemia. As early as 1950, DOS SANTOS, presenting angiograms of bone tumors one of which was taken in a case of knee-joint tuberculosis, provided the cautious commentary "there is hyperemia rather than vascular neoplasia."

It may be recalled that as a rule hyperemia is present besides exudate in both acute and chronic inflammations. Only the scar tissue which can form after abatement of the inflammation is usually rich in fibers and poor in vessels. The morphological reason for the accumulation of contrast medium in inflamed tissue is a dense network of dilated capillaries, most of which have a diameter of less than 100 microns. Arteriovenous shunts may also cause rapid perfusion of contrast material (DOERR, 1970).

LAGERGREN and coworkers (1958) were able to show that hypervascularization occurs not only in neoplasia but also in chronic inflammatory processes. The histological substrate is granulation tissue which contains dense capillary networks besides round cell infiltrations. Also, an inflammatory reaction of the local connective tissue in the vicinity of the tumor can render poorly vascularized tumors visible in the angiogram (WENZ et al., 1971).

For differential diagnosis it is necessary to distinguish tumor opacification not only from inflammatory hypervascularity but also from anatomic variants (e.g. accessory spleen) and peculiarities of contrast medium distribution, such as the tumor-like opacification of the gastric fundus (CHAVEZ et al., 1967).

Tumor opacification also encompasses the phenomenon of *contrast medium pooling*, which is caused by a localized widening of the vessels. In areas where this occurs, flow is slowed in accordance with the law

$$C = Vt/\pi r^2.$$

As a result, the phases of contrast material flow are displaced, that is to say, while the contrast medium has already drained from the normal vascular segments, blood containing the radiopaque material can still be found in the dilated vessels. Particularly the tumor vessels with their saccular protuberances can thus cause a retardation of contrast medium flow (Fig. 89). An extreme example is the hemangioendothelioma; here the contrast medium seems to remain in the venous phase owing to the localized vessel dilation.

5.2.3 Arteriovenous Shunts

A number of authors have called attention to the increased occurrence of arteriovenous shunts in tumorous tissue. In the angiogram they cause premature venous filling. Inasmuch as these anastomoses have a diameter of less than 300 microns (STAUBESAND, 1968), they are not individually discernible in the angiogram. By virtue of the shunts capillary resistance is bypassed and blood flow—hence the influx of contrast medium—is increased. Apart from an increased rate of tumor metabolism, this is probably the most important cause of the often enormous increase in the caliber of the main artery supplying the tumor region (MORINO et al., 1967).

5.2.4 Tumor Radiolucency

Cystic formations lacking vascularization may entail parenchymal radiolucency provided there is sufficient filling in the capillary phase (Fig. 88). Such cysts are therefore most readily recognizable in the kidney and the spleen, the two organs whose parenchyma is opacified best. A rounded, smooth-edged radiolucency is generally regarded as a true cyst; the "gore of parenchyma" at the margin is taken as an indication that the process is a benign one (Fig. 90).

Filling defects in the capillary phase may also reflect avascular areas resulting from tumors with central necrosis or prior hemorrhagic infiltration. Such zones of reduced blood flow are most difficult to visualize in the liver, not to mention the pancreas, since in these organs the contrast density in the capillary phase is comparatively low. This is true especially of poorly vascularized liver metastases, which also need to be differentiated from poorly arterialized regenerated nodules in cirrhosis of the liver (BÜCHELER et al., 1971).

5.2.5 Expansion and Infiltration

A *space-occupying lesion* can give rise to vascular displacements (Fig. 95a), that is, arcuate deviation, spreading, stretching, and clustering of vascular fascicles (Fig. 96). Diagnostic assessment of these indirect tumor indices presupposes exact knowledge of the anatomy, above all, of the range of physiologic variations. If only signs of displacement are present, it is not possible to estimate the size of the tumor, and localization of the organ, too, often proves difficult under these circumstances (Figs. 92, 93).

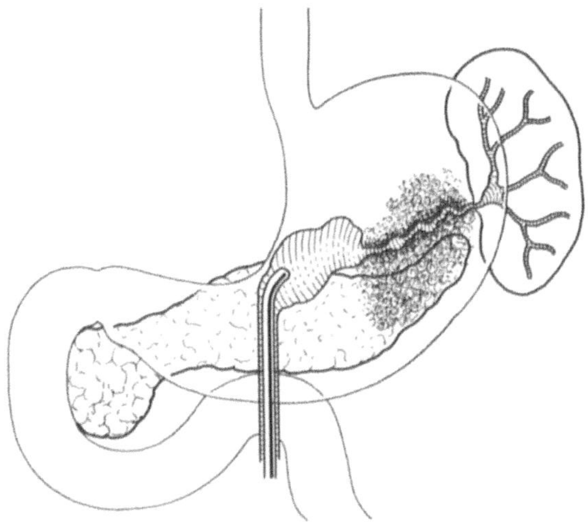

Encasement of the splenic artery by carcinoma of tail of pancreas

Infiltration—as a criterion of malignant neoplasia—can lead to penetration of the vessel wall (Figs. 95 b, 97). The tumor itself invades the vascular lumen, or intimal lesion results in formation of mural thrombi or in complete thrombotic obliteration. Typical signs are short-length arterial or venous stenoses or occlusions in the area suspected to be tumorous, with arterial stenosis usually showing a strikingly irregular—"nibbled at"—mural outline, as is shown by the example of the splenic artery in a case of carcinoma of the cauda pancreatis.

It stands to reason that the angiographer cannot attribute every vascular stenosis in the abdomen to a tumor. In fact, the small number of vascular changes caused by tumors are overshadowed by a host of arteriosclerotic vascular processes. In the majority of cases, of course, similar sclerotic vascular alterations will then be found at several other locations apart from the suspected tumor site. Even the less common angiitis mostly occurs in a generalized fashion. Tumor-related vascular stenosis further needs to be distinguished from an initially extravascular focus of inflammation which can spread to adjacent vessels and lead to thrombotic obliteration, as e.g. in the case of pancreatitis. We may mention further vascular spasm as a reaction to the injection of radiopaque material. Vascular infiltration is only possible, however, if the tumor spreads in the vicinity of the angiographically detectable major vessels (Fig. 97). Understandably, then, there will be "silent zones", mostly peripherally located, e.g. in the left lobe of the liver in which a tumor may escape angiographic detection for a long time.

Finally, attention should be called also to the "No. 1 enemy" of the angiographer, the relatively small, indifferently vascularized tumor which is not yet associated with any vascular infiltration and has not yet provoked any manifest displacements. Masked by its normal angiographic appearance, such a tumor escapes angiographic detection. It should be borne in mind whenever the findings are negative, and in such cases the global clinical picture should serve as a guide to further diagnostic and therapeutic measures.

5.2.6 Diagnostic Value of Angiographic Tumor Signs

A large tumor is detectable even by manual palpation, and angiography is therefore of value primarily in the *early diagnosis* of tumors and in the diagnosis of tumors that have not usually been detectable until now except by surgery. Examples are hepatic and pancreatic neoplasms. The "resolving power" of angiography is generally said to approximate 2 cm in tumor size (BOIJSEN et al., 1968). The determining factors are the opacifiability of the tumor as well as its localization and relation to the environment and, last but not least, the eye of the observer.

Nearly all of the aforementioned angiographic signs that may be used in the diagnosis of tumors can also occur—individually or in combination with other signs—in chronic inflammatory alterations, for which reason it is so exceedingly difficult to differentiate between chronic pancreatitis and carcinoma of the pancreas. It should be made unmistakably clear that *there is no angiographic sign that proves the presence of a malignant tumor!* In many cases, only a combination of a number of signs with other clinical, endoscopic and conventional radiologic alterations justifies the grave diagnosis of a malignant growth.

The ranking order of the value of the individual angiographic signs for the diagnosis of tumors is shown below in tabular form:

Neoplastic formation of abnormal vessels
Tumor blush
Vascular occlusion, stenosis and displacement
Tumor radiolucency
Arteriovenous shunts

Beyond the individual sign, it is the demonstration of tumor infiltration into adjacent tissues or organs as well as the visualization of metastases which proves the malignant character of a tumor.

We have thus sought to make it plain that angiographic diagnosis of tumors can only establish their probable presence and can never—even in the case of a "typical" hypernephroma—take the place of histological diagnosis.

6 Abdominal Angiography in Children

Only in recent years have angiographic examinations of the abdomen in children found increasing acceptance. Conventional radiologic methods such as plain x-rays, upper GI series, barium enema, and excretory urography are effectively supplemented by aorto-arteriography of the abdominal organs.

A total of 235 vascular examinations have been performed in children under 14 years of age at the Radiologic Division of the Heidelberg Surgical University Clinic since 1962; this number includes 101 abdominal angiographic examinations. It should be borne in mind that 75% of these examinations were carried out during the last 4 years. The children's average age was 9.4 years. The youngest child was just a few days old. Male patients accounted for two-thirds of the population.

PORSTMANN (1968), MCDONALD et al. (1968), DEBRUN et al. (1967), SCHIEFER (1967), KERK et al. (1969) and other authors have shown that angiographic examinations in children are no more risky than in adults. HALPERN (1968) found that postangiographic complications increase in frequency with age and are encountered least frequently in the youngest patients. According to our own experience, the rate of complications is not age-dependent. It depends mainly on the puncture technique and the examiner's experience. Excessive compression of a puncture site can be as harmful as the omission of a compression bandage after removal of the catheter. In the former case, a local thrombosis results, while in the other hemorrhage or hematoma may develop, though this is rarely seen in children.

Because of local thrombosis, a thrombus endarterectomy had to be performed at the site of catheterization of the femoral artery in a six-year-old girl three days after high translumbar aortography.

Apart from this one complication among 92 angiographic examinations, these results indicate that abdominal aortoarteriography may safely be performed in children as well (see also Chapter "Complications", p. 23).

6.1 Peculiarities of Angiographic Technique in Children

Abdominal angiography in children is complicated by the relatively small vessel diameter. However, the preparation and technical execution of angiography do not basically differ from what we have said about use of the method in adults. Using the simple equipment shown in Figure 39, we have been able to perform percutaneous aortic flush and selective angiography in patients as young as 2 to 3 years. Only in exceptional cases did we find it necessary to expose the femoral or brachial artery.

Impressive angiograms taken in neonates and infants were presented, for example, by FELLOWS at the Third Davos Course in Diagnostics in 1971. Needles and guide wires as well as the catheter material used at the Boston Children's Hospital Medical Center are listed in the table on p. 55.

With the aid of such sophisticated equipment, the percutaneous technique may also be used in children under 2 years of age if the following precautions are borne in mind:

The parents' written consent should be secured. Premedication should be adequate and safe positioning of the child on the examination table assured. A skin wheal should be set with 0.5% novocaine (without any epinephrine!); the local anesthetic is infused on both sides of the vessel, without suppressing the pulse. The incision in the skin is made slightly longer than in adults and the subcutaneous tissue is then pulled apart with the aid of surgical clamps. Guided by careful finger palpation, the needle held at a flat angle is then threaded into the vessel. *No pulsating outflow of blood is to be expected in children under 2 years of age on account of the narrow lumen.* It is the light red color of the emerging blood which counts.

The guide wire is carefully inserted and it should be possible to thread it, *without any resistance,* into the vessel to approximately the level of the first lumbar vertebra. Following removal of the needle, a dilator is needed to permit insertion of the selected catheter.

The catheter system has to be continuously washed with heparinized saline solution. In contradistinction to the adult, however, frequent aspiration of blood can lead to hypovolemic shock in the newborn.

Before withdrawing the catheter, it is necessary to make certain that there is no iatrogenic occlusion so that the indwelling catheter may be utilized for a possibly required angiographic examination to localize the occlusion. The following rules apply:

In children under 2 years of age, the skin temperature should be equal in both legs. In children over 2 years, the peripheral pulse should be palpable shortly before complete extraction of the catheter. In the event of iatrogenic occlusion or stenosis, an attempt should be made to correct it by intraarterial administration of a vasodilator. If this does not help, immediate excision of the thrombus has to be performed.

Postangiographic treatment begins with the slow withdrawal of the catheter and continuous injection of heparinized saline solution. Once the catheter tip becomes visible, the small quantity of blood may safely be allowed to emerge from the puncture site. This is followed by careful compression for 5 to 10 minutes, without complete suppression of the pulse. We attribute our only case of local thrombosis at a catheter entry site to unduly intensive compression.

The child is returned to the ward with a compression bandage, but without sandbag compression or the like, and should remain in bed for one day. The nurse is instructed to check on the puncture site and peripheral pulse—under the radiologist's supervision—every half-hour over a period of 8 hours.

Selective examinations (renal artery, visceral arteries) require between 3 and 25 ml and flush aortography up to 30 ml of a 60% contrast medium. The total dose should not exceed 3 ml/kg of body weight (BURGENER et al., 1971). We have been using Urografin 76% in children weighing more than 40 kg.

In young children the film speed should be somewhat higher than in adults. As a rule, 3 to 4 films in the first 3 seconds, and 1 film per second in the late phases, prove sufficient.

The technique described above may be adapted without any major change to venography and thus to visualization of the inferior vena cava. When the contrast medium is injected into both femoral veins, excellent visualization of the inferior vena cava can be accomplished in a child about 2 years old, with 10 ml each of a 60% contrast medium (Fig. 101).

For splenoportography in children, too—our experience now covers a total of 15 children under 14 years of age (WENZ et al., 1971)—we also use needles with the Longdwel plastic catheter. The only difference is that we carry out this procedure under general anesthesia in order to avoid abrupt respiratory movement when the needle is inserted into the spleen.

It is our impression that puncture of the spleen is easier in children than in adults since the organ can usually be very clearly delineated by fluoroscopy. We use 15 to 25 ml of Urografin 60%, and a film speed of 1 picture per second for 10 seconds.

Besides catheter examinations, direct puncture of the aorta may be necessary in a very few cases.

A boy now 7 years old had undergone a difficult nephrectomy for an infected cyst on the left kidney when he was 13 months old, and the operation caused an injury to the aorta. He was hospitalized for study of intermittent claudication with the suspected diagnosis of partial occlusion of the aorta. Translumbar aortography disclosed total occlusion of the abdominal aorta at the level of the intact right renal artery and an abundantly ramified collateral system which fully supplied the distal pelvic arteries by way of the lumbar, spinal and vertebral branches (Fig. 6).

6.2 Indications and Results

Of a total of 235 angiographies performed in children, 101 were designed for diagnosis of abdominal diseases. In addition to 7 translumbar aortographies, catheter flush aortography was carried out in 50 cases. Selective arteriography included 18 kidney examinations, 8 celiac angiographies, and 15 splenoportographies. A breakdown of the angiograms according to diagnosis showed a nearly even distribution of vascular and organ malformations, traumata and tumors among our patients. The group of postoperative examinations refers to x-rays taken after plastic vascular surgery. In the same category belongs preoperative angiography in kidney donors, an examination which has gained currency with the increasing use of kidney transplants. Precise knowledge of the arterial and venous systems of the organ to be transplanted is of crucial importance to the success of the operation (BEDUHN et al., 1970).

Let us now review the results of angiographic examinations of the abdomen as broken down into the categories of trauma, tumor, and vascular anomalies.

Abdominal tumors in children are, for the most part, neuroblastomas or Wilms tumors. In view of the poor prognosis of these diseases, efforts should be concentrated on early diagnosis. Angiography can make an important contribution by demonstrating pathological vessels, pooling of contrast medium, or radiolucent areas, and arteriovenous shunts (Figs. 101 to 106).

Tumor histology disclosed by abdominal angiography in children

MCDONALD et al. (1968)	58 arteriograms and cavograms: 14 neuroblastomas 12 Wilms tumors
HILLER et al. (1969)	100 abdominal angiograms: 28 Wilms tumors 26 neuroblastomas 7 hepatomas 7 cystic kidney changes 4 lymphosarcomas

Tumors other than those listed here are seldom seen in children; they are briefly enumerated according to their location in the table below.

Angiographically demonstrable abdominal tumors occurring in children

Kidneys, Retroperitoneum	Wilms tumors Neuroblastoma Cystic diseases of the kidney
Liver	Hepatoma Hemangioma, hemangioendothelioma Metastases (teratoma, insulinoma, etc.) Cysts and abscesses
Spleen	Neoplasms Splenic cysts Absent or supernumerary spleen
Pancreas	Cystadenoma Pseudocysts Insulinoma (possibly malpositioned)
Adrenal glands	Carcinoma

A 3-year-old boy exhibited unusually quiet behavior and tiredness. At the same time he suffered intermittent diarrhea. Apart from an enlarged liver, clinical and conventional x-ray examination yielded no pathological findings. Angiography disclosed a highly vascularized tumor with sizable areas of translucency throughout the liver. Numerous round areas of opacification were found in the capillary phase (Fig. 12). Histological examination uncovered a malignant metastasizing teratoma of the liver.

To an in creasing extent, angiography is becoming firmly established in the diagnosis of sequelae of intraabdominal injuries. In children, the kidneys are the internal organs most frequently injured (LAMESCH, 1964). The detection of ruptured kidney presents no difficulty in the presence of the three symptoms of pain in the flank, hematuria, and swelling of the flank. In many cases, however, it is uncertain whether the liver or the spleen was injured at the same time, and the precise extent of the renal lesion remains to be determined (Figs. 80, 99, 100). In such cases, a definite clarification of the situation is usually made possible by aortoarteriography. Particular attention must be paid to rupture of the spleen which, according to various surveys, occurs in cases of non-lacerating abdominal trauma at rates of 15–42% (AAKHUS and ENGE, 1964).

A 14-year-old boy was referred to us after a traffic accident, suffering from acute left-sided upper abdomen with hematuria. Selective renal arteriography revealed a transverse rupture of the organ. The subsequent celiac angiography uncovered the rupture of the spleen with enlargement of the organ, hematoma, a wedge-shaped avascular zone at the superior pole, and defective parenchymal filling.

The criteria applied to vascular and organ injuries in children are similar to those in the adult. Let us recapitulate the most important angiographic signs (Figs. 99, 100):

1. Occlusion, avulsion, stenosis or displacement of vessels.
2. Parenchymal perforation, extravasation of contrast medium, organ displacement.
3. Premature venous return.

Angiography not only provides objective evidence of the organ injury, but at the same time it determines the extent of the parenchymal defect and gives information about the arterial supply of the remaining organ segments. In the final analysis, the surgeon relies on the angiogram to decide whether the defect can be corrected by uniting the fragments, whether a resection should be performed, or whether, in cases of renal or splenic rupture, the entire organ should be sacrificed. In 70% of cases during recent years, it has been possible to save part of the injured kidney through organ-preserving surgery (POTEMPA and WENZ, 1968).

The 47 abdominal angiographies that we have in the meantime performed in children because of trauma (BEDUHN, 1972) may be broken down as follows:

16 selective renal angiographies
8 celiac angiographies
1 mesenteric angiography
14 flush aortographies
4 translumbar aortographies
4 pelvic arteriographies

All angiographically detected organ injuries were confirmed by subsequent surgery. In the remaining cases, the young patients were spared a laparotomy because organ injury was ruled out by the angiogram. Similarly favorable results attesting to the high diagnostic accuracy of angiography in abdominal trauma have been reported in the literature (see chapter on Abdominal Trauma, p. 43).

Vascular and organ anomalies (Figs. 107, 108) are rare indications for abdominal angiography in children. When such anomalies are demonstrated nowadays, there is no reason whatever for therapeutic resignation; on the contrary, extraordinarily effective surgical procedures are possible in the field of vascular malformations.

A striking example is offered by a 14-year-old boy with coarctation of the aorta at the thoraco-abdominal junction. Besides reduced arterial blood pressure in the lower extremities, the child suffered from digestive disturbances which remained unexplained for a long time. Aortography disclosed long stretches of stenosed aorta and massive collateral circulation leading via intercostal and lumbar branches to Haller's trunk. The stenosed superior visceral artery received much of its blood supply via Riolan's collateral from the inferior mesenteric artery (Fig. 108). The aortic stenosis was successfully bridged by means of a plastic prosthesis (Prof. VOLLMAR). Using this bypass, another prosthesis to the superior mesenteric artery provided for improved visceral blood flow.

One of the rare indications for visualization of the inferior vena cava in the presence of liver tumor in children is shown in Fig. 101, while indications for splenoportography with the special characteristics observed in early childhood are cited in the chapter on portal hypertension (p. 39).

Conventional methods of examination will continue to be given priority in abdominal diseases in children. Nevertheless, abdominal angiography may even today be considered a valuable addition to the radiological armamentarium in this stage of life.

Abdominal arteriography in pediatrics. (Technical suggestions from the Boston Children's Hospital Medical Center)

Injection and film sequence

Vessel	Amount of contrast medium	Rate of injection	Film sequence
Renal artery	3 to 7 ml	5– 6 ml/sec	4/2:1/10
Celiac and sup. mesenteric a.	10 to 30 ml	10–20 ml/sec	3/3:1/12
Aorta	15 to 35 ml	15–25 ml/sec	3/3:1/4

Total contrast medium per patient, max. 3–4 ml/kg body weight.

Catheter material for pediatric arteriography

FORMOCATH blue, thin-walled	Catheter size I.D. (mm)	Catheter size O.D. (mm)	Guide wire dia. in inches
RPX × 025	0.63	0.97	.021/.023
RPX × 037	0.44	1.22	.021/.025
RPX × 045	1.14	1.57	.025/.035
RPX × 055	1.40	1.90	.035
RPX × 062	1.58	2.08	.035
KIFA red			
thin-walled, red 1	1.15	2.20	.035
extra thin-walled, red 7	1.40	2.20	.035

Recommendations for cannulas and guide wires

Age of child	Needle (gauge)	Guide wire (inches)
3 days to 6 months	20 (Paul-New)	.021/.023
6 to 18 months	20/19 (Paul-New)	.021/.023/.025
18 months to 5 years	19/18 (Paul-New)	.025/.035
5 to 10 years	18 (Paul-New)	.035
10 years and over	18 (Paul-New)	.035

V Special Abdominal Angiography

1 Abdominal Aorta

The following pathological changes in the trunk of the abdominal aorta are clinically and roentgenologically important:
1. Anomalies
2. Occlusion and stenosis
3. Aneurysm
4. Aortocaval shunting

1.1 Anomalies

These involve mainly congenital aortic stenosis, which is called coarctation of the abdominal aorta. Suprarenal, interrenal, and infrarenal forms are distinguished according to localization (VOLLMAR, 1968).

The clinical picture has only recently become more familiar. In about 20% of the cases the constriction is hypoplastic and extended; most stenoses affect only a short segment.

The clinical disease pattern and the aortographically detectable collateral circulations, which are usually supplied by the intercostal arteries and the celiac trunk, depend on the localization. The blood flows caudad, principally through the superior and inferior mesenteric arteries, the lumbar artery, and the pelvic arteries.

In one case of typical coarctation of the abdominal aorta involving the celiac trunk and the superior mesenteric artery, collateral circulation utilized extraneous collateral vessels (Fig. 108). Fatigue of the lower extremities and postprandial abdominal pains were the predominant clinical symptoms.

The thoraco-abdominal aortic aneurysm in a six-year-old boy shown in Fig. 107 may also be interpreted as a deformity in the sense of an "aortic diverticulum". This interpretation is supported by the bud-like protuberance visible just above the aneurysmal sacculation.

Many aortic anomalies are discovered by accident. In most cases the technical procedure is percutaneous catheter aortography through the femoral artery. Stenosis necessitates high translumbar aortography or transbrachial survey aortography.

The typical angiographic findings are displacements of the aorta, cleanly demarcated segmental stenoses with collaterals, and absence of arteriosclerotic alterations or circumscribed aneurysmal sacculations.

1.2 Occlusion and Stenosis

A *suprarenal* occlusion of the abdominal aorta is consistent with life only if there is sufficient collateral circulation to the renal arteries. At our hospital, BEDUHN and HALLWACHS (1970) carried out successful experimental studies on renal blood flow after subtotal and total occlusion of the left renal artery, and on the effect of intrarenal implantation of the splenic artery after removal of the right kidney (Fig. 60).

Infrarenal obstruction of the aorta as a rule also involves the inferior mesenteric artery, whose territory is supplied via RIOLAN's anastomosis. From here, the iliac and femoral arteries can sometimes be supplied surprisingly well via lumbar branches and the arteries of the abdominal wall. In Figs. 57 and 59, an infrarenal aortic occlusion secondary to arteriosclerosis is compared with a postoperative iatrogenic occlusion of the abdominal aorta in a young child; in the latter case, the various collateral circulations are especially distinct. None of the cases of infrarenal aortic occlusion we have examined thus far presented any signs of insufficiency in the visceral vessel branches. In our opinion, the method of choice for the visualization of such stenoses and occlusions is translumbar aortography (Figs. 109, 110).

1.3 Aneurysms and Dissection

Aneurysms of the abdominal aorta are for the most part of arteriosclerotic origin. They often extend beyond the bifurcation into the iliac arteries (Fig. 111), and have a suprarenal localization in only 4–5% of cases (VOLLMAR, 1968). VOLLMAR also reports that about 40% of abdominal aneurysms are accompanied by clinical symptoms such as intermittent abdominal pain and throbbing sensations and, less frequently, chronic constipation, lack of appetite, nausea, vomiting, and bloody stools (HEBERER et al., 1966).

Usually, the diagnosis can be made by palpation. In obese patients, the detection of a calcific border may provide additional information. About 10% of all patients first see a physician at the stage of rupture (DE BAKEY et al., 1964), which is marked by intense, continuous pain. Either a retroperitoneal hematoma is formed or hemorrhages occur in the free abdominal cavity or in the gastrointestinal tract (duodenum!). Perforation into the inferior vena cava is infrequent (BEALL et al., 1964).

Not all surgeons are convinced of the necessity of an angiographic examination of a palpable aneurysm of the abdominal aorta. If, however, aortography is decided upon, the safest route is the transbrachial although we have never observed complications in either translumbar or femoral catheter aortography.

The objective of aortography is to localize the aneurysm as precisely as possible, to provide information on arterial inflow and run-off for surgical intervention, and to detect possible para-aortic tumors. In practically all cases only a very small portion of the aneurysmal lumen is visualized since thrombotic masses often close off all but a narrow residual lumen. Nevertheless, the surrounding aneurysmal sac is usually well outlined if the film is not too dark.

Acute, spontaneous dissection of the aortic wall is a rarity (Fig. 112) although its mortality is still high enough for a 1.1% ranking among pathological causes of death (MOTE and CARR, 1942).

Dissection usually arises from medial necrosis (GSELL, 1928; ERDHEIM, 1929; CELLINA, 1931; GORE and SEIWERT, 1952). Bleeding from the vasa vasorum occurs in the cystically altered media. Lacerations of the intima would therefore appear to be sequelae.

According to another pathogenetic interpretation, traumatic laceration of the intima is primary and leads to invasion of blood and destruction and dissection of the media. BRAUNSTEIN (1969) was able to show that perforation of the intima coincided with atheroma in more than half of his cases.

Since a pressure more than 10 times greater than the physiological systolic pressure is required to perforate the intima, hypertension can only play a secondary role.

DE BAKEY distinguished three clinical types of dissection according to their localization:

Type 1: Confined to the ascending aorta.

Type 2: Dissection of the ascending aorta extending distally beyond the aortic arch.

Type 3: Originating at the descending aorta in the region of the left subclavian artery and extension to the entire descending aorta.

Aneurysms (1959–1971). Radiology-Department of the University Surgical Clinic Heidelberg. 327 aneurysms in 230 patients (after NEUER, 1972).

Vessels	Total	Congenital	Arteriosclerotic	Traumatic	Iatrogenic	Others (mycotic, syphilitic, etc.)
Pulmonary artery	1	1				
Upper extremity	20	5	2	13		
Lower extremity and iliac arteries	185	8	111	15	44	7
Thoracic aorta with branches	35	1	11	13	2	8
Abdominal aorta	66		56	1	6	3
Celiac trunc	1		1			—
Splenic artery	8		7			1
Hepatic artery	4		2			2
Inf. mesenteric artery	1	1				—
Renal artery	5		4		1	—
Lumbar artery	1	1				—
Total	327	17	194	42	53	21

The following characteristic symptoms of dissecting aneurysm are invariably observed: Acute retrosternal pain, followed by ischemia of the right arm, transitory hemiplegia with loss of consciousness, visual disturbances, ischemia of the left arm, uncharacteristic intercostal pains, acute abdomen, anuria and, finally, symptoms of an acute iliac artery occlusion. Although about 50% of dissecting aneurysms extend to the abdominal aorta, an external rupture occurs in this area in only about 2%. At best, the outer channel may re-enter the true aortic lumen. This spontaneous healing is accompanied by the formation of a second aortic channel (double-barrel aorta), which later develops an endothelium or, in a few cases becomes thrombosed again. For visualization, we prefer catheter aortography, transbrachial if possible. The typical findings are tabulated below:

Angiographic criteria of dissecting aneurysm

1. Double-barrel aorta with distinguishable partition
2. Reduction and deformation of original aortic lumen
3. Elongated and tortuous course of aorta
4. Uneven and intermittent opacification of dissection
5. Widening of aortic wall by more than 5 mm (normal aortic wall width 2–3 mm) (HÄRTEL, 1971).

We should like to add a special form, *retrograde aortic dissection*, to DE BAKEY'S classification.

We had the opportunity to observe such a case presenting with acute abdomen (GRUSS et al., 1971).

Case report: A 77-year-old woman who had felt completely well before suffered an extremely severe attack of pain in the epigastrium, followed by a persistent boring pain, circulatory collapse, and temporary syncope. Myocardial infarction was ruled out first, and the patient was then transferred to the Surgical Clinic with the presumptive diagnosis of mesenteric or renal artery embolism.

Findings on admission: Very obese; diabetes mellitus; continuous arrhythmia; rigidity of upper abdomen; constant tenderness of epigastrium. Blood pressure 100/60 mm Hg; after treatment of shock 120/60 mm Hg. WBC 15,800; Hb 13.6 g/100 ml; hematocrit 39; 24-hour urine 400 ml, specific gravity 1026.

Catheter aortography: After injection of 40 ml Urografin 76% at the first lumbar vertebra, the abdominal aorta was strongly visualized with discrete arteriosclerotic changes in outline and slight kinking. In contrast to the dense opacification of the renal arteries, there was a slight filling delay in the celiac trunk. The distal thoracic aorta to a point just above the celiac origin on the left side of the vessel had a double contour. To determine the cause of the phase delay in the celiac trunk, the catheter was changed and a curved red ÖDMANN catheter was inserted into the celiac trunk. The origin at the first lumbar vertebra was atypically displaced leftward. The division into hepatic and splenic arteries and left gastric artery was normal. There was an irregularly outlined radiolucency at the origin of the celiac trunk from the aorta, with some of the contrast material refluxing into the aorta during the injection. Total occlusion of the gastroduodenal artery directly after its origin from the common hepatic artery. After injection of 25 ml Urografin 76%, a triangular extravasation of contrast medium above the celiac trunk remained visible from the late arterial phase until the end of the series 16 seconds after the injection. The contrast medium remained for several minutes. In addition, a delicate band-shaped opacification extended centrad for 15 cm along the descending aorta.

Angiographic diagnosis: Stenosis of the origin of celiac trunk, occlusion of gastroduodenal artery, dissecting aneurysm of descending aorta, obscure extravasation of contrast medium with persistence at origin of celiac trunk. Laparotomy did not confirm the dissecting aneurysm. An open endarterectomy of the proximal section of the celiac trunk was performed, but the patient died shortly afterwards from irreversible cardiac arrest. Autopsy disclosed a transverse triangular 2 × 1 cm laceration directly above the origin of the celiac artery. From this point proximally, the entire wall of the abdominal and thoracic aorta was torn and split open. The origins of the mesenteric and renal arteries were fully patent. All other large arteries displayed more or less pronounced atheromatous changes.

Angiographic findings and the results of histological examinations strongly suggest that the intimal laceration of the descending aorta constituted the port of entry of the bloodstream, hence the starting point of the dissection. We can only speculate why the dissecting aneurysm emanated from the abdominal aorta and the dissection occurred opposite the direction of flow of the bloodstream. The intimal laceration was precisely proximal above the origin of the celiac trunk; consequently, a distal pathway for the inflowing blood may have been blocked by the texture of the vessel wall. In addition, the localization of the intimal lesion directly below the diaphragm may have contributed to the fact that the suction effect of the low thoracic pressure at this point caused dissection in this atypical proximal direction. Although it is extremely rare, this observation shows that acute symptoms of occlusion of a visceral artery should also suggest the possibility of orthograde or retrograde aortic dissection.

1.4 Aortocaval Fistula

Violent pains in the stomach and back, increasing venous congestion in the lower half of the body with rapid onset of cardiac failure accompanied by signs of cerebral dysfunctions are symptoms of a rare complication of abdominal aortic aneurysm, namely, rupture into the vena cava, which BEALL et al. (1964) observed in only four of 130 cases of ruptured aneurysm of the abdominal aorta.

Our own case material includes only two traumatic aortocaval fistulas.

One case involved a female theater ticket seller who was shot in a holdup. The bullet remained lodged between the aorta and the inferior vena cava and a shunt was formed. The bullet was later removed by surgery along with the fistula.

The second case concerned a 43-year-old woman who had had her right kidney removed 19 years previously. Increasing signs of fatigue and a peculiar noise accompanying the pulse beat led the patient to consult her physician. Catheter aortography disclosed a wide shunt originating at the stump of the right renal artery, between the abdominal aorta and the aneurysmally dilated inferior vena cava (Fig. 113).

The changes were visualized very sharply in a color subtraction picture (Fig. 11) in which the arterial and venous phases appear in different colors (red and green). The zones of mixed venous and arterial blood and the fistula itself are distinguishable much better than on a black-and-white picture.

The shunt which formed after nephrectomy was found during the operation (Prof. LINDER) to be the result of mass ligature. Over the years, the ligature apparently worked its way through the vessel walls, thus forming a shunt. Shunts of this type are detected most readily by catheter aortography. After the fistula is localized, the shunt can in some cases be probed selectively (pressure measurements!).

1.5 Inferior Vena Cava

Aside from a few rare malformations, among which we may include obstruction of the pelvic veins (WANKE, 1957), the typical pathological changes of the inferior vena cava are:

1. Intravascular processes (thromboses)
2. Lumen constrictions of extravascular origin.

These are not always easy to differentiate by angiography!

Although thrombotic occlusions occur predominantly in the preceding pelvic veins, thrombi may occasionally extend to the vena cava or arise locally as a result of inflammatory or neoplastic processes (Fig. 114). These mechanisms also underlie the BUDD-CHIARI syndrome (endophlebitis hepatica obliterans), in which the inferior vena cava is not infrequently involved in the thrombotic process at the angle between the liver and the vena cava (see chapter on "Portal Hypertension").

An important task for angiography is the detection of tumor thrombi in hypernephroma. Drainage of the renal veins is usually not totally obstructed; the thrombus can prolapse into the venae cavae. These findings are crucial for the operative procedure.

CEN et al. have therefore proposed (1970) *indirect renal phlebography* by selective pharmacoarteriography with epinephrine (6–8 mcg epinephrine in the renal arteries) for richly vascularized tumors with arteriovenous shunts. In all other cases, including renal vein thrombosis of different pathogenesis, and for evaluation of the inferior vena cava itself, these authors prefer cavography: Injection of 50 ml Conray 70 into one or both iliac veins at a contrast medium injection rate of 11 ml/sec and a film speed of 2 frames/sec for the first 4 seconds and 1 frame/sec for the next 7 seconds.

There is always the danger that a thrombus will become detached during an angiographic demonstration! Such complications can be avoided by careful insertion of the catheter with "a steady hand" and injection of the contrast medium as far as possible from the suspected site of the obstruction. Trial injections with the tip of the catheter already in the iliac vein are even more important for preliminary orientation in these cases than in other investigations. The catheter end should also be perforated on the side to avoid too powerful a stream.

Along its course through the retroperitoneal space to the right of the aorta, the inferior vena cava is especially compromised by space-occupying processes in the directly adjacent organs, the para-aortic lymph nodes, the aorta, the right kidney and adrenal gland, the duodenum, the caput pancreatis, and the liver.

Extravascular alterations can usually be expected to give smoothly outlined impressions; however, the nature of the underlying spaceoccupying process cannot always be determined from the shape and contour of such impressions.

For example, Fig. 94 shows an egg-sized filling defect in the middle third of the inferior vena cava which surgery revealed to be an isolated metastasis of a teratoid carcinoma. Similarly, malignant generalized diseases of the lymph system can give rise to pathological phenomena, as in lymphogranulomatosis, for example.

If the caval wall shows irregular contours and partial destruction, a malignant infiltration is to be suspected (Fig. 103c, d).

Enlargement of the caput pancreatis and alterations in the duodenum can also cause displacement of the inferior vena cava. It is questionable, however, whether differentiation between benign and malignant processes can be accomplished by cavography in early cases.

We found a total obstruction of the inferior vena cava in a two-year-old child with a primary, extensive tumor of the liver (Fig. 101).

2 Liver

2.1 Anatomy

The liver is the largest organ in the body, weighing about 1500 g, and the major portion of it is situated in the right hypochondrium.

The falciform ligament, which marks the margin between the right and left lobes, begins at the diaphragmatic surface somewhat to the right of the median plane.

The fossae in the visceral surface are in the shape of an H. The transverse fissure, the porta hepatis, marks the entry of vessels and nerves and the exit of the hepatic duct and the lymphatic channels. The left, perpendicular fissure, the fissura sagittalis sinistra, separates the right and left lobes. and its anterior portion, the ligamentum teres hepatis, lodges the obliterated umbilical vein. The posterior half of the liver lodges the ligamentum venosum, the remains of the duct which in the embryo carried some of the blood of the umbilical vein directly into the inferior vena cava, bypassing the liver, by connecting the left branch of the portal vein with the left hepatic vein. The gallbladder is situated ventrally in the right sagittal fissure of the "H", while dorsally the sulcus venae lodges the inferior vena cava. The adjacent organs produce numerous impressions on the liver surface (kidneys, adrenals, stomach, duodenum, and colon). The pyloric portion of the stomach and the junction with the duodenum are contiguous to the quadrate lobe, while the pars superior duodeni produces the superficial duodenal impression on the neck of the gallbladder and the adjoining segments of the right liver lobe (Hafferl and Thiel, 1969).

2.2 Vasculature

Blood Circulation. The portal blood stream has a flow rate of 1000–1200 ml/min. About $^3/_4$ of the total blood supply to the liver passes through the portal vein, the other fourth passing through the hepatic arteries. Seventy percent of the O_2 requirement of the liver is supplied by the portal vein blood (Martini, 1970). Of the liver's two afferent vessels, the portal vein supplies the functional blood, and the hepatic artery the nutritive blood. The blood stream mixed in the liver sinus then drains through the hepatic veins into the inferior vena cava.

Artery. The hepatic artery—A. hepatica communis—arises from the celiac trunk and passes along the upper margin of the pancreas to the right as far as the hepatoduodenal ligament, where it divides above the pylorus into the gastroduodenal artery and the proper hepatic artery. The latter courses upward in the hepatoduodenal ligament to the left of the portal vein at the same level as the common bile duct, and usually bifurcates into left and right branches before reaching the porta hepatis. The left branch proceeds to the left lobe of the liver, while the right branch gives origin to the cystic artery, which leads to the gallbladder.

In its extrahepatic portion, the hepatic artery shows *anomalies in course and origin* in about 40% of cases (Schorn et al., 1957).

An accessory hepatic artery may course to the left lobe of the liver as a branch of the left gastric artery. But more important is the accessory hepatic artery which enters the hepatoduodenal ligament at the upper margin of the pars superior duodeni as a branch of the superior mesenteric artery, ascends between the common bile duct and the portal vein, and supplies the right lobe of the liver and the gallbladder if it takes that course. The proper hepatic artery then supplies only the left lobe. The accessory hepatic artery may also arise from the gastroduodenal artery instead of the superior mesenteric artery. The accessory hepatic artery from the superior mesenteric artery is the original hepatic artery, while the proper hepatic artery represents a neoformation. The hepatic artery opens via arterioles and arterial capillaries into the periportal sinus region and the centrizonal sinusoids as well as into the intermediate zones of the lobules.

Portal vein. The second afferent vessel, the portal vein, receives its blood from the large afferent veins—the superior and inferior mesenteric veins, the splenic vein, and the left gastric vein. The trunk of the portal vein enters the liver at the porta hepatis, where it forms two main branches, one for the left and one for the right lobe of the liver. Normal pressure in the portal vein is 3.5–13.5 mm Hg or 5–18 cm H_2O (MARTINI, 1970).

Shunts between the branches of the portal vein and the hepatic veins are usually to be found in the presinusoidal vessel segment (POPPER and SCHAFFNER, 1961).

Arterioportal anastomoses are formed only under pathological conditions. The portal vein bifurcates into its left and right branches quite near the porta hepatis.

Along its course in the hepatoduodenal ligament it receives only small veins, the gastric veins and—very close to the bifurcation—the cystic vein. In addition, minute paraumbilical veins, which originate at the navel and pass along the ligamentum teres hepatis, also empty into the portal system of the liver. The ligamentum teres may also lodge a residual venous channel which is important in umbilical portography. These veins dilate in portal hypertension.

Hepatic veins. The right lobe of the liver is drained via the right and median hepatic veins, while the left lobe is drained via the left hepatic vein; these veins open into the inferior vena cava directly below or within the diaphragm. Accessory veins also pass independently into the vena cava.

2.3 Conventional Radiography

Technique. The outward shape, the size, and the position of the liver can be determined by a two-plane *abdominal radiography*, sometimes combined with *tomography*, *G.I. series*, or *barium enema*. In addition, the neighboring organs (pancreas, kidneys, spleen) can be visualized in a *diagnostic retropneumoperitoneum* or *pneumoperitoneum* and their anatomical relation to the liver determined. The organ itself appears on survey films as a homogeneous shadow without any appreciable areas of densification.

Yield. By means of these techniques, it is easy to detect enlargement of the liver or anomalies of position (situs inversus abdominalis, Chilaiditi syndrome, prolapse, wandering liver, corset liver, atrophy of left liver lobe, etc.). Displacement of the liver into the thoracic space is of differential diagnostic significance in patients with a ruptured diaphragm. Simulated hepatomegaly due to atelectasis of the lower lobe or basal pleural effusion as well as diaphragmatic or adrenal tumors can also be ruled out by these techniques. Circumscribed radiolucencies caused by the accumulation of gas in liver abscesses or in the biliary duct or portal system should be considered pathological findings. Calcifications (liver stones, liver cysts, hemangiomas, metastases, etc.) are also visualized on the survey film.

Special radiologic methods. A modern technique for diagnostic examination of the liver is scintiscanning, which is especially suited for the detection of space-occupying processes and studies of liver function. In obstructuve jaundice, percutaneous or laparoscopic cholangiography has often proved valuable as an adjunct to oral, intravenous and intraoperative visualization of the biliary tract.

2.4 Angiographic Techniques

The hepatic artery can be surveyed by subdiaphragmatic aortography or catheter aortography. It can also be visualized without overshadows by selective celiac angiography. The left gastric artery and the splenic artery are then opacified at the same time provided there are no anomalies. Not infrequently, both inferior diaphragmatic arteries are filled simultaneously with contrast medium if their ostia are immediately adjacent.

The common hepatic artery can be superselectively visualized without great difficulty by using appropriate catheters.

In 70% of cases serial arteriograms of the hepatic artery will visualize fairly clearly the cystic artery and—in the late phase—the wall of the gallbladder besides the liver parenchyma. In the venous phase, sufficient pooling of contrast medium in the descending hepatic veins is extremely rare.

Celiac angiography has the advantage over selective hepatic angiography of visualizing the intra- and extrahepatic portal system owing to simultaneous filling of the spleen via the generally well-outlined splenic vein (arterioportography).

Visualization of the hepatic veins is necessary in only a few diseases. Unfortunately, neither arteriography nor portography yields sufficiently distinct pictures of the hepatic veins. The method of choice, therefore, is retrograde filling of the hepatic veins, either through the brachial veins or the femoral vein. The veins opening into the liver, which are usually multiple, are relatively easy to probe either via the inferior or the superior vena cava.

Hepatic vein thrombosis, which leads to the Budd-Chiari syndrome (loc. cit.), is the indication of choice. Most thrombotic filling defects within the venous lumen can be detected by retrograde injection of contrast medium (Fig. 76d).

Coutinho et al. (1967) recommend segmental hepatic angiography with a venous catheter inserted through the left median cubital vein past the right atrium into the peripheral portion of a branch of a hepatic vein. This technique should permit good visualization of presinusoidal changes in the liver parenchyma.

The same technique can also furnish evidence of portal hypertension.

Hepatic veins can further be visualized by percutaneous, transhepatic injection of contrast medium. Instead of the bile ducts—as in transhepatic cholangiography—branches of the hepatic veins may be punctured. We have not ourselves verified this, as in the Budd-Chiari syndrome, for example, but the indication seems plausible.

2.5 Angiographic Examination of Liver

General significance. Since radiology has so far contributed little of diagnostic value in primary liver diseases (with the exception of biliary tract disorders), we should not expect too much of angiography in this respect.

The following techniques are available:

1. Celiac or hepatic angiography for visualization of the arterial system and the liver parenchyma.
2. Portography for examination of portal system and liver parenchyma.
3. Retrograde angiography of hepatic veins.

We personally have had very little experience with angiography of the hepatic veins, and regard hepatic vein thrombosis in the Budd-Chiari syndrome and possible pressure measurements in portal hypertension as the principal indications. By contrast, arterial and portal angiography are considered for quite a number of indications in the following discussion.

Angiography cannot be expected to evaluate the stages of hepatitis or cirrhosis of the liver. Tried and proven laboratory techniques and the potential of percutaneous liver biopsy meet practically all diagnostic requirements. Of course, in clinically doubtful cases, as e.g. for differentiation between parenchymatous and obstructive jaundice, or in the presence of a tumor in a cirrhotic patient, angiography can be extremely valuable.

Indications. The following indications for angiography have been established and will be discussed individually:

1. Primary malignant tumors of the liver.
2. Liver metastases.
3. Benign liver diseases.
4. Parasitic liver diseases.
5. Subphrenic, intrahepatic and subhepatic abscesses.
6. Cirrhosis of the liver and portal hypertension.
7. Liver trauma.
8. Aneurysms of hepatic artery.
9. Arterioportal shunt.
10. Obstructive jaundice.

2.6 Arterial Collateral Circulation of the Liver

Occlusion of a main hepatic artery. Surgical ligation of a *principal hepatic artery* can give rise to a complex collateral blood flow through the organ via accessory hepatic arteries and interarterial anastomoses or bypass arteries. A marked dilatation of the branches proximal to the ligated main artery may also be observed.

According to Düx et al. (1966), ligation of a primarily well-developed main hepatic artery can be tolerated without subsequent necrosis of the organ. Retrograde filling of a centrally ligated principal branch will demonstrate the hemodynamic efficacy of the collateral vessels.

Occlusion of the celiac trunk and other visceral arteries: In contrast to the picture seen when a main branch of a hepatic artery is ligated, the angiographic findings in *central occlusion of the common hepatic artery* or the *celiac trunk* are relatively uniform. Blood is supplied to the liver via pancreaticoduodenal collaterals (see chapter on Chronic Visceral Blood Flow Disturbances, p. 27). When the *celiac trunk and the superior mesenteric artery are centrally occluded at the same time,* the necessary blood is supplied to the visceral abdominal organs by the inferior mesenteric artery via the aforementioned strongly developed Riolan's collateral and the pancreaticoduodenal arcade. The seriousness of the clinical symptoms is determined solely by the capacity of the new collaterals, so that clinical symptoms may be entirely absent.

2.7 Angiographic Pathomorphology

2.7.1 Primary Malignant Tumors of the Liver

General characterization of tumors. Primary malignant liver tumors do not loom very large in clinical considerations since they are quite rare in our part of the world. According to REIFFERSCHEIDT (1969), they represent only 1.5% of all tumors. They occur primarily in the 40 to 60 age group. Tumors generally develop secondarily to cirrhosis, and it is predominantly the right lobe of the liver that is affected. For a long time the tumors remain confined to the segment and lobe margins, and metastasize much later. Solitary, large-nodule growth forms and multilocular disseminated forms are distinguished. The most important histological types of tumors are:

Carcinomas

(a) Hepatocellular carcinomas
(b) Cholangiocellular carcinomas

Sarcomas

(a) Round-cell and spindle cell sarcomas
(b) Hemangioendothelial sarcomas
(c) Reticulum cell sarcomas.

Clinical diagnosis. The clinical symptoms of primary malignant tumors of the liver are uncharacteristic: Energy loss, anemia, epigastric tenderness, etc. If the tumor is palpable, it is already inoperable. Until quite recently, diagnosis was usually made on the operating table or in the autopsy room. An early, intravital diagnosis was first made possible by angiography and scintiscanning (Figs. 15, 115–118). Laparoscopy has also been of some value; however, tumors do not infrequently develop inside the liver, so that even in laparotomy they may escape the eye of the observer (DÜX, 1968; BOIJSEN et al., 1968).

Angiographic findings. While scintigraphy of the liver will disclose a space-occupying process, celiac angiography can to a limited degree determine the type of tumor (YU, 1967; STECKENMESSER et al., 1971). In contrast to metastases, which will be discussed later, primary malignant tumors of the liver are usually richly vascularized and therefore easily discernible in the angiogram (BOIJSEN and ABRAMS, 1965; BARTLEY et al., 1967). Hypervascularization, tumor vessels, contrast medium pooling, and arterioportal shunts are especially characteristic of hepatocellular carcinoma and sarcomas. All tumors produce displacement effects on the portogram. As a rule, a cholangiocellular carcinoma shows less contrast; it is characterized more by infiltrative growth and vascular occlusions (BIERMAN et al., 1951). However, even this type of tumor can have wide vessels, as we witnessed in a case of our own. An outstanding feature of these tumors is their occasional use of the basal membranes of the vessels as a matrix for growth of the tumor epithelium (WENZ et al., 1971).

Hemangioendotheliosarcoma (Fig. 117) bekame known as a Thorotrast-induced tumor. However, it occasionally develops in the liver without this radioactive carcinogen. The extremely late clinical manifestation of this tumor is noteworthy. We saw one patient who did not receive medical treatment until hemorrhage from a site near the liver capsule appeared in the abdominal cavity. Autopsy later disclosed that more than half of the liver was engulfed by the neoplasm (WENZ and OTT, 1965).

The angiographic picture is characterized by retention of the contrast medium past the venous phase in partly acinose, irregularly sized and often amorphous pools. Displacement and occlusion of arterial branches and, especially, early signs of portal vein branch diversion round out the angiographic picture.

In rare cases the radiologist may even discover the cause of a hypoglycemic disturbance by angiographic detection of a large liver sarcoma (HEGER et al., 1969).

2.7.2 Liver Metastases

Value of angiographic demonstration. The opinions expressed about angiographic visualization of liver metastases in the literature are rather disappointing, apart from a few especially impressive cases (Fig. 118). For the most part, this is due to the poor vascularization of most liver metastases. Richly vascularized metastases are exceptions; they include the few published cases of hormonally active tumors such as insulinoma, carcinoid, adrenal and thyroid tumors (LUDIN et al., 1966; HERNANDEZ et al., 1967; KIDO et al., 1968). Hypernephroma metastases are also well visualized.

Angiopathological background. Histologic studies of injection preparations in cases of primary and secondary liver tumor have shown that in both humans and animals 90–100% of the blood to the tumor nodules is supplied by the hepatic artery, even in animals in which tumors have been induced by inoculation of tumor cells into the portal vein. Failure of the portal vein supply was in most cases attributable to invasion of the radiating portal vein branches by the tumor. In contrast, the branches of the hepatic artery were rarely occluded. Accordingly, celiac angiography should theoretically provide good opacification of metastases. However, a study by BREEDIS and YOUNG (1954) showed distinctly less vascularization of metastases as compared with the surrounding liver tissue, so that the tumor metastases appeared as "cavities" in an arterial cast preparation. It is noteworthy that *regenerating nodules* receive 60% of their blood supply from branches of the portal vein. Thus, if they are sufficiently large, they may appear as filling defects in the parenchymal phase owing to their relatively reduced arterialization. We observed this in a female patient with a Thorotrast-damaged liver; a filling defect in the hepatogram suggesting a tumor turned out to stem from an extraordinarily large regenerating nodule upon laparotomy and histological examination.

Most secondary liver metastases from tumors in the gastrointestinal tract, the breasts, and the bronchial tree become noticeable only by divergence of arterial branches and an irregular distribution of contrast medium in the hepatogram phase. This explains the fact that, according to BOIJSEN (1965), metastases less than 2 cm in diameter located at the periphery of the liver cannot be visualized (BENNET et al., 1964; DEBRAY et al., 1965; NEBESAR et al., 1966; WEISSLEDER et al., 1966; STECKENMESSER et al., 1971).

BIERMAN et al. (1961), KAHN and CALLOW (1965), and STUHLBERG and BIERMAN (1965) recommended the use of vasoactive agents for improved results. According to BOIJSEN et al. (1968), the injection of very small quantities (5–10 mg epinephrine) into the hepatic artery appears to be useful.

The demonstration of richly vascularized liver metastases is a different matter. The more opaque area of the metastasis is set off in fairly dense contrast from the normal liver tissue, especially during the hepatogram phase.

We ourselves were able to detect angiographically numerous highly vascularized metastases in a two-year-old boy believed to have a liver tumor—a histological examination showed that these metastases represented a teratoid carcinoma (Fig. 102). The situation is similar for malignant, hormonally active tumors of the female genitalia, such as chorioepitheliomas.

2.7.3 Benign Liver Tumors

Benign neoplasms within the liver are rare, and have hitherto usually been incidental findings during laparotomy or autopsy. Their clinical significance is extremely low.

They have, however, acquired a certain importance in angiography since in many cases they simulate very closely the picture of a malignant tumor.

Benign liver tumors include hamartomas, adenomas, and hemangiomas.

According to SCHWARTZ (1964), it is not possible to assign one of these highly vascularized tumors to a specific histological type on the basis of angiographic findings. The detection of a tumor capsule, however, may make differentiation from a malignant tumor possible. Yet BOIJSEN et al. (1968) angiographically demonstrated distinct capsule formations also in metastases, so that this finding is not in itself diagnostic.

In cases of cavernous hemangioma, pools of contrast medium of varying size provide diagnostic clues. However, a definite differentiation from malignant hemangioendothelioma is possible only if sure signs of infiltration and invasion of adjacent tissues or organs have been observed (BERDON et al., 1969: Giant hepatic hemangioma with cardiac failure in the newborn; RANNIGER et al., 1963: Multiple arteriovenous anastomoses in familial telangiectasia).

Brief mention should be made of liver cysts which are usually congenital and which show only an avascular space on angiograms. In contrast to parasitic cysts—and also liver abscesses—the absence of capsule opacification is significant for differential diagnosis (CAPLAN et al., 1966: Nonparasitic cysts). BERT et al. (1968) recommend the combined use of splenoportography + scintiscanning or arteriography + scintiscanning in polycystic degeneration of the liver (UELNICK, 1955) for clearly visualizing round parenchymal filling defects.

2.7.4 Parasitic Liver Diseases

In our latitudes, only hydatid disease is of any practical significance among parasitic liver diseases. Arteriography is not necessarily required for the diagnosis of solitary or multiple Echinococcus cysts, but tomography as well as scintiscanning often yields astonishing results (MARTELLA et al., 1968). However, as soon as surgery is contemplated, the vasculature should be visualized and the site of the cyst localized by arteriography in addition to radiography of the intrahepatic bile ducts. Celiac angiography with filling of the arteries and the reflux phase of the portal vein system is of special importance (MCLOUGHLIN and HOBBS, 1971).

Our own case material includes angiograms of only three patients with liver echinococcosis, two of whom underwent surgery, one having the left lobe of the liver removed.

The pathomorphological picture is characterized by filled cavities which contain air only if connected with the biliary tract, adjacent to which the normal liver tissue has built up a richly vascularized, strong pseudomembrane. Angiograms will therefore reveal—in addition to signs of the simple space-occupying process—an avascular circular space surrounded by a relatively thick web of a membrane-like tissue rich in capillaries.

Precise angiographic localization is a prerequisite for surgical intervention (lobectomy, partial resection). There is a considerable risk of perforating the cyst and disseminating its contents into the abdominal cavity, especially if it is situated subcapsularly.

2.7.5 Subphrenic, Intrahepatic and Subhepatic Abscess

Not every abscess below the right subphrenic space reveals its presence by the typical air-fluid level, so that in many cases it is the pathologist who first makes the diagnosis of an abscess in the right hypochondrium or in the liver. The cause of sometimes abrupt temperature spikes, which are often masked by antibiotics, can sometimes be established by the angiographic detection of an abscess (JACOBS et al., 1969).

Liver abscesses typically appear as round radiolucencies during the hepatogram phase (Fig. 119). In addition, a hyperemic marginal zone may be visualized with adequate contrast.

The angiographic method of choice for the visualization of a liver abscess is celiac angiography or superselective hepatic angiography. However, the possibility of splenoportography should also be considered in view of the higher concentration of contrast medium in the portogram phase.

If no clinical information is available, it is practically impossible to distinguish a liver abscess from an echinococcus cyst on an angiogram.

2.7.6 Cirrhosis of the Liver and Portal Hypertension

See "Portal Hypertension" (p. 39)

2.7.7 Liver Trauma

In principle, liver trauma is very seldom an indication for angiography. In case of penetrating or blunt abdominal trauma, the clinical picture of acute abdomen is a vital indication for immediate surgery to prevent fatal intraabdominal hemorrhaging. It has so far hardly been possible to arrive at a detailed diagnosis of mild liver traumas toward which the surgeon adopts a wait-and-see attitude. But in contrast to the spleen, cases of so-called "two-phase" rupture are rather infrequent in the liver.

Our own experience has led us to believe that the advantages of arteriography in liver injuries are so great for the attending physician that arteriography is imperative.

The various possible sequelae to trauma and their pathomorphological correlates on an angiogram have been discussed in the chapter on "Abdominal Trauma". Changes are to be expected in both the hepatic vessels and in the hepatogram (Fig. 14).

A patient with blunt abdominal trauma in whom no pathological findings were made clinically—apart from a circumscribed area of tenderness to palpation above the porta hepatis—may serve as an example. Angiography alone indicated the need for laparotomy. Fig. 82 shows the traumatic perforation of the left hepatic artery, which only manifested itself intraoperatively by a small hematoma above the porta hepatis. The lesion was a throbbing arterial aneurysm which could have led to severe intraabdominal bleeding if the right hepatic artery had not been ligated.

Laparotomy permits easy detection of any lesion of the inferior aspect and the anterior portions of the liver. However, difficulties arise if a central hematoma is present or a lesion in the dorsocranial segments. Such localizations at times totally escape detection when laparotomy is performed in the usual manner, i.e. medially from above. Figs. 81 and 120 demonstrate the value of angiography in such central liver ruptures and in subcapsular hematoma.

Liver arteriography may also be indicated in cases of non-lacerating injury to the laterobasal thorax. Angiography is able to detect not only damage to the liver but also a concomitant rupture of the diaphragm (Fig. 84). To our knowledge, there has been hardly any reference to this indication so far in the literature (see chapter on ruptured diaphragm, p. 46).

The angiographic signs of liver rupture are the same as the vascular alterations, both intra- and extraparenchymal, described in the chapter on "Abdominal Trauma". It should merely be noted that angiography is indicated when there is even the slightest clinical suspicion of organ damage. If scanning facilities are available nearby, this should be done first, being a less drastic procedure, although it is unquestionably less precise and provides the surgeon with no information about the topographical location of the lesion and the condition of the supply vessels.

Tearing injuries to the liver can lead to pseudoaneurysms and disruption of small arterial branches. Arteriovenous fistulas may form between the hepatic artery and either the portal or hepatic veins. In the parenchymal phase of the angiogram, liver contusion causes mottled accumulation of contrast medium. Arterial collaterals may bypass arterial occlusions and fill branches peripheral to lacerations. The venous phase offers no further information; however, peripheral portal venous filling during the venous phase may be unusually well demonstrated in the presence of contusion (Boijsen et al., 1966).

Angiography following liver resection for trauma often shows vascular changes in addition to absence of the resected liver. After ligation of major hepatic artery branches, collaterals supply the liver distal to the ligation. Residual areas of traumatized liver may occasionally be present, such as intrahepatic hematomas, arteriovenous fistulas or pseudoaneurysms. Following a major liver resection, the remaining liver enlarges and the supplying arteries dilate and are spread as liver regeneration occurs.

At this point we may call attention to a rare complication, *hemobilia*, first described by the Swede Sandblom in 1948, because arteriography can make a decisive contribution to its diagnosis.

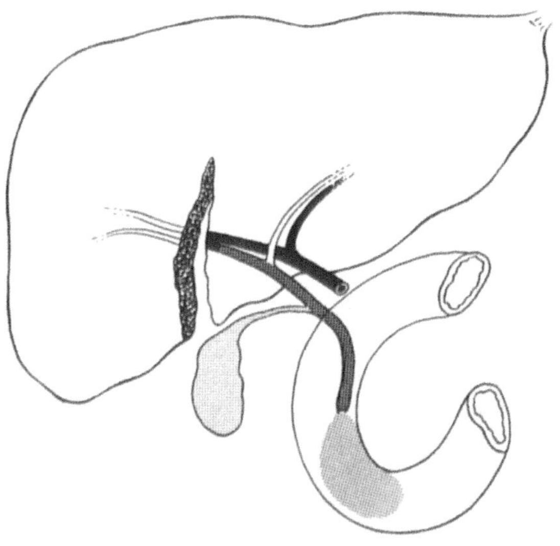

Hemobilia following rupture of liver

The principal sign of hemobilia is a relatively severe gastrointestinal hemorrhage due to hemorrhage into the biliary tract. Laceration of liver tissue, especially when the rupture is centrally located, is accompanied by disruption of the blood vessels, usually arterial branches, and the bile ducts, so that the pressure difference causes the blood to overflow into the duodenum via the bile ducts (GOERTTLER and HERFARTH, 1973).

The onset of gastrointestinal hemorrhage after a non-lacerating abdominal trauma with possible damage to the liver, or after confirmed rupture of the liver, must therefore immediately suggest such a hemobilia.

The method of choice for diagnosis is as selective as possible an angiographic examination of the hepatic artery, as illustrated by HERNANDEZ (1968) in a series of impressive pictures. The typical pathomorphological finding is filling of the biliary tract in the late arterial phase. In the same paper, HERNANDEZ presented examples of opacification of the gallbladder.

2.7.8 Aneurysms of the Hepatic Arteries

Frequency and cause. Aneurysms in the hepatic artery are much less important clinically than aneurysms in the splenic artery. According to BENNET and MUSSY (1970), a total of 160 aneurysms of the hepatic artery have been reported in the literature, and only 10 of these were detected by arteriography.

The most frequent cause of aneurysm in the hepatic artery is arteriosclerosis. Blunt abdominal trauma plays numerically a much less significant role (Fig. 82). An arteriovenous shunt is also a conceivable consequence of trauma (Fig. 12).

Clinical symptoms. There are no typical signs of the presence of an aneurysm in the hepatic artery. Nevertheless, such an alteration must be taken into account in differential diagnosis when intermittent, crampy, epigastric pains develop after meals. The symptoms resemble those encountered in abdominal angina and are pathophysiologically attributable to a similar mechanism. According to BENNET and MUSSY (1970), heobilia is one of the important clinical signs. These French investigators found a hemorrhage in the biliary tract in two out of six cases. In one of these, hematemesis, icterus, and pain in the right hypochondrium occurred as a result of aneurysmal rupture.

Angiographic findings. An annular calcific deposit may be seen radiographically and without the use of contrast medium. However, the method of choice is serial arteriography, which as a rule rapidly visualizes a large, saccular dilatation of a large hepatic branch, or also of a smaller peripheral twig (Fig. 121).

Sources of possible error are the points of ramification of the hepatic artery and superimpositions, which produce a picture quite similar to that of aneurysms. A misinterpretation is possible especially when angiography is performed in only one plane. However, persistence of the contrast medium in true aneurysmal dilatations is an important criterion for differential diagnosis.

Thrombi adhering to the vessel wall can conceal the true extent of an aneurysm. An inflammatory alteration may cause constriction of the lumen. Complete obstruction of the celiac artery due to a mycotic aneurysm has been described by ZEPPA et al. (1966), who also note filiform collateral vessels coursing over the aneurysmal sac.

The detection of an aneurysm in the hepatic artery is by no means of only theoretical interest since a favorable location of the aneurysm may well allow its resection or at least ligation of the afferent artery.

2.7.9 Arterioportal Fistula

Clinical significance. Pathological shunts between an artery and the portal vein region are uncommon but have been attracting more and more clinical interest since arterioportal fistulas represent the only surgically remediable form of portal hypertension (LINDER et al., 1968). Since WEIGERT first described it in 1886, 57 cases have been reported in the literature (BEDUHN and VOLLMAR, 1970). Intravital diagnosis of this vascular alteration was first made possible by the development of arteriographic vascular diagnosis (Fig. 12).

Etiology. Etiologically, congenital and acquired forms of arterioportal fistulas are distinguished. The former involve disturbances in differentiation of the primitive capillary plexus with persistence of arteriovenous shunts of varying morphologic design (VOLLMAR, 1967). Among the acquired forms, invasion of a satellite vein by a generally arteriosclerotic aneurysm of the splenic artery is the most frequent cause. Stab and gunshot wounds predominate among traumatic fistulas. Iatrogenic shunts also belong in this category; they account for 30% of the arterioportal fistulas reported thus far.

Etiology of arterioportal fistulas

I. Congenital
  1. Single-multiple
  2. Type I: Single transverse shunt (patent ductus arteriosus type)
     Type II: Multiple transverse shunts
     Type III: Longitudinal shunts

II. Acquired
  1. Spontaneous: Arterial aneurysm with secondary intrusion into vein
  2. Iatrogenic
  3. Traumatic

Pathophysiology. As a rule, a shunt between an artery and the portal low-pressure system leads to portal hypertension due to increased volume in the portal system; the degree of hypertension depends on the size of the arteriovenous fistula and the length of time it has been present. Just as in pre-, intra-, or posthepatic obstructive hypertension, a commensurate collateral circulation is developed entailing the danger of life-threatening hemorrhages from esophageal varices. In contrast to arteriovenous fistulas of the systemic circulation, remote effects on the greater circulation are rarely produced. Consequently, no enlargement of the heart, bradycardia, etc. ensues.

The reason for this is the interposition of a second capillary filter with relatively high flow resistance between the portal vein system and the vena cava. In arterioportal fistulas, too, the altered hemodynamics lead to a usually progressive dilatation of the afferent and efferent vessels included in the shunt with possible aneurysm formation (so-called arteriovenous aneurysm).

Clinical symptoms. Occasionally, arterioportal fistulas produce no clinical symptoms of any kind for several years. If the fistula is associated with fairly large aneurysm, pressure on adjacent organs may occur in rare cases, giving rise to uncharacteristic disturbances in the upper abdomen. The chief symptoms, however, are recurrent gastrointestinal hemorrhages, and usually also esophageal or fundus varices, whereas an enlarged spleen is not mandatory.

Clinical diagnosis relies mainly on auscultatory detection of a continuous machinery such as murmur which, together with other symptoms of portal hypertension, is presumptive evidence of an arterioportal shunt. In some cases, roentgenographic detection of an annular calcification in the region of the portal vein provides the first indication of localization. Gastrointestinal series, barium enema, cholecystogram, and an excretory urogram can provide further, if indirect, clues.

Angiographic diagnosis. The method of choice for the visualization of arterioportal fistulas and their exact localization is visceral angiography, specifically celiac and mesenteric angiography. The findings can be helpful in the planning of the surgical approach and the technical aspects of the operation.

Arterioportal fistulas are most frequently localized in the region between the splenic artery and splenic vein. Twenty-six of the 49 cases cited by LINDER et al. from the world literature (1968) were diagnosed angiographically, the first case, reported by STENER, dating back to 1955. Whereas initially most arterioportal fistulas were localized by aortography, selective visualization of such fistulas has become the method of choice in recent years (WENZ, 1966; BAYINDIR and GRAEBNER, 1966). Our own patient population included two characteristic cases of arterioportal fistulas that were detected angiographically.

Case Reports

Case I: A 27-year-old woman with massive hematemesis and melena, reduction of hemoglobin to 27%, and no previous abdominal illnesses. She had experienced pains in the left epigastrium for a year. The clinical findings were marked anemia, a large palpable spleen, and a loud bruit in the left upper abdomen. A plain film of the abdomen disclosed a ring-shaped egg-sized calcium deposit in the area of the splenic hilus. There were esophageal varices as thick as a pencil in the distal esophagus. Selective angiography of the splenic artery was performed. An arteriovenous aneurysm was found between the splenic vein and the splenic artery directly adjacent to the splenic hilus. The splenic artery was dilated and quite tortuous; the splenic vein showed funnel-shaped dilatation. Surgery (Dr.

Linder, 1965) confirmed the finding and consisted of extirpation of the arteriovenous aneurysm and the spleen. Since the operation the patient has had regular checkups and has been free of complaints (Fig. 136 and drawing below).

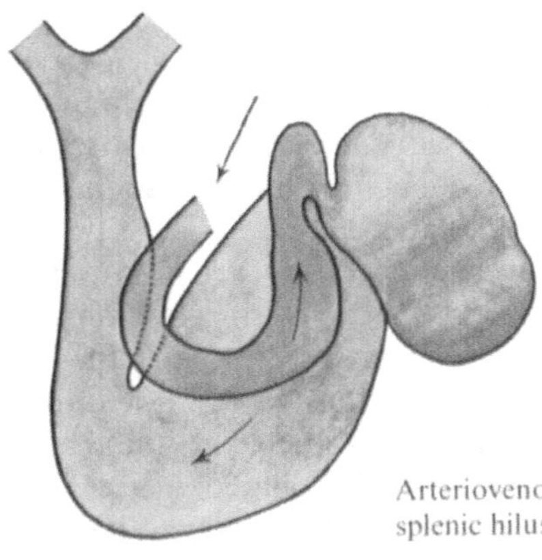

Arteriovenous fistula at splenic hilus with aneurysm

Case II: 65-year-old patient. In 1950, a perforated stomach ulcer had been oversewed. In 1964 a Billroth I resection of the stomach was performed because of renewed ulcer symptoms. A few months after this last operation the patient complained of occasional sensations of pressure in the upper abdomen. For 4 months he had had repeated tarry stools with occasional vomiting of small quantities of stomach contents resembling coffee grounds. Clinical findings: palpable thrill over a palm-sized area above the navel to the left. Auscultation revealed a systolic-diastolic bruit. The systemic blood pressure was 135/80 mm. There were small varices in the distal esophagus with a post-Billroth I stomach and an unremarkable anastomosis. Celiac angiography showed a considerably dilated common hepatic artery that extended in a U-shaped curve, without reduction in caliber, into the gastroduodenal artery and the gastroepiploic artery. Only the initial portion of the common hepatic artery was visualized, as a stump-like cone (pseudoocclusion!). Rapid passage of contrast medium from the terminal portion of the right gastroepiploic artery into the dilated and strictly parallel right gastroepiploic vein (Fig. 12) was already seen in the early arterial phase. Hereafter, the entire portal vein system was quickly filled, so that an arterioportal fistula between the right gastroepiploic artery and a branch of the superior mesenteric artery was diagnosed angiographically. The operation (Dr. J. Vollmar) confirmed the finding; the volume of blood shunted through the fistula was 40 ml/min. The arteriovenous fistula was extirpated and the afferent and efferent fistula vessels were individually ligated. Postoperative followup angiograms showed a distinct reduction in caliber of the common hepatic artery and the gastroduodenal artery. The left hepatic artery (initially regarded as proper hepatic artery) filled promptly since the steal effect was eliminated after extirpation of the fistula (Beduhn and Vollmar, 1970). Supplementary selective visualization of the superior mesenteric artery revealed an isolated right hepatic artery arising from it.

The combination of portal hypertension with the characteristic bruit in the upper abdomen should immediately suggest the possibility of arteriovenous shunting in the portal system. Such a shunt can be surgically corrected. The instantaneous elimination of portal hypertension can prevent the life-threatening hemorrhage from esophageal varices. The radiologist is thus faced with an exceedingly important diagnostic task, namely, timely angiographic detection of shunts in the portal system and their exact localization, permitting surgery to be planned.

Recently, Trinez et al. (1973) reported a case of congenital hepatico-portal fistula studied by celiac and upper mesenteric arteriography. The authors found a mesenteric ischemic syndrome together with a celiac steal and portal hypertension.

2.7.10 Obstructive Jaundice

Radiological diagnosis. In jaundiced patients the biliary tract can be visualized by transhepatic percutaneous cholangiography or laparoscopy. Endoscopic, retrograde opacification of the biliary and pancreatic ducts can be expected to provide important evidence in the future (Classen, 1971). The techniques make it possible to differentiate between parenchymatous and obstructive jaundice in clinically and biochemically ambiguous cases.

The nature and length of the obstruction cannot be definitively ascertained in all cases; moreover, the extent of a tumor and its encroachment upon adjacent organs can be determined only with difficulty. Diagnosis can be facilitated by using a combination of several investigative procedures (Swart et al., 1968).

In addition to plain radiography, GI series, barium enema, hypotonic duodenography and scintiscan, there are other possibilities for verifying angiographically detectable changes in obstructive jaundice by virtue of the close intrahepatic and extrahepatic proximity to the various vascular systems.

Relevance of angiography. Tumors in the liver, biliary tract and gallbladder, the papilla, and the pancreas can be detected by arteriography. Often, vascular stenoses or occlusions and irregular contours are the only indications of infiltrative tumor growth. Thus far, few clinical observations of cases of obstructive jaundice have been described in which celiac angiography was performed.

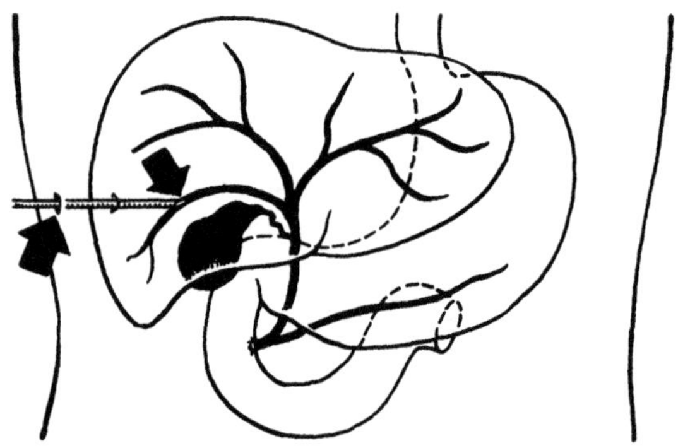

Percutaneous transhepatic cholangiography

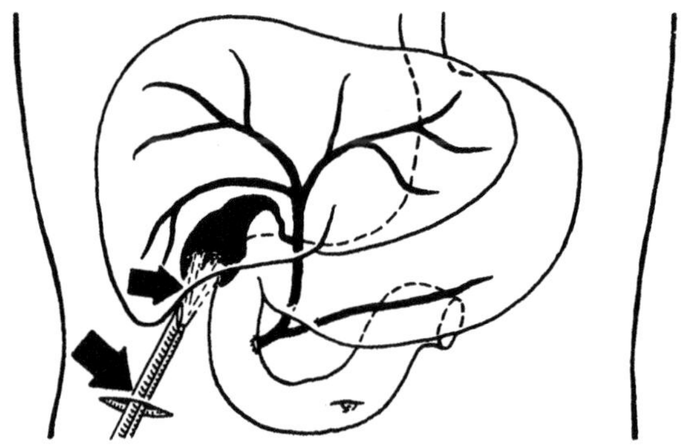

Laparoscopic cholangiography

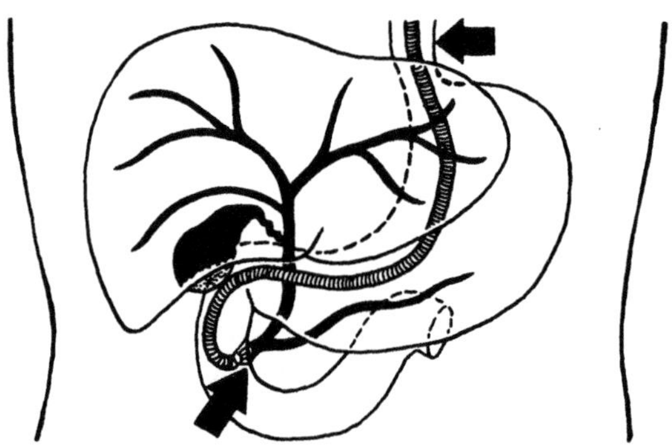

Duodenoscopic cholangiography

CHUDACEK reported in 1969 that no adverse effects of this examination were observed among his patients. Simultaneous visualization of arteries and bile ducts afforded BOIJSEN and REUTER (1967) an outstandingly clear view of the topographical relationships between the two systems. In our Department, this diagnostic investigation has not been found satisfactory so far because superimpositions hamper precise evaluation.

Angiographic findings in animal experiments. Changes in the bile ducts are not the only consequences of obstructive jaundice (BAYINDIR et al., 1968). In an experimental study we investigated the effects of surgical occlusion of the bile duct upon the vascular system in dogs. As the occlusion syndrome progressed, we employed selective hepatic arteriography at regular intervals to monitor the intrahepatic vascular changes.

In the liver, the hepatic arteries undergo dilation concomitantly with inflammatory structural rearrangements. At the same time increased vascularization may be noted in the peripheral segments of the liver. In the late phase, tortuosity of the dilated arteries may be interpreted as an inflammatory alteration, similarly to occasional variations in caliber and mural irregularities.

Changes in the portal venous system were systematically examined in the same manner. In dogs in which the common bile duct was surgically ligated, the changes, usually occurring in the second and third weeks after the operation, took the form of a moderate dilation of the central and peripheral portal vein branches, increasing inhomogeneity of the liver parenchyma as a result of structural changes, proliferation of connective tissue in Glisson's capsule, and dilation of sinusoidal capillaries (BEDUHN, 1970).

These structural changes closely resemble the patterns in human biliary cirrhosis (HANSER, 1930; KAUFMANN, 1960; GROSSE-BROCKHOFF, 1969). At the end of these study series a progressive portal vein thrombosis with development of extensive collateral circulations and ascites was a consistent finding at the stage of irreversible obstructive jaundice.

Splenoportography. Splenoportography has so far rarely been used in clinical cases of obstructive jaundice. By demonstrating compression effects and infiltrations, it can furnish important clues to the origin of a tumor of the pancreas, duodenum, or liver that can lead to obstructive jaundice.

Non-opacified areas of the liver, obstruction, and dislocation of individual portal vein branches are, according to CHUDACEK (1969), the most important radiographic signs of splenoportography in obstructive jaundice.

2.7.11 Gallbladder

Possibilities and limitations of radiologic techniques. Gratifying as the results of the x-ray visualization of the biliary passages are, it has not made possible the detection of gallbladder carcinoma.

The chances of diagnosing excretory insufficiency of the liver or obstructive jaundice have been significantly improved by the introduction of percutaneous transhepatic cholangiography and laparoscopic cholangiography.

Angiography has most recently also contributed to the visualization of poorly demonstrable or undemonstrable diseases of the gallbladder by conventional techniques prior to surgery. Initial intravital attempts at angiographic visualization of the gallbladder arteries have been described in papers by WENZ (1967) and DEUTSCH (1967).

Anatomy of cystic arteries. As a rule, the great cystic artery arises from the right hepatic artery. However, the large number of variations in the region of the portal vein vasculature includes variant origins of the cystic arteries (LEMAITRE et al., 1969):

Proper hepatic artery
Common hepatic artery
Left hepatic artery
Gastroduodenal artery
Celiac artery
Multiple origins have likewise been described.

The cystic artery usually divides into a right and left branch at the boundary between the neck and the body of the gallbladder. In its further course the left branch supplies the inferior aspect and the fundus, while the right branch supplies the anterior surface. There are numerous anastomoses between these ramifications and also transverse connections to the vascular regions of the subcapsular arteries, the gallbladder bed, the right lobe and the quadrate lobe of the liver, as well as to the vascular plexus of the cystic and hepatic ducts.

Cystic arteries in angiogram. In the postmortem angiogram (HABIGHORST et al., 1965) the cystic arteries are slightly tortuous, the windings depending on the state of distention of the hollow viscus. An arterial arcade is discernible at the transition between the body and the fundus and a second one, less consistently, in the middle of the fundus between the left and right main branches of the cystic artery. In patients, the cystic artery can be visualized by celiac angiography (OEDMAN, 1958; BOIJSEN and OLIN, 1964) (Fig. 122).

It should be borne in mind that the simultaneous filling of arteries that are not part of the hepatic circulation will visualize superimposed vessels, which greatly hampers proper differentiation.

In a total of 100 selective angiograms of the celiac or hepatic artery so far prepared, we have been definitely able to assign vascular branches to the cystic artery in 70 cases (36% by LEMAITRE). Selective probing of the proper hepatic artery yields better results. Beyond visualization of the arteries, it becomes possible by serial arteriography in the capillary phase to visualize the wall of the gallbladder in 26% (LEMAITRE 15%) of the patients examined (TJENG, 1971).

Indications for gallbladder arteriography. In the meantime, the indications for angiographic gallbladder visualization have been clearly established. Essentially, they are *gallbladder carcinoma* and *obstructive jaundice*.

Preoperative diagnosis of *gallbladder carcinoma* by means of conventional radiography is extremely rare. During the years 1943–1964 not a single gallbladder carcinoma was preoperatively diagnosed by x-rays at the Heidelberg Surgical University Clinic.

This situation was improved by the introduction of hypotonic duodenography, in which a compromise of the first and second portions of duodenum due to a spreading tumor could be demonstrated in a relatively early phase. In actual practice, of course, such a duodenal involvement usually means that the tumor is inoperable. By this time it has usually invaded the liver and the intrahepatic bile ducts in the form of a cirrhotically growing adenocarcinoma. Moreover, the tumor tends to spread across the surface of the peritoneum and not infrequently intrudes upon adjacent visci such as the duodenum and the small and large intestine.

Jaundice or a palpable tumor occur at a relatively late stage. The disease usually begins with uncharacteristic symptoms in a patient with a long history of gallbladder complaints. The presumptive clinical diagnosis is usually made too late. ABRAMS et al. (1970) succeeded in preoperatively detecting a gallbladder carcinoma by angiography in six cases. These are the angiographic criteria to watch for:

1. Dilatation of common hepatic artery.
2. Enlargement of cystic artery.
3. Stenosis or amputation of central or peripheral branch of cystic artery.
4. Neovascularity inside the gallbladder tumor.
5. Uneven thickness of gallbladder wall (thick wall sign).
6. "Vascular neoformations" within the liver are suggestive of metastases (4 of 5 cases, Deutsch; 5 of 6 cases, Abrams et al.) (Fig. 123).

The operable cases so far reported, by Wenz and Beduhn (1966), Deutsch (1967), and Abrams et al. (1970), provide the first ray of hope that a more timely diagnosis of this malignant tumor may become possible. More frequent angiographic examinations are therefore strongly recommended in female patients over the age of 50 suffering from chronic bile duct ailments. This applies especially to carriers of Thorotrast (Fig. 124).

At present, angiography has not yet found practical application in other diseases of the gallbladder. In celiac angiography, the organ is visualized during the investigation of other diseases of the liver, the pancreas, or the spleen. This opacification of the gallbladder wall is desirable in all those cases in which visualization of the hollow viscus has been precluded by a barrier to hepatic excretion of biliary contrast media. In many of these changes, however, the surgeon, at least for his part, would welcome information about the anatomy of the gallbladder even before the operation. The normal picture of the gallbladder obtained in selective hepatic arteriography is shown in Fig. 122.

Sato et al. (1969) believe that the gallbladder can be visualized angiographically whenever in celiac angiography at least 40 ml of a highly concentrated contrast medium is injected by means of a pressure syringe. In this manner a completely visualized enlarged cystic artery with a tortuous course and caliber irregularities was found in 9 out of 16 patients with gallbladder carcinoma. In the other 7 patients only the initial portion of the cystic artery was visualized, while atypical vessels were found at the level of the remaining gallbladder wall.

At the present time angiographic visualization of the cystic veins is still beyond our technical capabilities. Via choledochal veins they are closely connected to the drainage system of the head of the pancreas and are implicated in gallbladder-related inflammations of the head of the pancreas (Otto, 1971).

3 Spleen

3.1 Anatomy and Anomalies

The spleen develops in the dorsal mesogastrium and lies in a concealed position in the left hypochondriac region. Its diaphragmatic surface is in relation with the diaphragm, following the course of the 9th, 10th and 11th ribs. The anterior end of the spleen generally does not extend beyond a line that can be traced from the sternoclavicular joint on the left side to the apex of the 11th rib.

The visceral surface is in contact with the gastric fundus and is connected with the greater curvature via the gastrosplenic ligament. The colon is in more or less broad apposition with the spleen, depending on the position of the left flexure, which shows considerable individual variation. The tail of the pancreas is in contact with the spleen over a small area near the hilus. The dorsal surface of the organ, finally, is in relation with the upper and lateral margins of the left kidney.

In contrast to the liver, the spleen does not adhere to the undersurface of the diaphragm but is held in its position by peritoneal reflections. The position of the diaphragm, body posture, and the degree of filling of the adjacent organs, notably the stomach and the colon, greatly influence the position of the spleen (Hafferl and Thiel, 1969).

Small notches in the sharp anterior margin of the spleen (margo crenatus) are encountered in several variants; however, they may penetrate deeply into an otherwise smooth posterior wall or they may even completely divide the organ, so that an accessory spleen is formed. According to Lubarsch (1927), the following forms may be distinguished:

1. *Accessory spleen:* No relation to principal organ; dystopic primordium, or posttraumatic dispersion and implantation of splenic tissue.
2. *Succenturiate spleen:* Located in immediate vicinity of principal organ; developed owing to excessive indentation or lobulation (e.g. fissura genitalis).
3. *Lobate spleen:* Organ divided into several lobes; no principal spleen as such. Atavism?

The preferred localizations of the accessory spleen are the splenic hilus, the gastrolienal ligament, the lesser omentum, and the pancreas. Among malformations, alienia, though very rare, ought not to be forgotten.

3.2 Vasculature

The splenic artery, the left branch of the celiac trunk, follows the upper margin of the pancreas and divides into several branches near the hilus. The extreme tortuosity of the artery is peculiar. Small branches course to the pancreas, and near the spleen the left gastroepiploic artery branches off; it divides at the greater curvature, while the short gastric arteries continue to the gastric fundus.

The splenic vein arises near the splenic hilus and deviates to the right, caudad to the artery, so much that it is found above the pancreas only in the vicinity of the spleen but passes behind the pancreas in its further course. In its initial portion it receives the left gastroepiploic vein and the short gastric veins, which accompany its arteries.

3.3 Conventional Radiography

The spleen is visualized most easily with a plain abdominal film if superimposed organs do not prevent a clear differentiation. Generally, the contours of the spleen will stand out more clearly after inflation of the stomach and insufflation of air into the left colon. Normally, with the patient upright, the lower pole of the spleen is situated 3–4 cm lower than when the patient is in supine position (TESCHENDORF, 1964).

The spleen is always visible with retropneumoperitoneum or pneumoperitoneum. Even at normal size and particularly in the presence of a splenic tumor, spleen-induced impressions on the fundus and corpus ventriculi and on the left flexure of the colon are demonstrable upon visualization of these organs.

Scintiscanning of the spleen has been found particularly useful for determination of size in the case of positional anomalies and tumors.

Angiography may be described as the *method of choice for visualization of the spleen.* Above all, arteriography is adapted to the diagnosis of alterations in the afferent artery (tortuosity, aneurysms, arteriovenous fistula), for determining the position of the organ, and for detecting parenchymal changes. Technically, this can be accomplished in the course of celiac angiography or by superselective visualization of the splenic artery.

A polar artery of the spleen arising separately from the aorta is rare and little is known about it. As in selective renal angiography, it can cause an interruption of the splenic pulp on a splenogram, which can easily lead to a mistaken diagnosis when splenic rupture is suspected. When a polar artery is believed to be present, this can be confirmed only by a flush aortogram (WENZ et al., 1971).

The splenic vein and the portal vein are generally well visualized in the venous phase of splenography. For this purpose a sufficient amount of contrast medium (30–50 ml) has to be injected. If the enlargement of the spleen reaches extreme dimensions, venous drainage becomes so slow that no sufficient opacification can occur. In such cases, percutaneous or laparoscopic splenoportography is recommended, particularly when there is presumptive clinical evidence of splenic vein thrombosis or portal hypertension; the same examination, besides densely opacifying the efferent veins, also permits measurement of intrasplenic pressure.

The technique is described in detail on p. 16.

3.4 Indications for Splenic Angiography

1. Tumor of uncertain localization in left upper abdomen.
2. Splenomegaly of undetermined origin (tumor, cyst, splenic vein thrombosis).
3. Splenic trauma.
4. Accessory spleen and displacement of spleen (diaphragmatic hernia).

3.5 Angiographic Pathomorphology

3.5.1 Tumor in Left Epigastrium

The splenic tumor frequently developing in the wake of a septic or hematologic disease is not an indication for angiography since the cause of the splenomegaly may be found in the underlying disease. As a rule, angiography cannot clarify the pathogenesis of this spleen enlargement.

It is true that parenchymal filling defects, such as are seen e.g. in Hodgkin's disease, can be demonstrated (BACHMANN, 1967) but it may be assumed that such systemic diseases, especially leukoses, have previously been confirmed by hematological studies, lymphography, and lymph node biopsy. An exception is purely abdominal Hodgkin's disease with splenomegaly.

Angiography is required, however, if a tumor in the left upper abdomen cannot be definitely assigned to the spleen or if the cause of splenomegaly remains uncertain. In terms of the method, tumorous, cystic, inflammatory or vascular processes can be visualized most readily if they affect a circumscribed portion of the spleen. Generalized splenic alterations are more difficult to detect and interpret (Figs. 127, 128).

3.5.2 Malignant Splenic Tumor

Primary malignant tumors of the spleen are rare. Only 163 cases were reported in the literature up to 1954. In the same year EDSMAN reported the first angiographic demonstration. Dense opacification of the tumor can be expected in cases of hemangiosarcoma (RÖSCH, 1966).

In a patient with hemangiomatosis that was initially confined to the spleen we found a cottony accumulation of contrast medium distributed over the entire organ in the late arterial phase with prolonged persistence (Fig. 128). One year later an enlargement of the liver was noted. The diagnosis was not clarified until autopsy.

Metastatic involvement of the spleen is also seen infrequently (BENNET et al., 1966). Clear demarcation of such a metastasis can present clinical as well as angiographic problems, as we found in the case of a cystic metastasis of an ovarian carcinoma operated on a year previously (GRÖZINGER et al., 1968). The metastasis of a small thyroid carcinoma shown in Fig. 127 is also a rarity. A splenic metastasis with secondary splenic vein thrombosis had attracted attention much earlier than the inconspicuous, small struma. Splenography also makes it possible to detect a tumorous infiltration of the organ by malignant growths in the immediate environment emanating from the kidney, adrenal gland, or pancreas (BACHMANN, 1967).

3.5.3 Splenic Cyst

The most common benign "splenic tumors" include true cysts, 211 cases of which have so far been reported in the literature (POLLER et al., 1966). The angiographic indicators are spread-out splenic artery branches and smooth, round radiolucencies in the splenogram.

The localization of cysts in the spleen can usually also be accomplished by means of scintiscanning; however, attention may be called to an example (Fig. 129) in which angiography was required for full clarification.

The angiographic assignment of a space-occupying process to the spleen can be difficult if there are close anatomical relations to the splenic capsule, as e.g. in the presence of an old, organized extracapsular splenic hematoma or a chronic subphrenic abscess such as was studied by us (Fig. 125). In two cases the splenic capsule was not visible in any phase of arteriography and for this reason we had suspected a subcapsular inflammatory or neoplastic process.

As an accessory finding, we discovered multiple, evidently congenital splenic cysts in a patient with carcinoma of the tail of the pancreas. The demonstration of circular, delicate ring shadows is so characteristic of the picture of Echinococcus cyst inside the spleen (ROZMANN et al., 1962) that arteriography is seldom indicated. In most cases, however, celiac angiography is necessary for diagnostic confirmation of a calcific shadow in the left upper abdomen (POLLER et al., 1966). In differential diagnosis consideration has to be given to calcified cysts or tumors of the left epigastrium and also to splenic artery aneurysms. In rare cases tuberculosis of the organ (Figs. 131, 132) will simulate the picture of a splenic tumor.

Diffuse focal calcification of the splenic pulp is seen occasionally (miliary tuberculosis!) in patients who have had certain infectious diseases. An impregnation of metallic opacity, on the other hand, characterizes the Thorotrast spleen, but in such cases the abdominal lymph nodes and the liver usually show Thorotrast deposits. Angiography of the spleen will not prove diagnostic under these circumstances.

The rare hamartoma of the spleen is, according to WEXLER et al. (1964), characterized angiographically by large tortuous vessels, pools of contrast medium, and early venous filling.

3.5.4 Splenic Vein Thrombosis

The pathogenesis of a splenic tumor can be established if it involves an enlargement of the spleen related to obstruction of venous drainage.

In cases in which the spleen is enlarged considerably and it is distinctly visible beneath the left costal arch, the diagnosis of splenic vein occlusion by splenic arteriography is by no means always easy (Fig. 139).

We made a presumptive diagnosis, based on the findings at admission, in 3 cases but then, to be certain, followed up with the more reliable examination by splenoportography, and this revealed a patent vascular lumen.

The misinterpretation was due to the fact that the contrast medium was absorbed as by a large sponge and there was so little accumulation of it in the wide drainage vessels that the splenic vein trunk hardly stood out from its environment. In certain cases careful subtraction, especially color subtraction, can be helpful.

When splenic vein thrombosis is suspected, splenoportography is therefore most advisable, particularly since the measurement of intrasplenic pressure simultaneously provides information concerning portal hypertension (Fig. 138).

3.5.5 Splenic Trauma

The growing number of traffic accidents has greatly increased the importance of diagnosis in blunt abdominal trauma. The spleen is involved in about one-fourth of all such abdominal injuries (KLEINERT and ROMERO, 1961; FISCHER and SPANN, 1967).

Since the initial reports by NORELL (1957) and OEDMAN (1958) more than 60 cases of spleen rupture identified by angiography have been described in the literature (reviewed by VAN KAICK et al., 1970).

All investigators have emphasized the high diagnostic accuracy and the lack of discomfort for the patient. Adjacent organs can easily be visualized in the same examination (WENZ, 1970).

Splenic arteriography is indicated chiefly when a delayed or neglected rupture is suspected; complete ruptures require immediate surgical intervention. However, it has been found that in many cases angiography can rapidly be carried out preoperatively, thus providing the surgeon with valuable diagnostic assistance in planning the operation (multiple trauma!). In searching for splenic injuries, we did find also 7 ruptures of the left kidney and 1 rupture of the liver, not to mention the many patients who were spared a laparotomy.

The predominant pathomorphological features in the angiogram are vascular laceration and occlusion. Through *blood*

Splenic arteriography for suspected splenic rupture in 59 patients

Ruptured spleen ruled out included: 7 kidney ruptures 1 liver rupture	43 patients
Angiographically confirmed ruptured spleen	13 patients
Misdiagnosis	3 patients

Angiographic pathomorphology of splenic rupture

Pathology	Angiography
Vascular laceration	Extravasation of contrast medium (within pulp and subcapsular)
Traumatic arterio-venous shunt	Premature venous filling
Intrasplenic hematoma	Vascular splaying and smooth, rounded parenchymal radiolucency
Subcapsular hematoma	Vascular splaying, irregular margins and blurring of lateral margin of spleen
Pericapsular hematoma	Medial and caudal displacement of spleen; increased tortuosity of splenic artery
Vascular occlusion (thrombosis, severance, spasm)	Unsharply demarcated, partly cuneiform parenchymal filling defects, fading of contours
Broad laceration	Large parenchymal radiolucencies; fragmentation of organ

extravasation, individual multiple extravasates of contrast medium are produced within the pulp that in some cases persist beyond the venous phase (Fig. 13). Less frequently, the extravasated contrast material is distributed subcapsularly or extracapsularly (BAUM, 1965; RÖSCH, 1965).

The simultaneous opening of a neighboring sinus or vein creates a traumatic arteriovenous shunt causing premature venous filling (LOVE et al., 1968).

Hematomas situated in the pulp cause rounded parenchymal displacements which are visualized as smooth-contoured radiolucencies in the late capillary phase; the adjacent arteries are displaced and spread apart.

A subcapsular hematoma usually manifests itself by blurring or "fraying" of the lateral margin of the spleen. Identification of this pathological sign is particularly difficult because the lateral margin may be blurred in many cases even under normal conditions.

After laceration of the capsule and pericapsular bleeding the hematoma in the left hypochondrium can bring about a portal and medial displacement of the spleen with a spiral-shaped compression of the splenic artery (LOVE et al., 1968).

The loss of *blood flow* in a vascular segment is no less important than the consequences of vascular laceration. Traumatic vascular changes such as spasm, thrombosis, severance, and involution of the intima can be responsible for interruption of the blood supply. In the angiogram they are reflected in radiolucencies, particularly in the late capillary phase of contrast medium transit. They are mostly found in the marginal zones or at the poles, have unsharp, jagged outlines, and frequently are visualized more as breaks or interruptions of the splenic contours (Fig. 13). So far we have observed no case of total occlusion of a larger intrasplenic artery.

Angiographic findings in 13 cases of splenic rupture

Parenchymal filling defect	9
Extravasation of contrast medium	
intrasplenic	6
subcapsular	1
Mediocaudal displacement	4
Markedly splayed arteries	4
Premature venous filling	3

The gaping rupture site itself, filled with blood clots, is likewise characterized by a parenchymal defect. If there is broad laceration, the angiogram may also show a dislocation of the organ fragments (FONTAINE et al., 1968). A traumatic splenic cyst is shown in Fig. 130.

Possibilities of misinterpretation. In most of our patients a combination of the above findings was obtained. The reliability of the individual signs varies; in our experience extravasation of contrast medium and filling defect in the parenchymal phase are the most common and at the same time most dependable criteria.

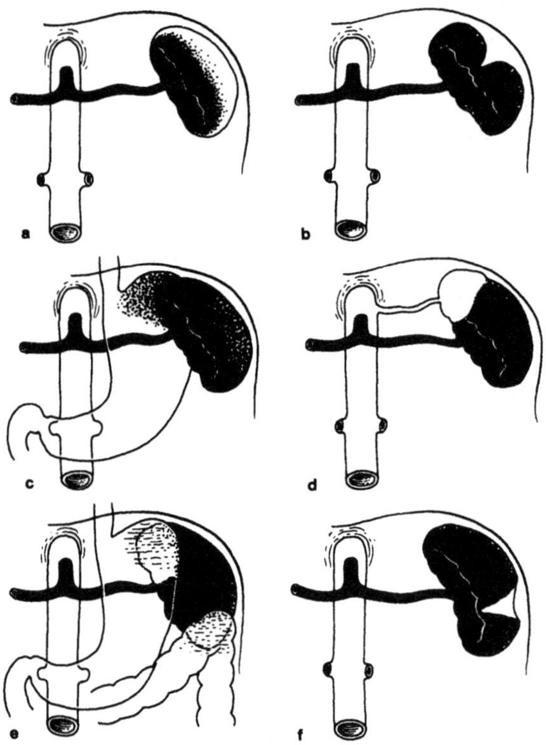

Possible misinterpretation of angiogram of splenic rupture

However, they, too, present certain dangers of misinterpretation. Even the normal spleen, because of its characteristic structure, may present a patchy parenchymal picture, which may appear even less homogeneous when filling is inadequate. The frequently encountered unsharpness of the lateral margin is due to the wide variability in the form and position of the spleen as well as to effects of x-ray scatter. This unsharpness may simulate or mask parenchymal filling defects at the lateral margin of the spleen (*a*).

Another source of possible error consists of sharply demarcated, arcuate lateral margin formations which occasionally extend deeply into the parenchyma and are usually due to abnormal lobulation or indentation. Attention may be called particularly to the dorsocranial lobe of the spleen which develops through persistence of the fissura genitalis and which lodged the gonad during embryonal development (PERNKOPF, 1941) (*b*).

A pseudotumorous opacification of the gastric fundus can mimic a diffuse accumulation of contrast medium or mask an extravasation in the region of the upper pole (*c*). Intrasplenic aneurysm, too, should be considered in differential diagnosis, although it is generally recognizable by its sharp outlines and its position. The extravasates we observed were clearly discernible in the different phases by increase in size and change in shape and invariably corresponded to a rupture.

Parenchymal filling defects can occur during celiac angiography or selective splenic arteriography if isolated polar arteries arise from the aorta. Such angiographic changes have to be differentiated by means of flush aortography from traumatic parenchymal radiolucencies (*d*).

By the same token, the superimposition of negative contrast (air-filled stomach, gas-distended colon) can conceal positive signs (*e*).

Recent or older splenic infarction can create true problems in differential diagnosis. In the absence of an unequivocal history, angiographic differentiation from a rupture is hardly possible (*f*) (WENZ et al., 1971).

Compared with signs of contrast medium extravasations and parenchymal defects, the other criteria are of relatively less importance. For example, the often described splaying of the arteries, if an isolated finding, is not sufficient as a basis for diagnosis (LOVE et al., 1968).

Evaluation of premature venous filling requires exact standardization of the examination technique with regard to timing, dose of contrast medium, and injection pressure. The time between the first appearance of contrast medium in the splenic artery and distinct opacification of the splenic vein averages 5 seconds. In the presence of a traumatic arteriovenous fistula this period never exceeds 2.5 seconds (LOVE et al., 1968). The degree of opacification of the splenic vein naturally depends on the size of the shunt and can be very low sometimes. It is necessary to determine the time span precisely to guard against false positive findings.

The situation of the spleen in the left subphrenic space varies considerably, which makes radiographic differentiation of these variations from a pathological organ displacement very difficult. For this reason BERK et al. (1969) attach little importance to this sign.

A perisplenic hematoma usually brings about a helical compression of the splenic artery as well as caudomedial displacement of the left kidney. In our patients, pathological displacement of the spleen was always associated with angiographically detectable changes related to a parenchymal lesion.

Pharmacoangiography has expanded the methodology of angiography and can contribute to the diagnosis of splenic rupture; intraarterial injection of epinephrine causes contraction of the intact intrasplenic arteries, but no such contraction occurs in lacerated arteries (STEIN, 1969). However, the object to be x-rayed has to be magnified if these differences in caliber are to be demonstrated.

We have obtained good results with electronic subtraction equipment. This not only furnishes a synoptic picture of the arterial and venous phases, but also makes for greater contrast in the capillary phase and eliminates interference from overshadows in the angiogram (ROTH and WENZ, 1969). We may also mention the method of color subtraction, which can provide impressive color differentiation of contrast medium extravasations, for example.

3.5.6 Accessory Spleen and Displacement of Spleen

The demonstration of an *accessory spleen* is of clinical interest in cases in which symptoms persist or could not be completely relieved despite splenectomy, e.g. because of hemolytic anemia (BRON, 1968). Again, scintiscanning as an exploratory method should certainly be given first preference. If doubts persist, angiography can be a decisive factor in visualizing the supply of the organ from the stump of the splenic artery or at least from the celiac trunk.

Occasionally, too, an accessory spleen may have to be considered in the differential diagnosis of obscure tumors in the middle or upper abdomen.

Thus, we found a splenomegaly of undetermined origin in a Greek worker. Medialward alongside the spleen, palpation revealed another tumor which fluctuated with the respiration but was evidently separate from the spleen itself. Besides a distinctly enlarged splenic shadow, the angiogram showed a second organ shadow that appeared in the same phases and was supplied by the same main vessel; we therefore described this as an accessory spleen. An operation which was performed because of concurrent portal hypertension confirmed this diagnosis and a detailed retrospective investigation then brought out the fact that the patient had a malarial spleen with accessory spleen. Owing to a linguistic misunderstanding the patient had previously denied having had such an infection (Fig. 133).

Evidence of displacement of the spleen is important in all cases in which a scheduled splenoportography could not be carried out. Most frequently, this occurs when the organ is small and medially or—e.g. after upper abdominal peritonitis—dorsally adherent. As Boijsen et al. (1968) were able to show, arteriography can also prove advantageous after splenoportography. The direct puncture of the organ can give rise to iatrogenic intrasplenic aneurysm. We have observed no such changes in surgically removed spleens among our patients.

Angiography of the spleen will also assume greater importance in displacements related to diaphragmatic changes such as congenital diaphragmatic defects, diaphragmatic rupture, diaphragmatic hernia, and paralysis. Since the inferior phrenic artery not infrequently arises with the celiac trunk from the aorta, splenic displacement and the state of the diaphragm can be assessed simultaneously.

Experience has shown that differentiation between hernia and eventration is very seldom possible without angiographic visualization of the muscle layer.

The conventional technique of simultaneous visualization of the stomach and colon yields an excellent overview of the location of these viscera in the presence of pathological diaphragmatic changes. Occasionally, however, we have failed to recognize a spleen displaced into the thoracic cavity, an observation which was also made by Haubrich in his monograph (1970) and which remains essentially true to date.

Preoperative differentiation between defect and hernia is possible only by means of a pneumoperitoneum, which is complicated and time-consuming and which fails if close adhesions have developed.

3.5.7 Aneurysm of the Splenic Artery

The course of the splenic artery sets it apart from other vessels. The lack of a supporting structure on its way to the spleen and the supply of an extremely plethoric organ account for the fact that the splenic artery runs a meandering course even in the young individual.

Rall (1972), working in our Department, demonstrated that this tortuosity increases with age. He employed for this purpose an index worked out by Springorum (1933) in an anatomic-morphologic study relating the true length of the splenic artery to the number of turns. Interestingly enough, a very high index, i.e. an extremely tortuous splenic artery, was in several cases associated with a clinical disease pattern that resembled chronic pancreatitis. No sharp line marks the transition from extreme vascular tortuosity to cirsoid aneurysm and angiographic differentiation is not always unequivocal.

Apart from arteriosclerosis, the most important causes of splenic artery aneurysms are congenitally weak vessel walls, trauma, inflammations, and pregnancy. Especially during pregnancy, splenic artery aneurysms rupture more often than aneurysms in other locations. Boijsen (1969) observed that splenic artery aneurysms occur more frequently in portal hypertension. He observed 9 cases of extrasplenic aneurysms of this artery among 192 patients. This incidence of nearly 5% among angiographic cases considerably exceeds the rate of 0.8% previously reported for autopsy material. In addition, six other patients had intrasplenic aneurysms with concomitant portal hypertension. Apparently, long-standing portal hypertension gives rise to degenerative changes in the splenic artery and its branches (Figs. 134, 135).

A branch of the splenic artery is often punctured in splenoportography. This may cause an aneurysm due to the changes in the arterial wall. Thus, Boijsen drew attention to the possibility of iatrogenic aneurysms after splenoportography in 1966 on the basis of six relevant cases among his patients. We ourselves have made no such observations.

A splenic artery aneurysm produces no characteristic clinical signs, unless an acute abdomen develops as a result of rupture into the free abdominal cavity. During pregnancy, therefore, the possibility of a ruptured splenic artery aneurysm must occasionally be considered in the differential diagnosis of acute abdomen. Angiographic localization is of considerable advantage for the surgery to be performed—usually extirpation of the spleen with resection of the aneurysm.

Whereas previously a roentgenogram without contrast medium permitted diagnosis only if characteristic annular calcium deposits were visible in the left epigastrium, the method of choice for the demonstration of splenic artery aneurysms today is celiac angiography or superselective splenic arteriography. If single or multiple, generally circular sacculations are seen, diagnosis is easy. On the other hand, orthograde kinks in the tortuous arteries make interpretation difficult. Delayed drainage of contrast medium from such pouches is an important criterion for identification of an aneurysm.

The patient with multiple extra- and intrasplenic aneurysms in Fig. 135 was subjected to celiac angiography because of portal hypertension. We detected no calcifications within the multiple aneurysms.

4 Pancreas

4.1 Anatomy

The pancreas, an oblong glandular mass, extends from the spleen in the left hypochondriac region to the right into the duodenal loop and curves around the lumbar vertebral column. The head of the pancreas, which is lodged in the duodenal loop, is distinguished from the body, which is situated at the level of the first lumbar vertebra and gradually tapers off to form the linguiform tail of the pancreas.

The shape of the pancreas is so adapted to its surroundings that the different organs are in precise apposition.

As a duodenal gland, the pancreas grows into the mesoduodenum in the embryo. The head of the pancreas fills the concavity of the duodenal loop and insinuates itself around the descending part of the duodenum. The pancreatic notch between the head and the body of the gland corresponds to the junction of the horizontal and ascending portions of the duodenum. Here, the superior mesenteric artery appears at the lower margin of the pancreas; the superior mesenteric vein ascends to the right of the artery. The arcades of the pancreaticoduodenal arteries are apposed to the anterior and posterior aspects of the head of the pancreas or to its margins bordering on the duodenum.

Behind the head of the pancreas, the superior mesenteric vein joins the splenic vein coming from the left, which has just been received by the inferior mesenteric vein. The union of these three veins, the so-called external portal vein roots, gives rise to the portal vein, which courses upward slightly behind the head of the pancreas, whence it runs to the liver.

The common bile duct courses downward, traversing the upper portion of the duodenum, and applies itself to the concavity of the duodenum from the left. It usually runs in a channel between the gut and the pancreas and is sometimes completely embedded in the glandular mass. Halfway up the descending portion of the duodenum the common bile duct receives the main excretory duct of the pancreas—the major pancreatic duct—and together they enter the major duodenal papilla. Craniad from this point, the accessory pancreatic duct passes from the head of the pancreas to the descending part of the duodenum.

The anterior surfaces of the body and tail of the pancreas are invested with the peritoneum of the omental bursa and separated from the posterior wall of the stomach by a crevice-like space. The posterior aspect faces the aorta and the second—sometimes also the first—lumbar vertebra. The caudal part of the anterior surface is covered by the root of the transverse mesocolon. The duodenojejunal flexure and the loops of the free small intestine approach this part of the pancreas from below.

The tail of the pancreas extends to the spleen and is covered caudally by the root of the mesocolon. A small portion of the left end is surmounted by the spleen. The splenic vein and artery are also in very close relation with the tail of the pancreas, the splenic vein appearing at the superior border of the gland.

4.2 Vasculature

The pancreas is supplied essentially by two major branches of the aorta, the celiac trunk and the superior mesenteric artery. However, these large aortic branches contribute four afferent arteries:

1. The gastroduodenal artery and the pancreaticoduodenal artery supply the head of the pancreas, especially the tissue areas surrounding the terminal pancreatic duct.
2. The right mid-colic artery supplies the right inferior half of the pancreas.
3. The splenic artery supplies the left superior half of the body and tail.
4. The left mid-colic artery supplies the left inferior half of the organ, so that even the inferior mesenteric artery supplies blood to the pancreas, though only to a very small extent. Additional branches arise from the celiac trunk and individual lumbar arteries (MICHELS, 1955).

This bewildering vascular architecture is further complicated by countless anomalies in origin and course, so that the textbook arrangement of the pancreatic vasculature can actually

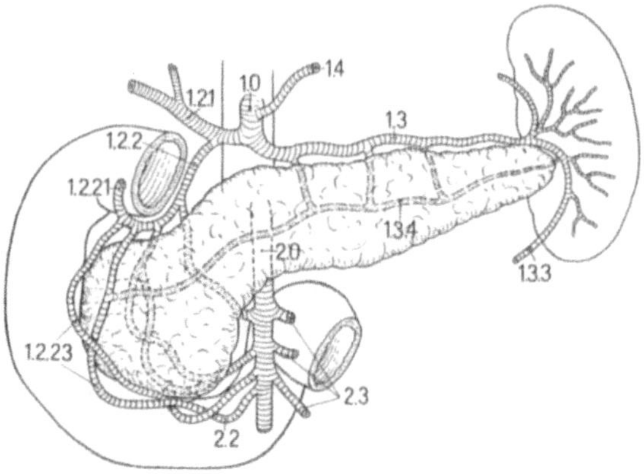

Pancreas: Vascularization (see page 6)

be considered an exception. At least that is the impression gained by anyone who views angiograms of the pancreas frequently.

Owing to its central location and elongated shape the pancreas has very close connections with numerous large vessels. The celiac trunk, which arises from the abdominal aorta directly above the body of the pancreas, immediately divides into its three branches, one of which, the common hepatic artery, courses along the upper margin of the pancreas, while another, the gastroduodenal artery, runs caudad between the head of the pancreas and the first part of the duodenum and gives off the two end branches, the posterior and anterior pancreaticoduodenal arteries extending into the right gastroepiploic artery. The branches of the pancreatic arcade are met by the inferior pancreaticoduodenal artery coming from the superior mesenteric artery, and the arterial arches along the duodenum are thus closed. The splenic artery is also in close relation to the pancreas. It runs leftward along the upper margin of the body and tail; in young individuals it is embedded in a short, fairly straight groove. In the elderly, on the other hand, it is usually very tortuous, the windings penetrating deeply into the mass of the pancreas and also running considerably beyond its superior border.

The superior mesenteric artery arises just below the celiac trunk behind the superior border of the pancreas, courses downward and somewhat to the right, and enters the mesenteric root together with the superior mesenteric vein between the horizontal part of the duodenum and the head of the pancreas.

4.3 Angiographic Technique

At first glance it seems that only aortography, either as flush catheter roentgenography or direct, translumbar aortography, is apt to provide a total view of all the pancreatic arteries (Figs. 18, 140). In fact, however, the usually extremely subtle vascular changes, particularly in carcinoma of the pancreas, are completely concealed by the vessels of the stomach and other neighboring organs, so that at best massive alterations in the large vessel trunks—we have seen elongation and tumor infiltration of a renal artery—are discernible. The desired early diagnosis of pancreatic tumors cannot even be approached by use of this procedure.

A plausible alternative consists in opacifying the two important afferent arteries simultaneously via two catheters. Boijsen was the first to call attention to this possibility in 1963, describing simultaneous celiac and mesenteric angiography as the method of choice for study of the pancreas. However, this technique has not found acceptance. One of the reasons undoubtedly is that the simultaneous introduction of two catheters increases the incidence of complications. Indeed, our only two cases of peripheral embolism occurred following a two-catheter examination. Sammons et al. (1967) confirmed the high risk factor involved. Moreover, it may be argued that in cases of occlusion or severe stenosis, e.g. of the pancreaticoduodenal or gastroduodenal arteries, the direction of flow and the true extent of the alteration cannot be determined. It then also becomes impossible to obtain any information about collaterals. Narrow segmental occlusions are easily concealed with this technique. Finally, mention should be made of the contrast background which, by opacifying the gastric and intestinal walls, almost completely obscures the pancreatic parenchymal phase, which is very faint in any event.

According to the literature, as well as our own experience, the method of choice appears to be sequential opacification of the celiac trunk and the superior mesenteric artery. First, the celiac trunk is filled with 30–50 ml contrast material (injection rate about 8 ml/sec), and then the superior mesenteric artery is visualized with the same quantity of contrast medium. The group working with Olsson in Lund,

Sweden, relies particularly on the preparation of additional oblique films.

We referred to the work of REUTER (1969) in the chapter on superselective techniques. This investigator attempted primarily to opacify the afferent arteries as selectively as possible for angiography of the pancreas. Thus, he sought out the splenic, common hepatic, or gastroduodenal artery, and even the dorsal pancreatic artery, injecting relatively small amounts of contrast medium (10–12 ml). Certainly, this procedure has the advantage of demonstrating discrete parts of the pancreas without superimposition and visualizing the parenchyma much more distinctly than is possible with the usual celiac or mesenteric angiography. Disadvantages are the additional time required to select the smaller branches and visualization of only part of the pancreas, necessitating laborious collation of the partial films of the pancreas during subsequent analysis of different serial angiograms.

Just as for the superselective technique, the pancreas is also the organ most frequently studied by pharmacoangiography. The substances most widely used are epinephrine, secretin, sodium nitroprusside and others. We ourselves made several attempts to increase the flow of blood to the pancreas—as had been done in animal experiments—by prior administration of highly concentrated dextrose infusions, which raised the blood sugar level to 350 mg/100 ml (Fig. 141).

However, this measure had no significant effect on our angiograms. Inflation of the stomach with air using an effervescent tablet helps to demarcate the pancreas from the gastric arteries which are generally visualized at the same time.

In the late phase of pancreatic arteriography, the superior mesenteric vein is opacified via the superior mesenteric artery, and the splenic vein via the celiac artery. Both veins, but especially the splenic vein, are in close relation to the pancreas and are originally important in the search for tumors and for diagnostic differentiation from inflammatory alterations in the pancreas.

Note that subtraction and color subtraction facilitate interpretation of the angiograms.

In some cases it is possible to opacify both major sources of supply of the pancreas through a single artery. Remarkably enough, all five of our cases of pancreatic insulinoma displayed this joint filling of the superior mesenteric artery and the celiac artery although the unprobed artery was not occluded. We suspect that the collaterals were extremely dilated —possibly owing to the pancreatic tumors—so that it made no difference whether the contrast medium was injected through the celiac or the mesenteric artery. In all cases both arteries were densely filled with contrast medium via the pancreatic arcades.

4.4 Angiographic Pathomorphology

4.4.1 Pancreatic Carcinoma

Carcinomas are the primary indication for pancreatic angiography, followed by pancreatic adenoma (insulinoma, cystadenoma, Zollinger-Ellison tumor), pancreatic cyst (pseudocyst and true cyst), and chronic pancreatitis. In rare cases, e. g. in acute abdomen, pancreatic arteriography can serve as an adjunct in the differential diagnosis of acute pancreatitis.

Two to three percent of all malignant tumors originate in the pancreas. They are five times more frequent in men than in women; their incidence reaches a peak between the ages of 60 and 70.

Localization:

Head	70%
Body	20%
Tail	10%

For a long time the tumors remain approximately walnut-sized and are tolerably well delimited, and they do not begin to show unlimited growth and diffuse infiltration until the terminal phase. There is an extremely strong tendency to metastasis (DOERR, 1970).

Cancer of duct epithelium	81%
Cancer of glandular epithelium	13%
Difficultly classifiable cancers	6%

The predominant form is adenocarcinoma, which is usually scirrhous and contains cystic as well as gelatinous deposits. The softer neoplasms originating in the acini, on the other hand, show necrosis and hemorrhage. Under these conditions it is understandable that traces of pathological vasculature should be completely concealed by necrosis, cysts, hemorrhages, and gelatinous deposits.

Clinical symptoms. The clinical symptoms of pancreatic carcinoma are ambiguous. It may be suspected if other upper abdominal diseases have been ruled out. As a rule, amylase values are not elevated; indeed, they are more often reduced. Pancreas-induced dyspepsia, in the sense of disturbed fat digestion, may occur. Migratory phlebitis is described in 30% of the cases. A malignant tumor in the body or tail of the pancreas is characterized by a marked paucity of symptoms. Unspecific abdominal pains on either the left or the right side, loss of weight, anemia, vomiting, constipation, and ascites (in the late stage) are the most frequent symptoms, in that order, in pancreatic carcinoma. In carcinoma of the head of the pancreas, obstructive jaundice may be an early symptom.

Conventional radiography. Because of the proximity of the tumor to the stomach and duodenum, it is relatively simple to detect a pancreatic carcinoma by means of a GI series or by duodenography to demonstrate secondary changes. However, this approach is suited primarily for tumors of the head or part of the body of the pancreas. Tumors in the tail of the pancreas are extremely difficult to detect with this conventional roentgenologic method. Not infrequently, when an impression and infiltrative tumor growth are present on the dorsal aspect of the stomach, a lateral view provides the first diagnostic evidence of the existence of a malignant tumor of the pancreas. Widening of the duodenal C-loop merely indicates an enlargement of the head of the pancreas; only destructive alterations in the contours of the inner wall of the duodenum are evidence of malignancy in the head. The Frostberg sign (epsilon-shaped impression on the interior surface of the descending duodenum) is typical of carcinoma of the head of the pancreas in only about half the cases; in all other cases it points to inflammatory swelling of the pancreas head.

Cholangiography and, occasionally, excretory urography revealing displacement of a kidney can provide additional information.

Angiographic findings. The frequent regressive alterations within a pancreatic tumor generally prevent its opacification so that diagnostic inferences can only be drawn by deciphering the intricate network of pancreatic arteries.

The principal vascular changes are displacement, stenosis, occlusion, or arteriovenous shunting (Figs. 143–145). But displacement and stenosis are just as likely to be caused by benign pancreatic alterations such as cysts or inflammatory edema or swelling (Figs. 19, 20). Generalized vascular diseases such as endarteritis obliterans (Fig. 49) or periarteritis nodosa (Fig. 52) can also cause multiple stenoses. The same is true of alterations in the venous system, especially in the course of the splenic vein or in the main trunk of the portal vein. An impression is merely an indication of a space-occupying mass, not a sign of a malignancy. Suspicion is warranted only when irregular mural defects point to infiltration of the easily deformed veins, or when the veins are completely occluded. In such cases, an extensive collateral circulation can develop, especially through direct communications to the veins of the gastric fundus, the body of the pancreas, the left kidney, or to retroperitoneal veins, in an apparently short time.

Curiously enough, we were unable to detect collaterals in a single case of extremely large pancreatic cysts producing pressure on the splenic vein and splenomegaly due to congestion, so that we consider bypass circulation from the spleen to the stomach in the venous phase of celiac angiography to be strong presumptive evidence of a tumor-induced occlusion of the splenic vein. Unfortunately, experience has shown that once the splenic or portal vein has become involved, the pancreatic carcinoma is usually inoperable.

The few observations of tumor opacification in cases of malignant growths in the pancreas (in 1 of a total of 61 pancreatic tumors among our own patients) have been due either to rare sarcomas with rich vascularization or to inflammation of the area surrounding the tumor. In one of our cases, microscopic examination of a frozen section made from the surface of a tumor in the tail of the pancreas led to an initial diagnosis of a chronic inflammation. Only a deep biopsy made possible the histological diagnosis of an adenocarcinoma.

More than in any other area of visceral angiography, the evaluation of an extremely complicated vascular architecture requires the discriminating analysis of at times minimal anomalies in the course and changes of lumen if the multiplicity of inconspicuous signs is to support the fateful diagnosis of pancreatic carcinoma. In the case of small tumors, no one could do this with a high degree of probability. Angiographic signs suggesting malignancy were present in only 13 of our 61 patients with pancreatic carcinoma.

Our statistical analyses (see p. 114) have shown that in cases of abdominal tumors—particularly pancreatic carcinomas—we tended to overrate angiographic findings as evidence of carcinoma. The following example is representative of other wrong diagnoses:

A 50-year-old patient was hospitalized on account of obscure disturbances in the upper abdomen and sharp weight loss. A palpable fullness or mass was found in the left upper abdomen that was difficult to localize. Conventional x-rays revealed no morbid changes. Angiography was performed under the presumptive diagnosis of a pancreatic tumor. The angiogram showed a slight elevation of the splenic vein and elongation of minute arteries in the tail of the pancreas region. These were criteria of an enlarged tail of the pancreas, which together with the clinical findings aroused suspicion of a malignant tumor. The patient refused surgery, was treated with a dietary regimen including pancreatic enzymes, and after three months was free of complaints. Weight increased, and a "tumor mass" was no longer palpable. This must therefore have been a localized pancreatitis—most likely with pseudocysts; in any case, pancreatic carcinoma was definitely ruled out on clinical evidence.

Let us review the angiographic signs of the presence of a malignant pancreatic disease:

1. Displacement of arteries and veins (splenic and portal veins).
2. Encasement of the arteries—eccentric stenosis—predominantly in the head and body of the pancreas. Encasement of veins mainly in the tail.
3. Total, tumor-induced vascular occlusion (gastroduodenal, pancreaticoduodenal, dorsal pancreatic and, less often, hepatic and splenic arteries; and among veins, especially the splenic vein and the trunk of the portal vein).
4. Tumor vessels and "tumor staining" (extremely rare).
5. Accumulation of contrast medium in the parenchymal phase due to concomitant inflammation.

Angiographic sources of error. Characteristic angiograms that make the presence of the malignant tumor highly probable (Figs. 143–145) contrast with angiograms in which vascular stenoses or occlusions are shown that are due to iatrogenic procedures (ligature of the gastroduodenal artery in a Billroth II resection of the stomach) and consequent inflammatory and primary vascular processes. They need to be considered critically in the differential diagnosis. As long, however, as a drug specifically acting upon cancer vessels has not become known, angiographic diagnosis has to be based, like it or not, upon these predominantly indirect signs.

With these nonspecific, indirect criteria there is a danger that occasionally pancreatic carcinoma will be diagnosed too frequently, the significance of individual signs being overrated. Yet this "overdiagnosis" is readily understandable since malignant tumors of the pancreas tend to metastasize early and therefore need to be discovered in the earliest possible stage if there is to be any chance for treatment.

Boijsen et al. (1968) are of the opinion that tumors with a diameter of less than 2 cm are not susceptible of angiographic detection in the pancreas. Among all of our cases the smallest diameter was 3.5 cm. The timely detection of pancreatic carcinomas in the angiogram depends to a not inconsiderable degree on the contrast density in unit time that is attained in the region of the vasculature supplying the pancreas. There are two possible ways of enhancing this contrast density: superselective injection of contrast media and pharmacoangiography.

Reuter in 1969 evaluated a total of 124 superselective catheter examinations in 76 patients with suspected pancreatic changes and found that certain areas of the organ can be visualized better by selective filling of the splenic, gastroduodenal, and pancreaticoduodenal arteries. Despite all the advantages of strong opacification of the catheterized arterial areas, the traditional techniques are, according to this author, by no means superfluous in exploring for carcinoma.

Great hopes have been placed in pharmacoradiography. According to optimistic reports of some authors, all the substances that have been tested appear to improve opacification of the pancreas; however, one gains the impression that more was read into some of the published angiograms than they actually had to offer. The drugs tested so far belong either to the epinephrine group, or represent bradykinin, or sodium nitroprusside, or the pancreas-activating hormone secretin. Their mechanism of action is based on a selective improvement of pancreatic blood flow (secretin), dilation of pancreatic vessels (epinephrine group), or a greater reduction in arterial as compared to venous blood pressure and a consequent prolongation of the retention of contrast medium within the parenchyma (sodium nitroprusside). Despite these refinements we are still a long way from the possibility of early diagnosis of pancreatic carcinoma by means of angiography.

4.4.2 Pancreatic Sarcomas

Sarcomas of the pancreas are extraordinarily rare. They occur in all forms and types:

Polymorphous sarcoma
Carcinosarcoma
Malignant endothelioma.

Sarcomas spread without limit into the retroperitoneal space and displace the abdominal viscera in a ventrocaudal direction. Not infrequently, the mesenteric root is also involved so that a blockade of the lymphatic channel with a secondary malabsorption syndrome is produced (DOERR, 1970). The special characteristics of lymphomas also should not be overlooked. They can spread from the parapancreatic lymph nodes to the pancreas itself.

There are no specific angiographic criteria for sarcoma. As a rule, a richly vascularized opacification of the tumor may be expected. As an exception we may mention the angiogram of a liposarcoma in which all that could be demonstrated was a vascular displacement.

In this case of our own, involving a 41-year-old female with liposarcoma of the pancreas, angiography merely revealed displacements of the arteries of the head of the pancreas, so that the diagnosis had to be confined to a space-occupying process and a malignant tumor at the head of the pancreas could not be established unequivocally (Fig. 46). In addition, the splenic vein was obstructed.

4.4.3 Cystadenoma of the Pancreas

Pathology. Cysts of the adenoma of the pancreas usually occur at several sites simultaneously. They are situated mainly in the tail of the pancreas and are generally related to the stratified epithelium of the duct. Adenomas and cystadenomas of the pancreas occur more frequently in women than in men (ratio 7:1).

A special form to be mentioned is the oncocytic metastasizing "adenoma". This exercises no endocrine function.

Clinical features. The tumor has hardly any clinical manifestations and is usally palpable as a round, immobile structure. Palpation findings and results of intensive conventional x-ray examination of stomach and duodenum usually do not permit the tumor to be distinguished from a pancreatic cyst or pseudocyst; an important retrospective criterion for the latter is prior pancreatitis. The principal sign discovered in a GI series is the rounded impression of the inner edge of the descending duodenum when the site is the head of the pancreas, or an impression on the dorsal aspect of the stomach.

Angiographic findings. Pancreatic cystadenoma is generally so richly vascularized that it can even be visualized in a flush aortogram, as has been shown by BIEBER and ALBO (1963) as well as by PYRAH and COWE (1957). However, as in carcinoma, the method of choice is selective angiography of the celiac and superior mesenteric arteries (BANG, 1965; SWANSON, 1963).

In the single case of cystadenoma that we saw, a tumor of the size of a billiard ball was located in the head of the pancreas and led in a twelve-year-old girl to moderate compression of the bile duct with distinct enlargement of the gallbladder. The principal angiographic sign was a massive displacement of the vessels without stenosis; increased vascularization was not demonstrable (Fig. 148).

The majority of cystadenomas are associated with the following angiographic characteristics:

1. Marked displacement of vessels without stenosis.
2. Increased vascularization.
3. Persistent capillary opacification with delayed drainage of contrast medium.
4. Strikingly distinct venous phase.

The same angiographic sign are seen with malignant cystadenoma and angiosarcoma so that histological clarification has to be preceded by differential diagnosis despite the demonstration of extensive cystic, avascular areas within the highly opacified pancreatic tumor.

4.4.4 Insulinoma and other Adenomas

Pathology. According to DOERR (1970), insulinomas are uncovered in 0.1% of all necropsies. In 85% of the cases single tumors are found; multiple insulinomas are found by pathologists in 15% of cases, with numbers of tumors ranging from 2 to 11 in the individual case. In more than half of the cases insulinomas have diameters of 1–3 cm and weigh 2–4 grams.

Localization:

Cauda	50%
Corpus	30%
Caput	20%

The majority of insulinomas are observed in patients between 40 and 50 years old. They may be broken down histologically into

"simple" islet cell adenomas	75%
islet-cell carcinomas	15%
disseminated adenomatous hyperplasias	10%

In 75% of cases islet cell tumors originate from beta cells. Of these, 85% are hormonally active. The 15% that are not include numerous tumors that are combined with adenomas of other endocrine organs.

Histological differentiation from islet cell carcinoma is extremely difficult and presents problems similar to those encountered in the diagnosis of metastasizing thyroid adenomas. Cancer of the islands of Langerhans is relatively mature and has a structure typical of the organ. Its growth is predominantly of a local destructive type and extremely slow. Individual cases with early metastasization have been described.

Clinical features. Signs of hyperinsulinism, namely, sudden sensation of hunger, hyperhidrosis, psychic and neurologic disturbances lead to the diagnosis of insulinoma. These symptoms occur in the early morning hours or 2 to 4 hours after meals. In the further course of the disease the hyperglycemic states are experienced with increasing frequency and severity, blood sugar values usually dropping below 50 mg/100 ml. These at times critical episodes can be aborted immediately by administration of glucose.

Localization of an insulinoma is not possible with conventional radiographic methods.

Angiographic examination. Since the first angiographic description of an insulinoma by OLSSON in 1963 numerous papers have been published in which the chances for angiographic visualization are evaluated in highly divergent ways. BOOKSTEIN and OBERMANN (1966) localized only two of 6 surgically confirmed insulinomas by means of selective angiography. In 1966, ZENKER et al. reported on the diagnosis of three out of a total of 5 insulinomas. Among our own patients, we succeeded in localizing 4 out of 7 insulinomas. MADSON and HANSON (1970), on the other hand, were able to localize correctly all 9 insulinomas in their series of cases; they called attention to the following factors that are important for successful visualization:

Kilovoltage should be kept as low as possible and in some circumstances the focal spot-to-film distance should be reduced. Superimposed shadows can be minimized by inflating the stomach with air. Finally, the arteriogram should be scanned very thoroughly so that pathological accumulations of contrast medium in the course of each artery belonging to the pancreas can be detected.

The authors make reference to 36 cases out of 48 reported angiographic tumor examinations in which insulinomas were exactly localized. Other authors attributed failures to technical errors in angiography (ZENKER et al., 1966; MCCONNELL et al., 1966; EMMRICH and FRERICHS, 1969); to small size of the tumor (ZENKER et al., 1966); superimposition of opacified spleen (OLSSON, 1965); low vascularization (HERNANDEZ et al., 1967), and absence or dilatation of sinusoids.

The main angiographic characteristics of an insulinoma are the dilated arterial branches leading to the tumor. In most cases the neoplasm shows increased vascularization and stores the contrast medium for an extended period so that a peak density is observed between the third and the eighth second after the beginning of the injection (Fig. 149). The contrast peaks are not always easy to recognize because of superimposed structures (spinal column). They can, however, be verified in a densogram. Moreover, insulinomas can be localized more readily by use of the subtraction technique (Fig. 21). In the differential diagnosis, very dense pools of contrast medium should bring to mind the possibility of an accessory spleen. If an afferent artery of sufficiently wide caliber is present, the origin of the vessels may conceivably permit correct localization and diagnosis.

There are no certain diagnostic criteria for a *malignant insulinoma*. The diagnosis can be established very rapidly only if celiac angiography demonstrates not only a primary tumor within the pancreas but multiple, richly vascularized rounded metastases within the liver. Such cases have been described by BOIJSEN et al. (1968) and LUDIN et al. (1966).

4.4.5 Zollinger-Ellison Syndrome

The subject of non-insulin-producing islet cell tumors with hypersecretion of a hyperacidic gastric juice and ulceration is also germane to the discussion of insulinomas. In contrast to insulinomas, these tumors produce no insulin but gastrin and thus cause the development of refractory ulcers which not infrequently show an atypical localization. Fifty percent of these islet cell tumors are malignant, representing fully matured islet cell carcinomas. Adenomas may develop at several sites simultaneously.

The Zollinger-Ellison syndrome may be suggested by demonstration of massive hypersecretion and atypical, continually recurrent and therapy-resistant ulcers in conventional x-ray examinations of the upper gastrointestinal tract; clinical diagnosis presents no difficulties. However, the pancreatic tumors producing this pattern are hardly detectable by means of a GI series or other conventional radiographic techniques.

Angiographic diagnosis is based on the same signs that we mentioned with regard to the localization of the insulinomas.

Some further considerations regarding angiographic pathomorphology have been offered by GAMMILL et al. (1971). They showed with reference to studies in 24 cases of islet cell tumors and carcinoids that the angiographic findings are completely identical for the two tumor types. Being peptide-producing endocrine tumors, they are believed to originate from a common stem cell. The observation that both tumors were able to produce insulin as well as serotonin is cited as clinical evidence.

4.4.6 Acute Pancreatitis

Pathology. The picture of acute pancreatitis is dominated by rapidly progressive inflammation with edema and tissue necrosis. When drainage is obstructed in the pancreatic duct or the distal biliary passages, this may readily be suspected as the cause but it rarely is. The hemorrhagic inflammation can lead within hours to large-scale necrosis of the entire organ.

Clinical features. The foremost clinical sign is upper abdominal pain, usually on the left side. The abdomen is only slightly rigid; there is diffuse tenderness with meteorism and subacute ileus. The face is flushed. Leukocytosis is a common finding. The urine and blood levels of amylase and diastase are usually elevated. Of late, increasing use has been made of the rapid lipase test.

The disease affects almost exclusively pyknic individuals, most of them women. Many have a history of gallstones.

Conventional radiography. Not infrequently the simple plain abdominal film is sufficient to make acute pancreatitis highly probable: Concomitant left-sided pleural effusion, circumscribed gaseous distention of stomach and duodenum and of parts of the transverse colon and, in left lateral decubitus films of the abdomen, discrete visualization of the descending duodenum with irregular contours of the inner wall bordering on the pancreas are nearly pathognomonic for acute pancreatitis according to SWART (1971). Occasionally it is possible to arrive at a presumptive diagnosis even without the use of a radiopaque agent.

Nevertheless there will always be borderline cases. They are familar to every internist and surgeon, and further diagnostic findings are appreciated particularly if the laboratory chemistry data yield no pertinent evidence.

Angiographic findings. Patients with acute pancreatitis seldom undergo angiographic examination (Figs. 150 and 151). We had occasion to observe an acute necrotizing inflammation of the pancreas with fatal outcome a few hours after the onset of the fulminant disease. As far as we know, the findings made have not been described previously:

A very obese man, age 55, who suddenly, without warning, fell ill with extremely severe upper abdominal pains was hospitalized immediately. His vital signs diminished precipitously and his abdomen was very rigid. The tenderness was greatest in the epigastrium. There was no evidence of perforation or ileus, and no history of gallstones. No elevation of amylase values. Angiography was performed to rule out a visceral artery occlusion. The celiac trunk could by quickly catheterized at the usual site; however, the contrast medium (25 ml Urografin 76%) did not drain but remained discernible in the arteries at the end of serial angiography and only disappeared slowly, several minutes later. The parenchyma was not visualized, and the veins could not be differentiated (Fig. 151).

The angiogram suggested a drainage obstruction, and because of the distinctly displayed arterial branches enlargement of the pancreas due to acute pancreatitis was assumed. We suspected a possible thrombosis in the portal vein system, and this was verified at autopsy. The prolonged retention of the contrast medium in the arterial phase, both in the splenic and the hepatic artery, can be explained only by intravascular clotting (consumption coagulopathy!).

Similarly to the widening of the duodenal C-loop reflecting an increase in the volume of the head of the pancreas, as revealed by barium enema, angiography in acute pancreatitis discloses a dilatation of the arteries leading to the pancreas and a moderate elongation or displacement of individual branches, and it generally fails to visualize the parenchyma.

If acute pancreatitis spreads to adjacent vessels, the splenic vein in particular and, from here, the mesenteric and portal vein trunks are compromised by thrombophlebitis with ensuing total thrombosis.

4.4.7 Chronic Pancreatitis

Pathology. The morphological pattern of chronic pancreatitis is extremely varied. Parenchymal necrosis is associated with inflammatory infiltration, connective tissue proliferation, and scirrhous contraction. Often the entire picture is dominated by a fairly large pseudocyst with chronic obstruction of the pancreatic duct. Scaly calcium deposits may be distributed over the entire pancreas.

Clinical features. Clinical diagnosis of chronic pancreatitis is exceedingly difficult since there is no satisfactory method of examination. However, a new diagnostic dimension is opened by opacification of the pancreatic duct through endoscopy using a fiber duodenoscope. As a rule, the diastase values are increased only during the acute episode. The intermittent course of the disease is characterized by anorexia, weight loss, persistent meteorism, and recurrent diarrhea. Not infrequently, such patients are treated for years for obscure upper abdominal complaints without clear evidence of ulcer, with uncertain biliary tract findings, and uncharacteristic hepatic and pancreatic laboratory data. Only very rarely do scaly calcific deposits on the abdominal x-ray point to calcifyng chronic pancreatitis.

Conventional radiography. Among our cases, abdominal roentgenograms and gastrointestinal series hardly ever disclosed pathological changes except in the form of calcifications. By contrast, hypotonic duodenography has proved very useful. It showed serrated irregularities of outline on the internal wall of the descending duodenum, cicatricial projections, or impressions due to pseudocysts of varying size.

Angiographic findings. The angiographic picture is extraordinarily variable. Specific changes are not to be expected in chronic pancreatitis either on the great vessels or on the intraparenchymal branches.

Some authors have linked celiac stenosis pathogenetically to chronic pancreatitis (REUTER and OLIN, 1965; BRON and RIDMAN, 1969; LECHNER and POKIESER, 1971).

While these authors cited incidence rates of celiac stenosis in pancreatitis of 2.5, 12.5 and 9.2%, respectively, we did not find a single case of celiac stenosis among our patients with chronic pancreatitis. In addition, ASANG and MITTELMEIER (1956) called attention to a causal relationship between chronic pancreatitis and deficient pancreatic blood flow due to occlusion of the major visceral arteries.

All authors agree that moniliform irregularities of caliber of the larger pancreatic arteries (REUTER et al., 1969) are seen invariably and that the small pancreatic arteries exhibit conical constrictions (HEPP et al., 1968).

In terms of differential diagnosis such vascular stenoses are very difficult to differentiate from vascular systemic diseases. Therefore, the diagnosis of chronic pancreatitis requires additional angiographic evidence (Fig. 153). Examples are the displacement of peripancreatic vessels and adjacent organ arteries by cysts (Fig. 154), abscess formation (Fig. 19), or inflammatory organ enlargement. Of importance, too, is the detection of larger arteries in the cyst wall since dangerous erosion hemorrhages may develop at this location.

Arteriography performed in a 35-year-old patient in an attempt to find evidence of acute gastrointestinal hemorrhage yielded as the only finding a localized pancreatitis in the area of the tail. The surgical specimen showed an erosive hemorrhage with invasion of the duodenum.

In our own case material, the detection of outstandingly well-vascularized areas in the pancreas seems to us the most important indicator of the presence of chronic pancreatitis. Reports regarding zones with increased vascularization mentioned highly divergent rates of incidence: NEBESAR and POLLARD (1967) 20%; REUTER et al. (1969) 27%; LECHNER and POKIESAR (1971) 33%; RÖSCH and BRET (1965) 75%. The explanation for this considerable variance is easy: the pathomorphological substrate varies in individual cases of chronic pancreatitis. It is understandable that in cases with extensive necrosis or pseudocyst formation, areas of hypervascularization are much smaller in number than they are in cases of chronic inflammation with more or less acute recurrence. In the latter type of case hyperemia and dilatation of pre-existing vessels as well as newly formed capillaries in the granulation tissue can contribute to the increased vascularity.

Angiographic pathomorphology of pancreatitis

Acute	Chronic
Arteries	*Arteries*
Straight to arcuate course	Hypervascularization
Dilatation	Constriction
No stenoses	Possible stenoses
Parenchyma	*Parenchyma*
No visualization of organ	Strikingly good organ opacification with possible cystic filling defects
Veins	*Veins*
Unremarkable	Cicatricial distortions of major vessels (rare)
Delayed drainage of contrast medium if portal vein is thrombosed	

Pancreatic rupture. Isolated pancreatic injuries are decidedly rare observations owing to the concealed situation of the organ and its "envelopment" by neighboring organs and the spinal column. There is no typical clinical symptomatology. Even conventional x-ray examination of cases of recent pancreatic injury have done little more so far than to raise an uncertain suspicion by demonstrating functional or anatomical changes in adjacent viscera.

By contrast, angiography can provide more precise evidence of involvement of the pancreas in blunt abdominal trauma. The first published paper on the angiographic diagnosis of pancreatic rupture that came to our attention was written by CHVOJKA (1970), who found a filling defect in the gastroduodenal artery during celiac angiography in a 44-year-old accident victim. Selective angiography of the superior mesenteric artery produced a retrograde opacification of the pancreatic arcades and revealed no streaming phenomena of any kind in the venous phase at the opening of the splenic vein into the portal vein. This led to the presumptive diagnosis of traumatic rupture of the gastroduodenal artery with thrombosis of the splenic vein. Both findings, besides crush injury to the head of the pancreas as well as laceration of the liver and the spleen, were later verified at autopsy.

Our own observations were made in a 15-year-old girl who had been struck in the upper abdomen by a hoof and in a man of 27 who suffered a blunt abdominal injury in a traffic accident. The angiographic signs of pancreatic injury in the first case were broad splaying of the gastroduodenal and right gastroepiploic arteries, indicative of enlargement of the pancreas as well as accumulation of contrast medium around the organ, in addition to which a splenic rupture was discovered (Fig. 80). The young man had suffered an incomplete detachment of the right hepatic artery arising from the superior mesenteric artery, as evidenced angiographically by an annular stenosis and persistence of the contrast column in this vessel, besides which—as in CHVOJKA's case (1970)—the gastroduodenal artery was not visualized (Fig. 155). Surgery disclosed an extensive rupture of the head of the pancreas and a detachment of the indicated vessels and the common bile duct.

Insofar as conclusions can be drawn from these sporadic angiographic examinations, the following criteria for *pancreatic injury* in nonlacerating abdominal trauma may be proposed:

1. Rupture or stenosis of one or several arteries of the pancreatic region.
2. Occlusion or stenosis of efferent veins directly adjacent to the pancreas (splenic and mesenteric veins and portal vein).
3. Displacement of arteries accompanying the pancreas, with extravasation of contrast medium.

4. Detection of injuries or hemorrhages in adjacent organs (splenic, hepatic rupture, retroperitoneal hematoma).

REUTER and REDMAN (1972) examined 3 patients with pancreatic trauma. One, who had a complete transection of the pancreas, had no angiographic abnormalities in or around the pancreas. The second had a traumatic pseudocyst, which was demonstrated by angiography. The third had a hematoma of the tail of the pancreas, in addition to a splenic laceration. No abnormal angiographic signs were present in the pancreas.

5 Stomach and Duodenum

5.1 Anatomy

Three-fourths of the stomach are situated in the left hypochondriac region, while one-fourth is situated in the epigastric region. The fundus is in apposition with the inferior surface of the diaphragm to the left of the esophageal hiatus. The cardial portion shows little change in position when the stomach is filled; the position is also unaffected by the movements of the diaphragm. The pylorus is found at varying levels but usually anteriorly to the first lumbar vertebra. In asthenic individuals, radiography not infrequently localizes it at the level of the fourth or fifth lumbar vertebra.

The lesser curvature and the pylorus are not in apposition with the anterior abdominal wall; the inferior margin of the liver comes between both. The greater curvature, however, reaches the anterior abdominal wall and is displaced downward and to the left when the stomach is filled.

The shape of the *duodenum* varies to an extraordinary extent. It may be divided into four portions: the superior horizontal portion, descending portion, inferior horizontal portion, and ascending portion. Like the shape, the position of the duodenal segments varies considerably.

As they enter the root of the mesentery, the superior mesenteric artery and vein traverse the inferior portion of the duodenum on its ventral side. Pressure from the weight of the root and its vessels can lead to arteriomesenteric occlusion of the duodenum in the supine patient.

Similarly to the stomach, the duodenum has numerous relations to contiguous organs, which lie mostly in the retroperitoneal space, namely, the kidney and the adrenal gland, as well as the inferior vena cava. On the other hand, it is in contact with the liver, the gallbladder, the head of the pancreas, the transverse colon, and the jejunum.

While the superior portion of the duodenum is surmounted by the right lobe of the liver and in contact with the quadrate lobe as well as the neck of the gallbladder, the common bile duct passes downward, with the portal vein on its left. The common bile duct is lodged in the furrow between the head of the pancreas and the descending portion of the duodenum, where it joins, just before its entry into the wall of the duodenum, the pancreatic duct, opening into the duodenal papilla midway up the descending portion (HAFFERL and THIELE, 1969).

5.2 Vasculature

The major supply vessel for stomach and duodenum is the celiac trunk (Fig. 156). From its branches the *left gastric artery* passes upward and courses along the lesser curvature, giving off branches to both surfaces of the stomach. The left gastric artery anastomoses with the *right gastric artery*, which arises from the proper hepatic artery and meets it from the pyloric end of the stomach. Thus, an arterial arcade is formed at the lesser curvature receiving its main supply from the left gastric artery, which together with its esophageal branches also supplies the inferior end of the esophagus and along this route frequently communicates with its thoracic vessels.

The second vessel of the celiac trunk is the *splenic artery*. Besides a number of pancreatic branches, it gives origin to the short *gastric arteries* in the vicinity of the splenic hilus. Here, too, a larger terminal branch of the splenic artery, the left *gastroepiploic* artery, originates and runs to the right in the gastrocolic ligament along the greater curvature of the stomach. The artery gives off gastric branches to both surfaces of the stomach and epiploic branches to the greater omentum. Its end anastomoses with the *right gastroepiploic artery*, which comes from the pyloric end of the stomach. Thus, a vascular arcade is also formed at the greater curvature, receiving its main supply from the right gastroepiploic artery.

The third vessel of the celiac trunk, the *common hepatic artery*, divides above the pylorus into the *proper hepatic* and *gastroduodenal arteries*. The latter courses downward along the superior portion of the duodenum near the pylorus, appears caudally to the duodenum next to the pylorus, and divides here into two terminal branches: The *right gastroepiploic artery* follows the greater curvature, while the *anterior superior pancreaticoduodenal artery*, which is considerably smaller, enters the concavity of the duodenum, supplying this and the adjoining head of the pancreas.

The *gastric veins* carry blood to the *portal vein*. Their course closely corresponds to that of the four gastric arteries. To be noted is a venous arc consisting of the right and left gastric veins (vena coronaria ventriculi). As a small gastric vein of topographical significance we should mention the prepyloric vein, which courses in the pyloric sulcus and marks the border line between the stomach and the duodenum.

5.3 Conventional Radiography

At this point we need not give a detailed description of the visualization of the stomach and the duodenum with the aid of a radiopaque meal and its diagnostic value. It may simply be pointed out that the double-contrast method (application of contrast medium and air inflation) and pharmacoradiography yield considerably more detail—also with respect to neighboring organs (pancreatic changes)—than is obtainable with the customary mucosal technique and full-stomach pictures. The double-contrast method in particular has proved extremely useful for the early diagnosis of gastric carcinoma. The same is true of the detection of early changes of the head of the pancreas with the aid of so-called hypotonic duodenography, which we use routinely in our Department whenever pancreatic alterations are suspected.

Since this examination is by no means familiar to all radiologists, we will give a brief outline below.

5.4 Hypotonic Duodenography

(Technique used at the Radiological Department, Surgical University Clinic, Heidelberg.) Following introduction of a duodenal catheter, the tip of which had best be placed near the inferior duodenal flexure, 1–2 ml of Buscopan (Boehringer Ingelheim) is injected intravenously and immediately thereafter 10–20 ml of a dilute barium suspension is administered, being evenly distributed over the entire duodenum by careful inflation with air. The injection of Buscopan produces a marked hypotonicity of the intestinal wall, with the peristalsis generally ceasing within one to two minutes, and the duodenum can then be visualized without any overshadows. Anteroposterior views

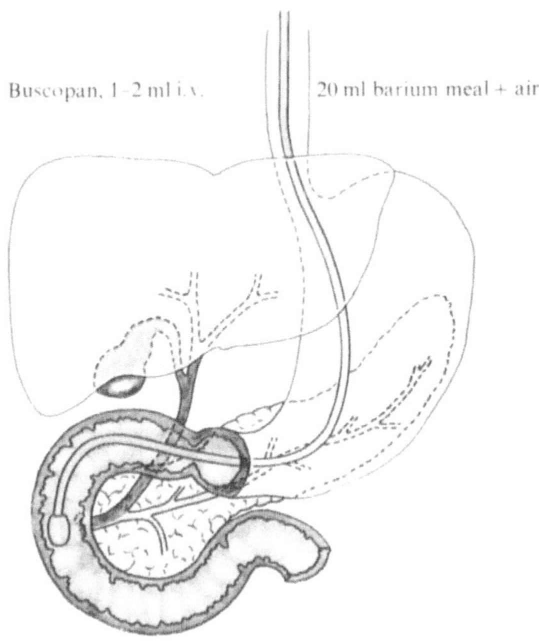

Hypotonic duodenography

and oblique projections, particularly with the patient in prone position, will quickly disclose any swelling of the papilla and changes at the inner margin of the descending portion of the duodenum due to pancreatic changes.

5.5 Angiographic Technique

The access route for the vessels of the stomach and the duodenum are the aorta, the celiac artery, the superior mesenteric artery, the inferior vena cava, and the portal vein.

Flush aortography is of value only for the approximate localization of space-occupying processes in the gastric and duodenal regions. The method of choice is selective visualization of the celiac artery and, depending on the location of the suspected lesion, superselective filling of the left gastric artery (Sundgren, 1970). Changes at the inferior duodenal flexure, the inferior horizontal portion of the duodenum, and its descending portion can be detected via the branches of the pancreaticoduodenal artery arising from the superior mesenteric artery.

5.6 Angiographic Pathomorphology

5.6.1 Vascular Changes

Angiography is most likely to be diagnostically successful in elucidating alterations in the vascular system of the stomach and the duodenum, whether this be in the form of reduced or increased blood flow. A pathogenetically more interesting example of *reduced blood flow* in stomach and duodenum is coarctation of the abdominal aorta, with stenosis of the afferent celiac artery and numerous collaterals, some of which communicate via intercostal and vertebral arteries (Fig. 108). It is understandable that, as a result of the deficient blood flow, upper abdominal pains should develop after each meal.

An extremely rare observation made in one of our cases was stenosis of the celiac artery associated with an atypical course of the left gastric artery. The vessel *wound* around the trunk and compressed it at the same time. Clinically, the patient had for years suffered from upper abdominal complaints, and the assumption made on several occasions on the basis of radiographic findings that they were due to a duodenal ulcer with an intact bulb proved to be baseless.

This group of vascular constrictions includes ulcers associated with a chronic circulatory deficit which have long been known to pathologists (WANKE, 1969), and were observed repeatedly in celiac artery stenosis by SCHIMANSKI and SCHMIDT (1971).

Increased blood flow may be expected when there is a local vascular dilatation or a shunt to the venous side. An arterioportal shunt of this type which formed after collective ligature following a Billroth II resection of the stomach between an artery on the greater curvature and a mesenteric vein is shown in Fig. 12. The angiographic picture is dominated by dilatation of the afferent artery and the portal vein. The clinically most prominent sign was a vascular bruit, detected by the patient himself, in addition to marked portal hypertension with bleeding esophageal varices.

5.6.2 Gastroduodenal Hemorrhage

Acute hemorrhage is one of the most important indications for angiography of the stomach. The difficulties experienced in the localization of sources of bleeding by means of conventional methods are well known: a niche lined with clots, the frequent occurrence of fist-sized clots; these are difficulties that are just as familiar to the endoscopist.

The previously customary practice of waiting for diagnostic signs ought to be abandoned in the patient's interest since failure to determine the cause of a hemorrhage may cost him his life. Even laparotomy fails to localize the source of bleeding in 6–8% of cases! Since an immediate upper GI series does not yield the desired results in a great many cases, we have adopted the practice of at once performing angiography in cases of subacute hemorrhage.

It is a rule of thumb that the chances of detection increase with the severity of the hemorrhage; in practice this means that angiography is always associated with the continuous administration of blood transfusions (WENZ et al., 1969).

Even when laparotomy has been unproductive, angiography can still establish the localization of the hemorrhage. In the example shown in Fig. 161, the contrast medium has drained just below the cardia via the selectively catheterized left gastric artery and is retained in the stomach.

The second laparotomy performed immediately after this angiography can demonstrate a spurting vessel at this very site during gastrotomy. The bleeding can be controlled by means of a purse-string ligature.

The changes involved here are among those sources of bleeding that have tremendously increased in incidence, along with peptic ulcer, in recent years. To us, three syndromes involving gastric hemorrhage appear particularly significant (see p. 92).

The angiographic examples cited attest to the high information yield of which this technique is capable. Nevertheless, angiography and emergency endoscopy should not compete with one another. *Recourse should be had to whichever method is available in an acute emergency, presents no unusual technical problems, and does not impose more strain on the patient than is absolutely necessary.*

Occasionally, the endoscopist will be able to stop a hemorrhage by sclerosation. This may also be feasible during angiography. Thus, ROESCH et al. (1971) in an extensive review

Syndromes with acute hemorrhage from cardial portions of stomach

1. Boerhaave syndrome (1724)	Atraumatic, complete rupture of esophagus or stomach in the vicinity of the cardia. Clinical features: Violent pain in upper abdomen, mediastinal or dermal emphysema, mediastinal empyema. *Moderate bleeding* (Fig. 159).
2. Mallory-Weiss syndrome (1929)	Atraumatic, incomplete rupture of esophagus or stomach in vicinity of cardia. Clinical features: *Massive gastrointestinal hemorrhage* after severe vomiting, usually accompanied by hematemesis, as the dominant symptom. Like 1, this syndrome usually affects alcoholics (Fig. 160).
3. Dieulafoy ulcer (1897)	Acute gastric erosion and ulceration, usually in the cardial region; dominant symptom: *Massive gastrointestinal hemorrhage* (stress situation?) (Fig. 161).

paper reported on the possibilities of controlling acute gastrointestinal hemorrhages after use of a mixture of vasopressin, epinephrine and propanol on the superior mesenteric artery in animal experiments had led to rapid reduction of mesenteric blood circulation to 10–30% of normal values.

In 12 patients with arterial or capillary hemorrhages, injection of 10 to 16 mcg epinephrine/min into the hepatic artery, or 8–10 mcg epinephrine into the left gastric artery, proved so successful that the hemorrhage could be stopped in 10 cases. The injection of 0.3 unit of vasopressin/min proved effective over a period of 2 hours in severe bleeding from the esophageal varices.

The mechanism of this specific pharmacologic hemostasis is a localized narrowing of the vascular pathway and reduction of blood flow leading to stable thrombotic plug formation. In arteriosclerosis, of course, the chances of success diminish rapidly as vessel wall elasticity decreases.

Who would ever have thought in the days before angiography that roentgenologists would play a diagnostic, let alone a therapeutic, role in gastrointestinal bleeding!

A massive extravasation of contrast material at the level of the gastroenterotomy just after a Billroth II stomach operation, with life-threatening hemorrhage, is illustrated in Fig. 64. The source of the bleeding was a vessel stump in which a suture in the anastomosis had opened up.

The investigative techniques employed to localize a source of bleeding in the gastrointestinal tract are discussed further in the chapter on "Gastrointestinal Hemorrhage" (p. 34).

5.6.3 Gastroduodenal Tumors

Logically, more or less profuse extravasation of contrast material in the case of a bleeding stomach would be followed in pathomorphological order by a richly vascularized tumor, especially a vascular tumor of the stomach or duodenum. However, such tumors are rare, and the paramount question for the clinician, namely, is a tumor malignant or benign, can hardly be answered by means of angiography.

BOIJSEN et al. (1968) emphasize that the diagnosis of a malignant gastric or duodenal tumor requires extraordinarily broad experience and a highly painstaking evaluation of the angiograms.

BERT et al. (1968) believe that the angiographic differentiation between a malignant and a benign gastric tumor is extremely difficult.

CHAVEZ et al. (1967) report on three angiographic misdiagnoses of tumors, all in the stomach:

1. Simulation of a circumscribed area with hypervascularization at the level of the spleen, which turned out to be an inflammatory alteration of the greater omentum.
2. A localized finding suggestive of a tumor in a celiac angiogram; laparotomy disclosed a discrete chronic pancreatitis with left-sided subhepatic abscess.
3. Presumptive angiographic diagnosis of a retroperitoneal tumor in celiac angiography, which showed a zone of distinct hypervascularization at the level of the duodenum. Surgery, however, only uncovered a chronic duodenal ulcer with an old perforation and considerable adhesions in the vicinity.

One of our own observations belongs in the same category. A patient with a long history of duodenal ulcer was admitted because of considerable weight loss and severe upper abdominal complaints. An upper GI series disclosed marked duodenal deformation suggestive of a neoplasm. Celiac angiography, showing displacement of branches of the gastroduodenal artery and areas of irregular hypervascularization, seemed to confirm this diagnosis. However, surgical demonstration of a chronically penetrating duodenal ulcer refuted it.

Since the diseases with by far the highest incidence, carcinoma and ulcer, essentially involve the surface of the mucosa, it seems plausible to apply ideally suited investigative methods of extremely high diagnostic accuracy for such cases. It then only remains for angiography to find the primary site of very large tumors, to detect liver metastases, and to determine the extragastric spread of a tumor. The number of vascular examinations required in this part of the upper digestive tract is thus reduced, particularly since highly productive techniques such as the double contrast method, hypotonic duodenography, pharmacoradiography, cinematography and, last but not least, modern endoscopy are available.

Therefore we believe that owing to these morphological characteristics, angiography is necessary only in exceptional cases of gastric tumor (Figs. 157,158). A comparable situation exists in bronchial carcinoma, which is unquestionably much easier to diagnose by bronchography than via visualization of the pulmonary vessels. Moreover, the opacification of a gastric tumor is not clearly distinguishable from an inflammatory reaction in the vicinity of a scirrhous ulcer. The differentiation between a malignant and a benign mass should also be made with the aid of the above-mentioned methods, particularly by means of biopsy during endoscopy.

Nevertheless—in line with the discussion in the chapter on angiographic diagnosis of abdominal tumors—vascular displacement, stenoses, and ruptures are important clues to the presence of a gastric tumor (Fig. 137), especially when similar alterations, notably thromboses, are detectable in the accessory veins.

Tumor-suggesting filling defects in the cardia of the stomach can be identified as varices with the aid of *splenoportography* or *arterioportography*. Besides, these methods often make it possible to determine the size of tumors when a gastrointestinal series has failed to do so.

In this context we should also mention the use of ascending lumbar venography, introduced by Düx et al. (1968), for detecting retroperitoneal expansion of gastric carcinoma. Obviously, however, this method has not yet been used to any large extent.

Arteriography can be eminently useful in the determination of the primary site of a large tumor. Let us take a look at the massive radiolucencies in the anterior and posterior stomach walls of a 40-year-old female patient (Fig. 158) from whom a cylindroma at the left angle of the mandible had been removed one month previously. Epigastric complaints and increasing vomiting occasioned a GI series which led to the provisional presumptive diagnosis of a possibly sarcomatous gastric tumor. However, detailed evaluation of the celiac angiogram showed the left hepatic artery to be the afferent vessel. Laparotomy disclosed a fist-sized cylindromatous metastasis in the left lobe of the liver that was readily operable.

On the other hand, a giant gastric neurinoma—with quite similar findings obtained by barium meal—remained undetected on a flush aortogram, even when the site of the operation had been determined. Nor did endoscopy show whether the neoplasm originated in the stomach or elsewhere.

Gastric carcinoma, gastroduodenal ulcer, and gastritis are, and in our opinion will remain, the domain of conventional radiography and endoscopy.

This is true notwithstanding Sundgren's excellent monograph (1970) on the left gastric artery with its many richly detailed angiograms. In a retrospective survey of their own cases, Shibata and Iwasaki (1970) cited 31 visualizations of tumor vessels and 22 instances of tumor opacification among 34 gastric carcinomas, with angiography yielding no more information than conventional radiography, let alone histological evaluation. In ten cases of gastric ulcer, the angiographic picture was "not so greatly different from that of a normal stomach."

The observation of Pinto et al. (1970) in a case of gastric tuberculosis demonstrates how little information pertinent to the diagnosis of a malignant tumor is provided by hypervascularization alone. In this case, hypervascularization was accompanied by mural thickening but there was no infiltration into neighboring organs.

Therefore, it is our opinion that angiography is superfluous when the localization, extent, and histological characteristics of a malignant growth are known. It has no place in the routine evaluation of gastroduodenal illnesses. There are, however, good reasons to consider angiography for the following indications when conventional methods and endoscopy do not achieve the desired results, or when the information obtained by these methods is incomplete:

1. Primary vascular diseases with involvement of stomach and duodenum.

2. Gastric hemorrhage.
3. Tumors of undetermined origin.
4. Arteriomesenteric compression of the duodenum, positional anomalies, and paraduodenal hernia.

5.6.4 Arteriomesenteric Compression of Duodenum

The root of the mesentery with the large mesenteric vessels passes over the horizontal portion of the duodenum, producing—even physiologically and easily detectable by a GI series—a furrowed, perpendicular impression.

Since the duodenum is attached to the posterior abdominal wall alongside the pancreas, it cannot move under pathological conditions and is compressed by the mesenteric vessels. Bilious vomitus and loss of fluids and minerals dominate the clinical pattern of acute arteriomesenteric compression of the duodenum. Chronic intermittent occlusion is encountered mostly in emaciated youths, who not infrequently complain of recurrent colicky pains in the upper abdomen.

Generally, a careful upper GI, series is sufficient for diagnosis. It will show distention of the stomach and duodenum as far as the site of obstruction, which is marked by a ribbonlike, vertical impression about an inch wide. Generally, pharmacoradiography with metoclopramide and cinefluoroscopy permit differentiation from an annular pancreas and obstruction due to rotation anomalies of the intestine (LENZ et al., 1971).

By opacifying the mesenteric vessels, visceral angiography cannot only validate the diagnosis but can provide clues to the pathogenesis. HEARN (1966) showed for the first time on an angiogram of the superior mesenteric artery how the angle between this vessel and the aortic wall can be reduced, with the result that the subjacent duodenum is compressed.

Duodenal compression due to reduction of the angle of bifurcation may be congenital or acquired. Malformations of the mesentery or the supporting connective tissue as well as anomalies in the course of the mesenteric artery are possible congenital causes. According to LENZ et al. (1971), the compression syndrome first becomes manifest in adolescence or adulthood when mechanical factors restricting the flexibility of the root of the mesentery enter into play. Examples are marked weight loss with enteroptosis and depletion of adipose tissue in the root of the mesentery, inflammatory, traumatic, and cicatricial-adhesive alterations.

In an anteroposterior view the simultaneous visualization of the duodenum through a duodenal tube and filling of the superior mesenteric artery will show the identity of the duodenal impression and the corresponding vascular fascicle (Fig. 162). However, under no circumstances should one neglect to follow up with lateral angiography since it provides a far more distinct picture of the compressive effect of the vascular root by demonstrating the acute angle at which the large visceral artery arises from the abdominal aorta (Figs. 162 a–c).

Just as angiography can be valuable in detecting positional anomalies of the gastrointestinal tract (Fig. 162), so it can be useful in rare cases for the diagnosis of *paraduodenal hernia* (Fig. 163).

In 1970 MEYERS was able to show that such a hernia must be considered in postcholecystectomy and postgastrectomy syndromes. If visualization by means of an opaque meal reveals a slight median displacement of the duodenojejunal flexure, the contrast medium remains in the duodenum for a relatively long time, and the upper jejunal loops appear oddly ovoid, arteriography can verify the presumptive diagnosis of paraduodenal hernia by demonstrating that the jejunal branches first take the normal leftward course but then turn to the right in a short arc.

6 Small Intestine and Right Large Intestine

6.1 Anatomy

The small bowel loops which are surrounded by the large intestine are widely displaceable. Topographically, the loops of the small intestine are distributed over the jejunum and ileum in such a way that the horizontal and vertical loops to the left as well as some of the loops in the umbilical region belong to the jejunum, while the ileum loops to the right of the spinal column may be expected in the area of the lower abdomen and in the true pelvis. Here they extend to the floor of the pelvis when the pelvic viscera are empty. Only two parts of the small intestine cannot change their position, the duodenojejunal flexure and the ileocecal junction.

The junction between the ileum and the large intestine is situated in the right iliac fossa; the ileum ascends from the space of the true pelvis, in which its last loops are located, passing upward to the right, crossing the right psoas muscle and the common iliac artery and vein as well as the ureter. At its junction with the ileum it is invaginated into the cecum, as it were, so that folds are formed in the interior of the intestine that involve all the coats of both intestinal segments with the exception of the tunica serosa, which is the only one bridging the invagination.

The cecum is lodged in the right iliac fossa on the iliac muscle but it can also cover the psoas muscle and will not infrequently extend beyond the margin of the latter into the pelvis minor. Its mobility is determined by the attachment of the intestine to the posterior abdominal wall. When filled with gas, it generally adheres to the anterior abdominal wall. In very rare cases, when the embryonal growth of the large intestine is terminated prematurely, the cecum cannot be found in the right iliac fossa. The ascending colon is then short or entirely lacking and the cecum will accordingly be situated more craniad and occasionally on the inferior side of the liver. The appendix may hang down freely, it may be situated medialward, laterally between the abdominal wall and the cecum and, finally, it may be directed upward behind the cecum.

In contrast to the ascending and descending colon, the transverse colon has a fairly long mesocolon which makes possible its mobility. The right colic flexure lies further caudad than the left flexure so that the transverse colon ascends from right to left in an arcuate course. On the right side it is surmounted by the liver and on the left by the spleen. The transverse colon is connected with the stomach via the greater omentum which extends downward from the greater curvature. There are direct relations between the right colic flexure and the descending portion of the duodenum and the head of the pancreas (Hafferl and Thiele, 1969).

6.2 Vasculature

The small intestine and the right large intestine are supplied by the superior mesenteric artery. This is the vessel of the umbilical cord and gives origin to branches both for the small intestine and for the large intestine to a point near the left colic flexure (for details see chapter "Radiologic Anatomy," p. 3).

The branches of the superior mesenteric artery supplying the small intestine, the jejunal and ileal arteries, arise from the left side of the trunk. Only a right branch, the ileocolic artery, participates at the same time in the supply of both the small and the large intestine by giving origin to a small branch going to the lower part of the ileum. The small bowel arteries are interconnected by numerous anastomoses that form two or three arcades from which the terminal branches approach the intestine. The arcade formation is designed to assure the blood supply of the intestinal loops even when their positions and degrees of filling vary.

The arterial supply of the right portion of the large intestine is mediated via the ileocolic artery, which in its ascending branch extends to the beginning of the colon. The right colic artery arises from the superior mesenteric artery where it intersects the inferior portion of the duodenum; alternatively, it may also appear as a branch of the ileocolic or middle colic artery. At the colon it divides into an ascending and a descending branch. The middle colic artery leaves the superior mesenteric artery somewhat craniad to the right colic artery and turns upward into the transverse mesocolon, where it is usually located to the right of the midline. The area it supplies extends to the vicinity of the left colic flexure (Fig. 2).

After reaching the intestinal wall, the branches of the superior mesenteric artery spread around the intestine and ramify into innumerable twigs which are profusely anastomosed. Some are ramified within the serosa itself, while the remainder penetrate the tunica muscularis, giving off afferent branches to it, and subsequently form a strong, widely spread-out network in the submucosa. The vessels of the mucosa develop within this submucosal network, penetrating first the tunica muscularis mucosae and then forming a new, plane network at the base of the gland crypts (Rauber, Kopsch, 1955).

The veins of the small intestine are disposed like the arteries; they, too, form arcades. These arcades give origin to vessels that follow the course of the arteries, passing above or below them. The jejunal and ileal veins also approach the trunk of the superior mesenteric vein from the left; only the ileocolic vein comes from the right. The trunk of the superior mesenteric vein is situated to the right of the artery, crosses the duodenum together with this artery from the front, and disappears at the inferior margin of the pancreas. Here the vein lies in the pancreatic notch and behind the head of the pancreas joins the inferior mesenteric vein and the splenic vein to form the portal vein. A similar pattern is shown by the veins of the large intestine. As ileocolic, right colic and middle colic veins, they form arcades parallel to the arteries and follow their course.

6.3 Conventional Radiography

In contrast to the largely standardized examination of the upper gastrointestinal tract, there are many special techniques available for visualization of the small intestine. This in itself is an indication that there is no one ideal method for complete detection of all, including minor, changes in the small intestine. Non-selective survey films that give information on edema, hypermotility, transit time, and the function of the ileocecal valve are recommended. Fractional opacification according to PANSDORF is aimed at visualization of more subtle morphologic alterations; so-called "intestinal transit accelerators" all have the disadvantage of irritating the mucosa of the small intestine and have not been found acceptable for routine use.

How unsuccessful the conventional small intestine series is may be demonstrated by the fact that all of our five last cases of benign small bowel tumors were overlooked during routine examination. Malignant tumors, too, can be overlooked. This is due not only to the superimposition of different small bowel loops and the impossibility of continuously monitoring the head of the contrast column but also to the tendency of most malignant tumors of the small intestine to grow extraluminally, as a result of which stenoses and the attendant, easily detectable prestenotic dilatation of small bowel segments appear at an extraordinarily late stage.

In one case, for example, we were unable to localize a necrotizing sarcoma of the ileum in the small intestine although the sarcoma was unmistakably palpable. Several ileal loops were adherent so that, in the absence of lumen constriction, an inflammatory conglomerate tumor was assumed to be present.

BERT et al. (1968) therefore recommend that whenever a tumor is suspected in the gastrointestinal tract and the GI series is unproductive, the superior mesenteric artery be visualized so as to rule out a neoplasm in the area of the small intestine. Retrograde opacification of the colon using WELIN's modified technique has been found very satisfactory for examination of the large intestine. This permits detection of even the smallest polypoid alterations down to a diameter of less than 0.5 cm. Conditions in the distal ileum can thus be readily surveyed through reflux via the ileocecal valve, which is easily produced in most cases.

6.4 Angiographic Techniques

The large celiac artery is clearly visualized both in aortography and in selective catheterization. Its trunk, however, is very frequently concealed by the aorta itself in an anterior-posterior film obtained by aortography. Selective exploration of the generally wide ostium at the level of the first lumbar vertebra presents no difficulty if an appropriately curved catheter is utilized.

Catheterization with the patient in lateral position or with a lateral x-ray beam from an image-magnifier television system is rarely necessary. As a rule, it is sufficient to inject 30–40 ml of a highly concentrated contrast medium. The intestinal wall is opacified 45 seconds after the start of the injection, while the veins are filled 5–8 seconds later, with the medium collecting in the superior mesenteric vein and finally in the portal vein (see Chapter "Arterioportography," p. 17).

6.5 Angiographic Pathomorphology

6.5.1 Pathology and Clinical Aspects of Intestinal Tumors

The *malignant epithelial* tumors are invariably adenocarcinomas. They occur in 5 principal forms (DOERR, 1970):

1. Polypoid-papillary, exophytic.
2. Bowl-like ulcerated.
3. Scirrhous, constricting.
4. Mucigenous, gelatinous.
5. Mat-like spread, partly polypoid, partly ulcerative.

Primary sarcomas of the bowel wall are preferentially localized in the vicinity of the ileocecal valve and in the lower part of the small intestine. They are generally solitary and can occur in every age group but more commonly in children. The following histologic types have become known: Reticulum cell sarcoma, spindle cell sarcoma, round cell sarcoma, leiomyosarcoma, melanosarcoma, and lymphosarcoma (the most frequent).

Among *epithelial* small bowel tumors, the adenomas are known as *benign* neoplasms. The term "polyps" may denote tumors of widely varying histological origin. Generalized polyposis usually has a hereditary basis (PEUTZ-JEGHERS syndrome and polyposis coli). Flat, mat-like polyps generally are suggestive of a carcinoma. The malignancy rate of polyps at the preferred sites—flexures of the colon and the rectum—ranges up to 50%!

Non-epithelial benign tumors include lipomas, fibromas, leiomyomas, neurofibromas, neurinomas, vascular neuromas, ganglioneuromas and, less frequently, lymphangiomas. All these tumors can develop simultaneously in several locations. Hemangiomas are very easily detectable by angiography:

1. Simple capillary hemangioma.
2. Cavernous hemangioma.
3. Arteriovenous hemangioma.

Multiple neurofibromas and neurinomas can occur primarily in RECKLINGHAUSEN's disease. Vascular neurinomas are of angiographic interest as sources of severe hemorrhage.

Owing to their rarity, the clinician usually does not think of the possibility of a neoplasm in the small intestine. The clinical symptomatology is not very specific, comprising anemia, occult bleeding, abdominal pains, vomiting, and recurring states of subacute to acute ileus. Occasionally, small bowel tumors can also lead to intussusception, hence to ileus. At times, obscure gastrointestinal bleeding is the only clue to the presence of a small bowel tumor. In the past the diagnosis was in many cases first made on the operating table.

6.5.2 Malignant Tumors

Angiographic detection of the typical adenocarcinoma is fairly difficult. The entire vasculature is usually very densely opacified, so that at times vessel displacements and also delicate newly formed vessels can be found. Not infrequently, too, one finds areas of poor vascularization within a strongly opacified wall during the parenchymal phase that are suggestive of a poorly vascularized tumor (Fig. 8).

In a patient with surgically detected canalicular metastases and a typical tumor filling defect in the jejunum visualized by a small-bowel series, we were unable to make any pathologic findings in a technically perfect arteriogram of the superior mesenteric artery.

Although the number of cases we have seen is very small, we view the angiographic diagnosis of small bowel carcinoma with due reserve.

Angiographic demonstration of small bowel carcinoid is a different matter. Typical examples have been reported by BOIJSEN et al. (1968), REUTER and BOIJSEN (1966), and VIAMONTE (1966). Star-shaped vascular neoplasms with sharp outlines characterize these tumors (Fig. 165). According to REUTER and BOIJSEN (1966), metastatic small bowel tumors and reticulum-cell sarcomas have an extremely sparse vasculature and are difficult to localize by angiography (Fig. 167). By contrast, neurosarcomas, myosarcomas, and other richly vascularized small bowel sarcomas—like those in other abdominal regions—are easily recognized by their bizarre vascular architecture and accumulation of contrast medium in the neoplastic tissue.

6.5.3 Benign Tumors

Benign tumors of the small intestine usually lend themselves readily to angiographic visualization. While a homogeneous opacification is produced in the parenchymal phase in cases of neurinoma and myoma, a more lattice-shaped disposition of tumor vessels is seen in the presence of hemangioma. Hemorrhage into the intestinal lumen produces an intraintestinal pool of contrast medium that remains discernible beyond the venous phase, and can finally visualize the mucosal relief. Intraluminal pools of contrast material of this type may be considered the most important characteristic of a bleeding intestinal tumor.

A tumor can occasionally be localized by means of mesenteric angiography when even careful laparotomy fails to uncover the cause of an obscure severe gastrointestinal hemorrhage (WENZ and KREBS, 1967).

A few striking clinical reports from our case material may be cited for illustration.

Case 1. This 40-year-old patient for the first time observed tarry stools in 1960; they were seen again a total of 3 times. Radiography failed to locate the source of the bleeding. Subsequently, a small duodenal ulcer was detected by radiography. A new gastrointestinal hemorrhage occurred at the beginning of 1967 and a bleeding duodenal ulcer was suspected and laparotomy performed. It was decided to perform a Billroth I gastric resection but no source of bleeding was found in the resected specimen. The small intestine, like the colon, was filled with blood. The focal site of the hemorrhage was not visualized despite two follow-up examinations of the intestine.

Massive intestinal bleeding occurred in the course of the following day. Despite intensive transfusion therapy (5 transfusions in 24 hours) the hemoglobin fell to 8.2 g/100 ml, the blood pressure dropped, and tachycardia developed. The patient, now gravely ill, was referred for angiography and further treatment in our clinic. During continuous blood transfusion the superior mesenteric artery was visualized and a smoothly outlined tumor 2 cm in diameter at the level of the topmost jejunal artery was opacified. A pool of contrast medium bordered the superior margin of the tumor (Fig. 66). Angiographic diagnosis: Small bowel tumor with extravasation of contrast medium.

Immediate repetition of laparotomy uncovered a nodule with dimensions of 3 × 2 × 3 cm that was concealed between the aorta and the small intestine; it was resected. It was histologically identified as a neurinoma. Fourteen days later the patient was symptom-free and could be discharged.

Case 2. In this 45-year-old female a skin tumor over the right buttock had been removed 4 years previously. She had suffered severe gastrointestinal hemorrhages for a month. More than a dozen x-ray examinations and endoscopies failed to localize the source of the bleeding. When referred to our clinic the patient had already received numerous blood transfusions; a visceral angiography was performed immediately. Mesenteric angiography: Arachnoid accumulation of contrast material in ileum projected onto the right lower abdomen, which persisted beyond the venous phase.

Angiographic diagnosis: Richly vascularized, small tumor in ileum. Laparotomy: Small, highly vascularized tumor interpreted as hemangioma and resected. Histological examination surprisingly led to the diagnosis of a metastasis of a gemmangioma, the tumor on the right buttock that had been removed four years previously (Fig. 168).

Mesenteric angiography is also useful in patients with known generalized diseases in whom the source of a life-threatening hemorrhage needs to be located.

Case 3. This 40-year-old patient was known to have a Peutz-Jeghers syndrome. He experienced his first gastrointestinal hemorrhages during puberty. Marked pigmentary anomalies were found on the labial and buccal mucosa. Acute hospitalization became necessary because of a life-threatening gastrointestinal hemorrhage. At the time of admission the patient was known to have polyps in the stomach as well as in the small and large intestines. The source of the bleeding could be localized by means of mesenteric angiography during which a persistent accumulation of contrast medium in one of the uppermost jejunal loops could be demonstrated. At surgery, a large-sized cluster of polyps in this segment was removed and a fresh hemorrhage from one of the tumors detected. After removal of the hemorrhagic source the patient recovered very rapidly. He has now been followed up for three years and has experienced no serious gastrointestinal bleeding during that period (Fig. 7).

6.5.4 Enteritis and Regional Enteritis

Enteritis, which is characterized by great etiologic and pathogenetic diversity, is diagnosed and classified by the internist. Its extent can be determined with adequate accuracy by means of opaque meals and the histological changes can be evaluated with the aid of modern suction biopsy. In addition, functional analysis by cinefluoroscopy will prove enlightening. Pharmacoradiography, too, has gained more and more prominence in recent years in the diagnosis of small bowel disorders (Sielaff, 1970). Angiography can hardly be expected to add any further diagnostic clues. Much of the same is true of local enteritis although a whole series of papers dealing with angiographic characteristics of this disease have been published (see below).

Moreover, the changes of inflammatory disease can be mimicked by normal variations. Food passing through the small bowel increases the vascularity to the segment containing the bolus of food at the time of angiography.

Terminal ileitis. This is an unspecific, chronic, inflammatory intestinal disease and also the most common. In patho-anatomical terms a chronic, inflammatory sclerosing of lymphatic channels is followed by a wall thickening and narrowing of the lumen ("elephantiasis of intestinal wall"); later on, granuloma formation sets in.

The clinical picture is dominated by diarrhea, difficultly localizable abdominal pains, subfebrile temperatures, weight loss and fistula formation. Four stages are distinguished:

1. *Acute stage* (edematous, phlegmonous inflammation of lower ileum).
2. *Subacute stage* (ulceration).
3. *Development of scar stenoses.*
4. Fistula formation.

Pathogenesis. Suggested causes of regional enteritis include blood flow disturbances in the area supplied by the mesenteric artery in association with ischemic necrosis of the intestinal wall, allergic-anaphylactic vessel wall inflammations, thromboangiitis, as well as thromboembolisms in patients with acute cardiac failure or congenital heart defect.

Dingendorf et al. (1971) have looked into the question of transition from acute regional enteritis to chronic Crohn's disease. Acute regional enteritis can heal without resection; so far, apparently, no transition from the acute stage of the disease to chronic regional enteritis has been observed. FAHRLÄNDER and GLOOR (1967) doubt that the acute stage could even be described as an early form of regional ileitis.

On the other hand, DINGENDORF et al. (1971) were able to show on the basis of observations in a 55-year-old patient that he had an acute regional enteritis due to thromboembolism. They noted two typical embolus radiolucencies in the angiogram of the superior mesenteric artery. A chronic regional Crohn's disease showing all the macroscopic and microscopic characteristics associated with this illness developed within about three months. Laparotomy in the acute stage ruled out an acute exacerbation or recurrence of a pre-existing regional enteritis. Remarkably, the arteriogram showed that contrast material surrounded the emboli and that the partially blocked supply area still received an influx from the environment; therefore, intestinal gangrene could not develop.

Angiographic findings. The full-blown picture of Crohn's disease (Fig. 170) encompasses dilated intestinal vessels, dense accumulations of contrast material in the capillaries, and early, vigorous reflux. (BOIJSEN and REUTER, 1966; BRAHME, 1966; LUNDERQUIST and LUNDERQUIST, 1967; DOMBROWSKI et al., 1970; ERIKSON et al., 1970).

LAGERGREN et al. (1958) believe that arteriovenous shunts develop in ulcerative colitis. Conceivably, it is these shunts which also produce the heavy venous reflux in regional enteritis.

We ourselves have seen tortuosity and narrowing of the rarefied vessels inside the intestinal wall in late stages of the disease (Fig. 169); these changes, of course, do not betray their primary vascular or primary inflammatory origin. In such late stages, therefore, it is not possible to determine on the basis of angiography whether the Crohn's disease has a vascular or an inflammatory cause. The pathologico-anatomically proposed role of circulatory disorders in regional ileitis can be elucidated angiographically only if we succeed in demonstrating more frequently vascular changes in the form of thromboembolic processes, inflammatory or arteriosclerotic vessel wall alterations, or arteriosclerosis with blood flow disturbances of the intestinal wall (BOLEY et al., 1963).

The angiographic findings of regional enteritis are related to both the activity and duration of the disease. The early findings are those of acute inflammation and are nonspecific. During periods of activity, prominent hypervascularity is accompanied by dilated arteries and early, dense venous filling. Increased parenchymal contrast medium accumulation may reveal a thickened bowel wall. When the inflammation becomes quiescent, the vascular abnormalities usually return to normal. In the later stages of progressive and recurrent disease, fibrosis may cause irregularities of the vasa recti, some of which may be occluded. The arterial branches in the mesentery may show areas of narrowing and the vasa recti tend to arise at right angles from the mesenteric branches instead of at the usual acute angle. A severely diseased and fibrosed segment of bowel may have a decrease in the number of vasa recti. REUTER and REDMAN (1972) made the experience that these angiographic abnormalities which accompany long-standing regional enteritis are specific.

In general terms it may be said that mesenteric angiography throws no light on the nature of the underlying inflammatory process; it does at times facilitate evaluation of its size by comparison with visualization of the small bowel with the aid of an opaque meal. Specifically in regional enteritis, it will contribute to a better assessment of the possible effect of primary vascular disorders.

6.5.5 Protein-Losing Enteropathy

In rare cases, mesenteric angiography can help to determine the pathogenesis of the protein-losing enteropathy syndrome. According to WAGNER and WENZ (1969), there are two possible interpretations of the phenomenon:

1. The bleeding.
2. A mechanism that may be linked to the development of ascites in Meig's syndrome.

A disproportion between the arterial blood supply in the area of polyps and the return transport of blood and interstitial fluid by the venous or lymphatic route could explain the fact that an increased amount of interstitial fluid is "squeezed off" into the intestinal lumen despite the intactness of the surface epithelium. A hemorrhage is rarely accepted as a cause of a chronic protein-losing enteropathy with hypoalbuminemia.

Such angiographic findings as opacification of only moderately voluminous polyps and rapid filling of veins from the polypoid intestinal segments can be explained only by more intense and more rapid blood flow relative to the surrounding intestinal wall. As is true in arteriovenous anastomoses, the increased pressure on the venous side may hamper reabsorption of the interstitial fluid, causing increased seepage of the fluid into the intestinal lumen.

6.5.6 Blood Flow Disturbance

The small intestine bears the main brunt of acute and chronic blood flow disturbances of the visceral arteries. Indications, techniques, and accuracy of angiographic examination are discussed in the chapter "Visceral Blood Flow Disturbances" p. 27.

TOMCHIK et al. (1970) carried out a very critical study of a total of 67 unselected confirmed cases of intestinal infarction and found that conventional methods such as plain abdominal radiography and a small-intestine series permitted retrospective diagnosis of infarction in only 19% of the cases. In arterial thrombosis and so-called non-occlusive infarction, radiographic clues to the disease were found in only 11 and 8% of cases, respectively.

It may be noted that in the special case of the small intestine, occlusion of the main trunk of the mesenteric artery by thrombosis or embolism can be detected very easily and rapidly. However, difficulties are presented by smaller emboli which not infrequently cause a spastic narrowing of adjacent vessels. AAKHUS and BRABAND (1967) succeeded in correcting such spastic alterations by local administration of 0.04 g of the vasodilator tolazoline (2-benzyl-2-imidazoline).

As the same authors noted and we ourselves were able to demonstrate angiographically in several animal experiments as well as in the course of severe gastrointestinal hemorrhages, vasoconstriction can also be caused by shock (CZEMBIREK et al., 1971).

It seems that intestinal infarction with no vascular occlusion demonstrable at necropsy, such as has been described by a number of authors (SOLHEIM et al., 1963), is attributable in some cases to improper dissection technique, to fibrinolysis, or to spastic factors. Also to be borne in mind is the possibility of intestinal gangrene in cardiac failure and arrhythmia or myocardial infarction (MING and LEVITAN, 1960; CORDAY et al., 1962).

Vasoconstriction in the area of the viscera may serve as a protective mechanism in heart failure designed to maintain adequate circulation in the more vital organs of heart and brain. When there is concomitant vascular disease, e.g. in arteriosclerosis, such a vasoconstriction can lead to circulatory inadequacy of the small bowel. Much the same can be said about vasoconstriction due to drugs such as pressor agents (BROWN et al., 1959), morphine (KATZ, 1959), and digitalis (GAZES et al., 1961).

We never observed vascular spasms due to introduction of a catheter. In one case we noted a so-called string-of-pearls phenomenon affecting several branches of the superior mesenteric artery (Fig. 53).

Examination following a subintimal injection of contrast medium in a trial of mesenteric angiography (Fig. 44) which we performed in the infancy of our angiographic research revealed no objective or subjective sequelae. The lumen was only slightly constricted after withdrawal of the tip of the catheter and a short waiting time. No delayed symptoms occurred.

To sum up our experience, the decision to proceed to mesenteric angiography when circulatory disorders are suspected should be made quickly, and the diagnostic findings so obtained are undoubtedly extremely valuable.

In chronic blood flow disturbances, even occlusion of the main trunk of the mesenteric artery may not cause any symptoms if adequate collaterals have formed which course either from the celiac artery via the pancreatic arcades or via the inferior mesenteric artery by way of Riolan's anastomosis. Details regarding the various collateral pathways may be found in the chapter on "Visceral Blood Flow Disturbances", p. 27.

6.5.7 Angiodysplasia of the small and large intestine

A convenient designation for the group consisting of arteriovenous malformation, small hemangioma, or hereditary telangiectasia is *angiodysplasia*. Pathologists have a great deal of difficulty in differentiating these entities histologically and to attempt to do so radiologically is of academic interest (REUTER and REDMAN, 1972).

Most of the arteriovenous malformations in patients with chronic recurrent bleeding occur in the cecum, ascending colon and the sigmoid (Fig. 173). Occasionally, angiodysplasia involves a small segment of the large or—rarely—the small bowel. The surgeon often sees and feels nothing abnormal in the bowel wall. Therefore, the area which includes the angiographic abnormality with localized hypervascularity and early venous return must be resected even in the presence of a negative exploration. Dilated submucosal veins are each time seen by the pathologist.

6.5.8 Positional Changes of Small and Large Intestine

A characteristic shared by different positional anomalies of the small and large intestine usually is a mesenterium commune. According to the ultimate position of the intestine, we distinguish several major groups, the most important of which are nonrotation, malrotation I, and malrotation II.

While positional anomalies of the colon may not be important for the individual, they can make a differential diagnosis very difficult in some circumstances. CZEMBIREK and GRÖZINGER (1970) have published a report on a case in point witnessed at our Department (Fig. 164).

A man of 28 had been complaining for two days of sudden gastric pains with vomiting. Examination of the abdomen yielded the palpation finding of a fist-sized tumor in the left upper or middle abdomen. The tumor was extremely tender but was not definitely assignable to any organ. For this reason a selective angiography of the left kidney, the celiac artery, and the superior mesenteric artery was carried out. The left kidney was found to be intact and the branches of the celiac artery were unremarkable. A mirror image of the usual ramification of the superior mesenteric artery was found, with the small bowel arteries diverging to the right. The ileocolic artery passed caudally leftward and communicated with the right colic artery, which was likewise situated on the left. Both arteries surrounded a space-occupying process and ended in a highly vascularized marginal zone. Surgery revealed a double fist-sized conglomerate tumor in the left upper abdomen which was identifiable as the ileocecum upon inspection. The terminal ileum entered from the right by way of nonrotation, and an acute appendicitis with appendiceal abscess involved it in an inflammatory conglomerate tumor.

This proves that such a malformation can be diagnosed also through the vascular distribution in the mesenteric region. However, angiography cannot be regarded as the method of choice for the diagnosis of rotational and fixation disorders of the intestine. As a rule, barium enemas and GI series are entirely adequate for unequivocal verification of the diagnosis.

Displacements of the small and large intestine due to hernia should also be mentioned in this connection. Fig. 163 presents a diagram illustrating the possible angiographic diagnosis of a paraduodenal hernia (MEYERS, 1970). ENCKE et al. (1972) of our Department have reported on mesenteric angiography in an individual with a large sacral hernia following sacroabdominal extirpation of the rectum.

7 The Left Colon

7.1 Anatomy

The descending colon is firmly adherent to the posterior abdominal wall, which distinguishes it from the sigmoid colon with its extensive mesentery. As a rule, the sigmoid extends caudad to the point where the dorsal mesentery of the intestine finally ends, namely, at the junction between the second and third sacral vertebrae. Here begins the rectum, which is primarily adherent to the anterior wall of the sacrum (HAFFERL and THIELE, 1969).

7.2 Vasculature

Blood is supplied to the left large intestine through the inferior mesenteric artery. The territory supplied by this artery begins at the left colic flexure and comprises the descending colon, the sigmoid colon, and the major portion of the rectum. The artery arises from the aorta below the renal artery and after a short distance gives off the left colic artery, whose ascending branch passes toward the left colic flexure, while its descending branch runs toward the caudal portion of the colon. The next branches are the sigmoid arteries; they often originate from a common trunk. The superior rectal artery (superior hemorrhoidal artery) supplies only the most distal end of the sigmoid; it is the last branch of the inferior mesenteric artery and represents its extension. The arteries of the large intestine are distinguished from those of the small intestine by the fact that they form a single row of arcades, which lies near the intestine. Consequently, the arterial supply of the large intestine is not as secure as that of the small intestine, so that ligation of one of the large trunks will cause necrosis of the bowel.

The course of the inferior mesenteric vein in its peripheral segment is similar to that of the arteries. The peripheral branches accompany the arteries of the same name. The inferior mesenteric vein arises from the sigmoid and superior rectal veins, runs peripherally to the left of the trunk of the inferior mesenteric artery but continues cranialward beyond it. It receives the left colic vein and reaches the superior duodenal fold to the left of the duodenojejunal flexure. Finally, it empties into the splenic vein or superior mesenteric vein behind the pancreas, forming the portal vein.

7.3 Conventional Radiography

The method of choice for examination of the large bowel is a barium enema, which may be filmed both at extreme filling and after evacuation of the contrast medium using a mucosal technique. A.W. FISCHER'S double-contrast method (1925) as modified by WELIN (1955) has found general acceptance. We will not discuss the technical details of a barium enema.

Evaluation of the colon with the aid of an orthograde barium meal also yields functional data. However, we do not attempt any detailed diagnoses without a (retrograde) barium enema.

7.4 Angiographic Technique

General diagnostic significance. Barium enemas and endoscopy meet most diagnostic demands. The accuracy of both methods exceeds 90%, so that the use of angiography is limited to a few special problems. For example, angiography is generally unnecessary when trochoscopy or endoscopy have detected a malignancy unless the size of the tumor or possible metastases are to be demonstrated.

Technique. The left colon may be demonstrated by flush aortography, with the contrast medium also passing into the inferior mesenteric artery, which seldom arises above the third lumbar vertebra. *Selective visualization* of the vessel, which often has an extremely narrow lumen, is technically difficult and quite time-consuming compared with celiac angiography or visualization of the superior mesenteric artery.

However, we have made the observation that when there are inflammatory changes in the territory of the artery its lumen widens considerably. The exploration is done with a specially curved catheter directed ventrally and usually to the left. As a rule, 15–20 ml of a highly concentrated contrast medium is sufficient for good visualization of the inferior mesenteric artery.

7.5 Indications

For pathological changes—especially tumors of undetermined origin in the pelvis, for which the rectum, sigmoid, or the descending colon has to be considered by way of differential diagnosis—flush aortography is recommended initially and should be focused below the origin of the renal arteries so that the inferior mesenteric artery and the pelvic arteries as well as the lumbar branches are visualized as well. Quite often the very dense opacification of these vascular regions makes it possible to determine the nature of the underlying lesion and also its origin and extent (cf. BREIT, 1967, and MUSSGNUG and PORTMANN, 1965).

WHOLEY et al. (1965) have advocated more frequent use of selective angiography of the inferior mesenteric artery. They point out that this technique has by no means been generally accepted and is most suited to the following indications: Differential diagnosis of space-occupying lesions in the region of the inferior mesenteric artery; vascular status; operability and assessment of tumor recurrence after partial resection of the colon; selective use of drugs; and chemotherapy of tumors. They do not state how often they have performed inferior mesenteric arteriography. The study by KAHN and ABRAMS (1964) also deals to a large extent with aortography in addition to selective opacification of the inferior mesenteric artery.

7.6 Angiographic Pathomorphology

7.6.1 Carcinoma of the Colon

Digital examination, endoscopy, and radiopaque enemas, especially with use of the double-contrast technique, are highly likely to yield a correct diagnosis of a colonic tumor. Differentiation from an inflammatory conglomerate, for example, in sigmoid diverticulitis or at the pole of the cecum following a pericecal abscess, does present problems. We know of no angiographic study to date that has dealt with this problem on the basis of significant numbers of examinations.

A colonic carcinoma is generally opacified. Fig. 172 shows pathological vascular neoplasms and atypical vascular courses. Increased vascularization is also present, however, in an inflammatory conglomerate. The different reaction of tumor vessels to drugs may in the future facilitate differential diagnosis.

The rectosigmoid and the cecal pole are sites at which the origin of a tumor may be in doubt. An example is an extensive ovarian carcinoma involving the cecal pole. It may be completely encased in a barium examination. Under certain circumstances selective renal arteriography can be useful for visualization of the ovarian artery in such cases.

We are of the opinion that in suspected carcinoma of the colon angiography can provide additional information only regarding the size of the tumor and on the origin of extensive space-occupying masses, and that ultimately only histological study can determine if such a growth is malignant or benign.

7.6.2 Colonic Polyposis

Diagnostic role of angiography. With WELIN'S technique, polyps, even those measuring only a few mm in diameter, can be demonstrated by means of radiopaque enema.

Moreover, observations of the course of an illness are a reliable indicator of the malignant or benign nature of a growth so that angiography is needed, if at all, only in cases of larger polyps to obtain evidence for or against malignancy.

Angiographic findings. Colonic polyps are distinguished by a well-developed vascular supply. Thus, in the parenchymal phase, dense vascular fascicles in the fungiform polyps accumulate contrast material in the form of sharply outlined shadows that produce a very striking, dense opacification of the colonic wall in an angiogram, particularly in generalized colonic polyposis (Fig. 171). The picture resembles the findings in a barium enema except that instead of the usual negative filling defect the polyps are positively visualized.

Indications. One of the advantages of angiography in the diagnosis of colonic polyposis is that it may furnish clues to the localization of true tumor development within a potentially precancerous region.

In severe gastrointestinal bleeding requiring surgical intervention, selective arteriography can lead to life-saving surgery by localizing the bleeding polyps (see chapter on "Angiography of Gastrointestinal Hemorrhages," p. 34).

The significance of polyposis in protein-losing enteropathy and the role of angiography in determining pathogenesis have already been discussed in the chapter on the small intestine.

7.6.3 Ulcerative Colitis

In this disease, too, clinical signs and careful endoscopic examination with biopsy of the rectosigmoid mucosa afford sufficient diagnostic clues.

Contribution of angiography to pathogenesis. Angiography is of interest with regard to the much-debated pathogenesis of this disease. Whereas WARREN and SOMMERS (1949) and WARREN and BERK (1957) believe that causative factors in ulcerative colitis include vasculitis with necrosis, thrombosis and perivasculitis, SPJUT and MARGULIS (1965) were unable to confirm this view in microangiographic studies of two ulcerative colitis preparations. They report finding dilated and proliferated vessels and vascular changes mainly within the mucosa. Only when the mucosa was altered were changes also found in the submucosal vessels. On the whole, vascularization of the colonic wall was markedly increased. Numerous measurements revealed that vessels in the diseased area were larger in diameter than those in normal segments of the colon.

In one of our own cases (Fig. 176) we compared preoperative mesenteric angiography findings, a surgical specimen injected with contrast material, and the untreated specimen. Whereas the distally situated small-bowel vessels in this case of ulcerative ileocolitis with pseudopolyposis were fully extended and showed no caliber variations, the vessels in the diseased portions were dilated and kinked with irregular accumulations of contrast medium in the pseudopolyps.

Venous return was more rapid than in the normal areas.

It can thus be shown that angiography may be used to assess the true extent of a process in ulcerative colitis; it can also help to rule out a primary vascular lesion as the cause of the disease. Still, the value of angiography for the clinical diagnosis of ulcerative colitis is quite limited.

7.6.4 Circulatory Disturbances and Ischemic Colitis

Circulatory disturbances are less frequent in the colon than in the small intestine. So far, only a very few authors have dealt with the diagnosis and pathogenesis of these disturbances in the radiological literature.

A case history recorded in our Department and published by VOLLMAR (1967) in his monograph may be called a "classic": Segmental sigmoid stenosis after operative ligation of the inferior mesenteric artery as part of a bifurcation bypass.

Doubtless, such cases, also of a non-iatrogenic nature, arise more frequently but fail to be diagnosed. In 1966, FARMAN reported on a total of six cases in which occlusion or stenosis of the inferior mesenteric artery or peripheral embolization or thrombosis had resulted in a syndrome of which the main symptom was diarrhea with mucous and bloody stools without any detectable causative factor. According to the authors, the possibility of a vascular cause should be considered if vascular surgery has been performed, or if there are signs of severe, generalized arteriosclerosis.

A barium enema disclosed either fairly long "narrow segments" or—as a reflection of discrete mucosal swelling—fingerprint-like impressions when the colon was distended.

Among (YOUNG et al.'s 1962) 800 patients, eight showed signs of colonic insufficiency after surgery on the abdominal aorta. MARSTON (1964), SHANNON (1962), SHANAHAN and STEDMAN (1962), and HANNAN et al. (1964) reported on thrombosis of the inferior mesenteric artery associated with aneurysm of the abdominal aorta, while YATES and CLAUSEN (1960) have described ulcers of the colon, and SCHWARTZ et al. (1964) pseudotumors related to disturbances in colonic circulation.

Low perfusion state by decreased cardiac output or occlusive vascular disease in which the collateral circulation is not adequate to maintain complete bowel wall integrity may cause *ischemic colitis*. The decreased blood flow causes mucosal devitalization with resulting bacterial invasion and an inflammatory response with granulation tissue. Mucosal edema and hemorrhage, which may be prominent, are seen as "thumbprinting" at barium enema. If the arterial blood flow is restored before the muscle layers are damaged, the bowel wall generally heals completely; however, with more severe damage, fibrosis and stricture occur. If blood flow is not restored, necrosis, perforation and death ensue.

Angiographic findings after the onset of symptoms are usually normal unless a vascular occlusion is present. As the inflammatory process progresses, dilated arteries, prominent parenchymal contrast medium accumulation and dense early venous drainage appear. With healing, the angiogram returns to normal unless fibrosis has been significant, in which case the vascularity to the involved segment may be diminished.

The nonspecificity of the angiographic changes in ischemic colitis does not allow differentiation of the disease from ulcerative colitis, which it may also resemble both clinically and histologically (REUTER and REDMAN, 1972).

8 Mesentery and Omentum

8.1 Anatomy and Clinical Significance

Following the discussion of pathological changes in the great vessel trunks and the viscera, it is appropriate to inquire about the value of angiography for mesentery and omentum. These are peritoneal folds through which the major vascular trunks course towards the organs they supply.

Along their course they may be displaced or constricted by space-occupying masses which, for example, as mesenteric sarcomas, can originate in one of these mesenteric leaves. Since experience has shown that the incidence of these tumors is extremely low, the diagnosis is rarely made preoperatively.

In differential diagnosis it is most important—and often decisive for the patient—to distinguish a primary malignant tumor from an inflammatory "omental" tumor of the type occasionally discovered as a palpable and usually very tender mass after an operation.

8.2 Vasculature

The most important vessel supplying the mesentery is the superior mesenteric artery; by contrast, the territory of the inferior mesenteric artery is relatively small since it supplies only the mesentery leading to the left colon. In the lesser omentum, between the lesser curvature of the stomach and the liver, both the left and the right gastric artery and the vessels of the porta hepatis may be compromised by pathological changes in this region.

Blood is supplied to the greater omentum through the right gastroepiploic artery and, to a lesser extent, through the left gastroepiploic artery. These two arteries give rise to the omental arteries which run a straight caudal course and quickly taper so that their lateral ramifications can seldom be differentiated.

An arcade is usually observed between the two gastroepiploic arteries at the level of the greater curvature; the contrast medium usually reaches this arcade first from the right side rather than from the left gastroepiploic artery.

The presence of a few, filiform omental branches is a normal feature of the omental vasculature. Opacification of thick vascular trunks over 1 mm in diameter in addition to collaterals from the splenic artery indicates an abnormal condition (BENKÖ, 1971).

8.3 Angiographic Pathomorphology

Space-occupying processes are the only pathological changes within the mesentery and the omentum that are of clinical importance. Inflammatory processes such as SCHLOFFER'S tumor as well as discrete abscesses are associated with large-caliber afferent vessels, usually in a reticular arrangement, with obstructions or arteriovenous shunts.

In accordance with the criteria applied in tumor angiography, malignant tumors, particularly sarcomas, are distinguished by neovascularity, usually displaying corkscrew-shaped shoots. The tumor is often "stained", but here again angiography cannot anticipate the histological findings.

In four surgically detected cases of generalized peritoneal carcinosis, with its predominantly small-nodule metastases, we found no angiographic evidence—even retrospectively—of the existence of these lesions.

The case illustrated in Fig. 174 is an exception. A conventional x-ray of the gastrointestinal tract disclosed multiple, irregular impression defects that suggested peritoneal carcinosis associated with an unidentified primary tumor.

A tuberculous abscess in the anterior abdominal wall can also be detected by mesenteric angiography. The lateral view shows a central lucency with opaque soft tissue and a slight inflammatory marginal reaction, providing—together with an outwardly visible localized erythema without appreciable hyperthermia—presumptive evidence of a tuberculous abscess.

Thus, the value of an angiographic examination in the rare diseases of the mesentery and omentum is rather limited although in individual cases, e.g. by demonstration of a well-opacified tumor, both the origin and the extent of such growths may be established preoperatively (Figs. 174–177).

9 Retroperitoneal Space

9.1 Anatomy

The retroperitoneal space contains several organs the anterior aspects of which can come into contact with the parietal peritoneum: the kidneys, adrenal glands, ureter, the great vascular trunks, and the sympathetic trunk.

The retroperitoneal space is bounded ventrally by the posterior wall of the peritoneal sac, dorsally by the musculature of the back, cranially by the diaphragm, and caudally, on both sides, by the inguinal ligament (HAFFERL and THIELE, 1969).

9.2 Vasculature

Blood is supplied through the lumbar arteries. They have a relatively narrow lumen and, compared with the organ arteries, they have to supply a relatively extensive area. There are collaterals between neighboring lumbar arteries but under normal conditions they are as a rule not angiographically visible. The great vessel trunks themselves—above all, the abdominal aorta—and their course have been described in the introductory chapter on topographic anatomy.

Venous return takes place through the lumbar veins which run parallel to the arteries. These veins open into the inferior vena cava and communicate with one another via a longitudinal anastomosis. This is called the ascending lumbar vein, it communicates caudally with the common iliac vein, and continues craniad into the azygos and hemiazygos vein, which ends in the superior vena cava.

The lymphatic vessels and their lymph nodes are of special radiologic interest in the retroperitoneal space. The efferent lymph vessels from the lower extremities, the pelvis, the peritoneal cavity, and the abdominal wall come together at this point. Three larger lymph vessel trunks, the intestinal trunk and the right and left lumbar trunks, arise from the retroperitoneal lymph vessels near the aortic hiatus and unite behind the aorta to form the thoracic duct.

9.3 Conventional Radiography

Abdominal radiography without contrast medium and excretory urography are indispensable for the diagnosis of diseases in the retroperitoneal space inasmuch as the kidneys, adrenals, and ureters as well as the urinary bladder, which are all situated retroperitoneally, are usually affected by pathological changes at a rather early stage. Radiography in two planes permits localization of calcifications in the retroperitoneal space. They may be diagnostically differentiated as neurogenic, notably sympathicogenic tumors, but also as calcified abscesses, hematomas, and as calcium deposits in the vasculature.

Opacification of the urinary tract can make it possible not only to localize but also, on occasion, to define the nature of a process by visualizing displacements, impressions, and areas of destruction.

Tomography, possibly combined with excretory urography (nephrotomogram), can be very informative.

Pneumoretroperitoneum has lost much of its importance since the distribution of air in the retroperitoneal space is dependent on an extraordinarily large number of factors and cannot be reliably regulated. It often gives rise to false interpretations, so that its use has been limited to very few indications, particularly after angiography began to be routinely employed. We have not diagnosed a single case of pheochromocytoma, for example, by means of pneumoperitoneum in the last ten years; we always used angiography.

9.4 Angiographic Technique

Diagnostic significance. We have dealt with the retroperitoneal space in this book only to the extent that it has a bearing on differential diagnosis of tumors of undetermined origin; such tumors are not infrequently palpable from the retroperitoneal space and the radiologic changes they induce in adjacent organs may also make it appear that they are of intraperitoneal origin. Therefore, in the present context only neoplastic changes in the retroperitoneal space will be considered. It should be noted that despite technical excellence aortograms may be extremely difficult and at times impossible to interpret in the search for a tumor in the retroperitoneal region.

Technique. Angiographic examination of the retroperitoneal space is best carried out by flush aortography, in particular, translumbar aortography or cathether aortography (BÜCHELER et al., 1965).

The inferior vena cava can be clearly visualized by simultaneous puncture of both femoral veins at the level of the inguinal ligament or by catheterization of a single iliac vein followed by injection of contrast material (FUCHS, 1961; DÜX et al., 1967).

9.5 Angiographic Pathomorphology

Blood is supplied to retroperitoneal tumors through the small-lumen lumbar arteries and, in the pelvis, from the branches of the internal iliac artery. For this reason, only sparse and small-caliber arterial tumor vessels and merely moderate opacification are generally visible in the capillary phase. In contrast to the diagnosis of tumors in organs, the angiographic differentiation between benign and malignant tumors in the retroperitoneal space is possible only to a very limited extent, especially in the case of large and necrotic tumors (BÜCHELER et al., 1967) (Figs. 177–182). Moreover, because of the scanty vascularization tumor necroses can develop relatively rapidly. Mistaken aortographic diagnoses of a benign tumor, retroperitoneal abscess, or hematoma are consequently possible. Another uncertainty factor is introduced by overshadowing of the smaller visceral arteries and the intrarenal ramification. Nevertheless, it is usually not possible to dispense with a survey aortogram, for while some authors consider selective arteriography of lumbar branches completely harmless, others view it as the cause of grave transverse myelitis and paralysis (see p. 24).

Conclusions regarding the origin of retroperitoneally situated tumors can be drawn only with considerable reservations. Cavography and lymphangiography can be very useful in this respect (VON KEISER and MÜLLER, 1963; LINDBOM, 1964). This combined technique is becoming increasingly important for presurgical evaluation (Fig. 178). With the wider range of operations now available, tumors once regarded as inoperable on account of venous changes or caval infiltrations are now fully operable in some cases or can at least be partially resected.

It is of course a necessary precondition that the opening of the renal veins is free of thrombotic or tumorous alterations so that the patency of the collateral communications between the pelvic veins and the retroperitoneal venous system is assured.

Lymphangiography is, as the method of choice, necessary for the diagnostic evaluation of lymph node enlargements in the investigation of retroperitoneal tumors. When a generalized disease of the lymph nodes is suspected, it takes precedence over aortography and cavography. Cavography is superior to lymphangiography only if the lymphatic channels are completely blocked.

VI Frequency of Use and Diagnostic Value of Abdominal Angiography

The diagnostic significance of abdominal angiography is not difficult to document in the individual case. The range and diversity of the indications described in the preceding chapters, however, are ample testimony that the roentgenologic visualization of the vascular system represents a new and important diagnostic technique in the clinical management of abdominal illnesses.

Yet neither the rare syndrome successfully diagnosed by angiography nor the sizable number of examinations on which the present book is based should make us lose sight of the fact that angiography is just *one* of many possible, proven methods of disease detection.

We therefore think it fitting to present in this final chapter the quantitative data that have supported our remarks.

During the ten-year period between 1961 and 1971, 7091 angiographies were performed in our Department, to which must be added 4000–5000 cerebral angiographies, which are beyond the scope of this book.

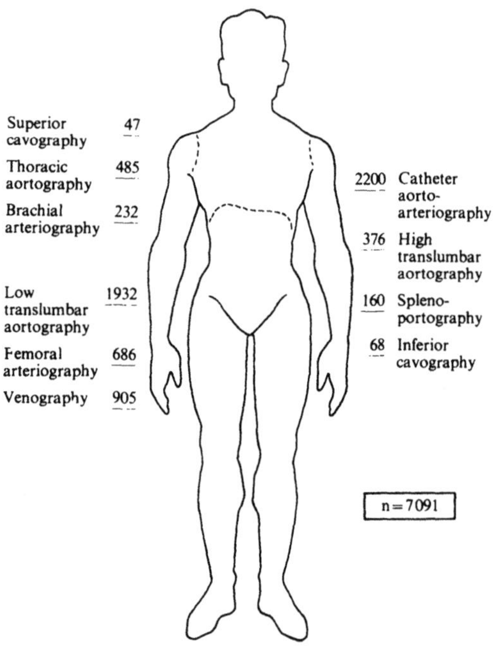

Angiographic techniques in 7091 examinations

Abdominal angiography (1961–1971)

Techniques	
Catheter aortography	786
Translumbar aortography (subdiaphragmatic)	376
Celiac artery and branches	572
Superior and inferior mesenteric arteries	411
Renal arteries	431
Splenoportography	160
Inferior vena cava and branches	68
Total	2804

Leaving out translumbar aortographies, splenoportographies, and cavographies, we are left with *2200 catheter examinations in a total of 1950 patients*. The age distribution shows a distinct peak during the sixth decade of life. Over half of the patients examined were between the ages of 40 and 69. The youngest catheter patient was less than one year old; angiographies of the umbilical vessels are not included in the present list. Our oldest patient, a 94-year-old Ukrainian in an enviable state of general health, had an aneurysm of the abdominal aorta.

Considerably more men than women were examined angiographically. The ratio of 64% men to 36% women was no doubt at least partially attributable to the higher incidence of degenerative vascular diseases in men.

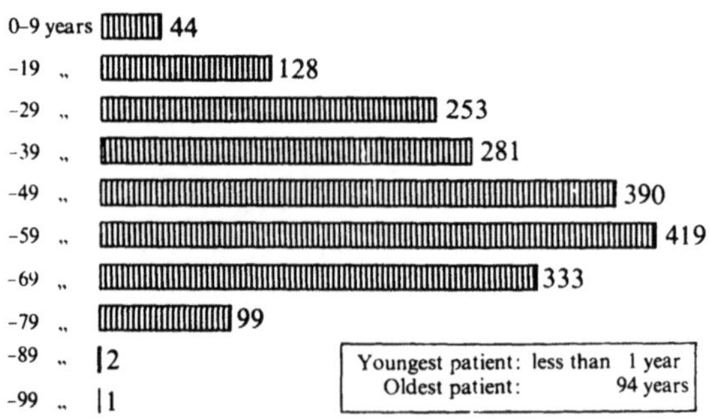

Age distribution in 2200 catheter angiographies

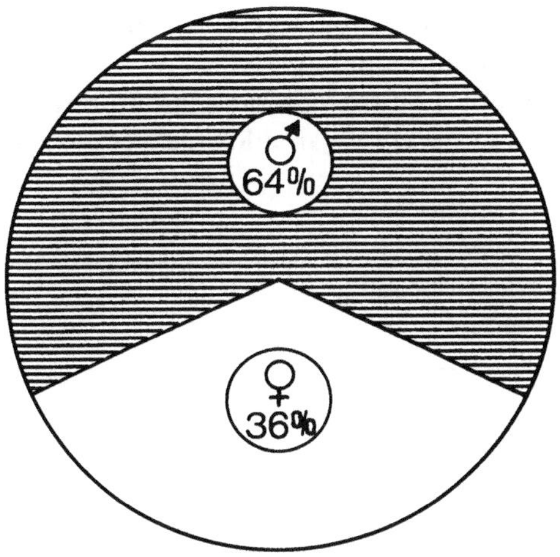

Sex distribution of 2200 angiographed patients

The preceding tables provide information on frequency of use, indications, and diagnostic yield of the individual investigative techniques.

A critical note is in order about the first table. Selective arteriography was not infrequently preceded by catheter aortography, especially when the organ in which the suspected lesion was localized was not known, or when disturbances in visceral circulation were involved. During the first few years of our angiographic activity we made more frequent use of aortography, but now we rely more and more on selective and superselective techniques. Forty-seven patients could not be examined on account of kinking, stenosis, or occlusion of the iliac arteries. They were subjected to translumbar aortography instead.

The surprisingly large number of kidney disease cases among the indications for translumbar aortography all go back to the first few years. At present the method of choice is selective renal arteriography.

A major portion of the direct aortographies involved obliterating vascular processes

Abdominal catheter aortography (n = 786)

Indication	Total	Confirmed	Ruled out	False		?
				+	–	
Gastrointestinal						
hemorrhage	8	–	–	–	8	–
tumor	18	6	6	–	4	2
inflammation	3	–	–	–	–	3
Liver						
tumor	16	5	4	–	7	–
echinococcosis	1	–	–	–	–	1
rupture	2	–	–	–	–	2
Spleen						
tumor	2	2	–	–	–	–
rupture	15	3	8	–	–	4
Pancreas						
inflammation	6	2	–	–	3	1
neoplasm	26	5	13	–	3	5
cyst	7	4	–	–	1	2
Adrenal glands						
hyperplasia	15	–	5	–	5	5
neoplasm	3	2	–	–	1	–
pheochromocytoma	24	16	7	1	–	–
Retroperitoneal tumor	56	30	14	–	–	12
Occlusion of portal vein	3	–	–	–	–	3
Arterial occlusion, stenosis	64	30	32	–	–	2
Rupture or diaphragmatic hernia	3	3	–	–	–	–
Diaphragmatic tumor	1	1	–	–	–	–
Total	273	109	89	1	32	42
Kidney diseases	431					
Data missing	35					
Catheter aortography technically not feasible	47	(Stenosis of aorta or pelvic artery followed immediately by direct aortic puncture)				
n	786					

and—in a hospital where much vascular surgery is performed—the postoperative results of vascular reconstruction. Less common indications are retroperitoneal lesions when access via the femoral arteries is blocked and vascular surgery is contemplated.

The tables on mesenteric angiography and celiac angiography should be considered

Translumbar, subdiaphragmatic aortography (n = 376)

Indication	Total	Confirmed surgically	Ruled out	False		?
				+	–	
Kidney diseases	127					
Postoperative bypass control	71	71	–	–	–	–
Aortic aneurysm	37	33	4	–	–	–
Aortic occlusion or stenosis	38	36	2	–	–	–
Occlusion or stenosis of visceral arteries	34	19	15	–	–	–
Aortocaval fistula	1	1	–	–	–	–
Retroperitoneal tumor	5	2	2	–	–	1
Pheochromocytoma	6	2	3	–	–	1
Pancreatic neoplasm	6	–	–	–	–	2
Pancreatitis	4	–	4	–	–	–
Total	329					
Data missing	45					
Angiography not practicable	2	(anesthetic problems)				
n	376					

Angiography of celiac trunk and its branches (n = 572)

Indication	Total	Confirmed	Ruled out	False		?
				+	–	
Pancreatitis	40	26	1	2	7	4
Pancreatic neoplasm	133	30	86	2	5	10
Islet cell tumor	15	5	5	–	1	4
Pancreatic cyst	24	15	7	–	1	1
Pancreatic trauma	2	2	–	–	–	–
Splenic tumor, enlargement	24	22	2	–	–	–
Splenic cyst	10	6	1	–	2	1
Splenic rupture	59	13	43	2	1	–
Liver abscess	2	1	1	–	–	–
Subphrenic abscess	4	3	1	–	–	–
Liver rupture	21	4	12	–	4	1
Liver echinococcosis	7	5	2	–	–	–
Liver tumor and metastases	44	16	26	1	–	1
Liver tumor due to Thorotrast	4	2	1	1	–	–
Gallbladder tumor	3	2	–	–	1	–
Gastric tumor	6	1	3	–	2	–
Peritoneal carcinosis	5	1	–	–	4	–
Diaphragmatic rupture	3	1	1	–	1	–
Gastrointestinal hemorrhage	36	16	–	–	16	4
Occlusion of portal or splenic vein	62	18	39	1	2	2
Splenic aneurysm	2	2	–	–	–	–
Arterioportal fistula	2	2	–	–	–	–
Occlusion of visceral vessels, or stenosis	32	20	11	–	–	1
Total	540	213	242	9	47	29
Data missing	24					
Angiography impracticable	8					
n	5/2					

Angiography of superior and inferior mesenteric artery (n = 411)

Indication	Total	Surgically confirmed	Ruled out	False +	False –	?
Liver tumor	26	8	17	–		1
Liver echinococcosis	2	1	1	–	–	–
Gallbladder tumor	2	1	1	–	–	
Pancreatitis	40	32	1	–	4	3
Pancreatic cyst	17	12	3	–	1	1
Pancreatic neoplasm	118	23	81	1	5	8
Islet cell tumor	11	1	4	–	3	3
Small-intestine tumor	10	6	2	–	1	1
Large-intestine tumor	15	10	4	–	1	–
Arteriomesenteric compression	4	4	–	–	–	–
Arteriovenous malformation	1	1	–	–	–	–
Abdominal abscess	1	1	–	–	–	–
Peritoneal carcinosis	7	1	3	–	–	3
Mesenteric tumor	8	5	2	–	–	1
Gastrointestinal hemorrhage	29	11	–	–	14	4
Occlusion or stenosis of portal vein	31	13	15	–	1	2
Arterial occlusion or stenosis	45	21	23	–	–	1
Traumatic vascular changes	6	1	4	–	–	1
Total	373	152	161	1	30	29
Data missing	29					
Angiography not practicable	9					
n	411					

Splenoportography (n = 160)

Indication	Total	Confirmed	Ruled out	False +	False –	?
Occlusion of portal vein	115	23	88	–	–	4
Occlusion of splenic vein	16	11	3	–	–	2
Aneurysm of splenic vein	1	1	–	–	–	–
Budd-Chiari syndrome	3	3	–	–	–	–
Cruveilhier-Baumgarten syndrome	1	1	–	–	–	–
Liver carcinoma	1	1	–	–	–	–
Total	137	40	91	–	–	6
Technically unsuccessful	23 (14%)					
n	160					

Inferior cavography (n = 68)

Indication	Total	Confirmed	Ruled out	False +	False –	?
Obstruction, stenosis due to tumor	33	13	20	–	–	–
Thrombosis	34	9	25	–	–	
Total	67					
Failures	1					
n	68					

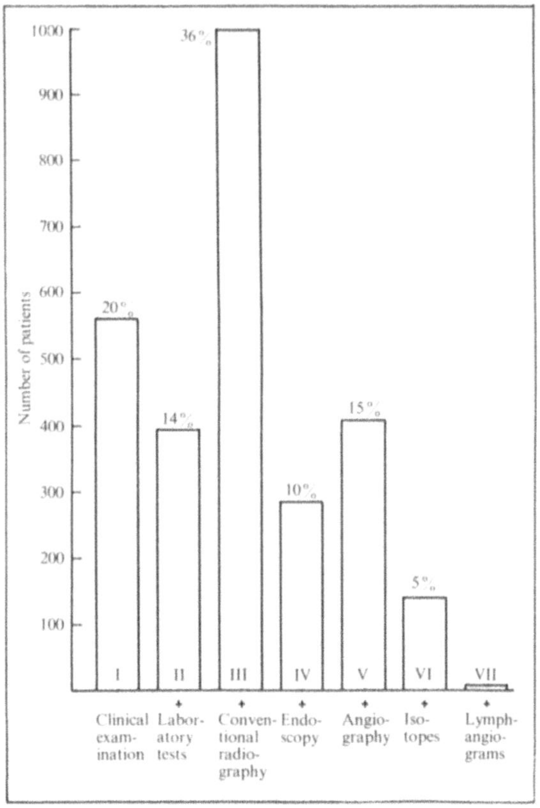

Frequency distribution of diagnostic procedures in 2784 patients

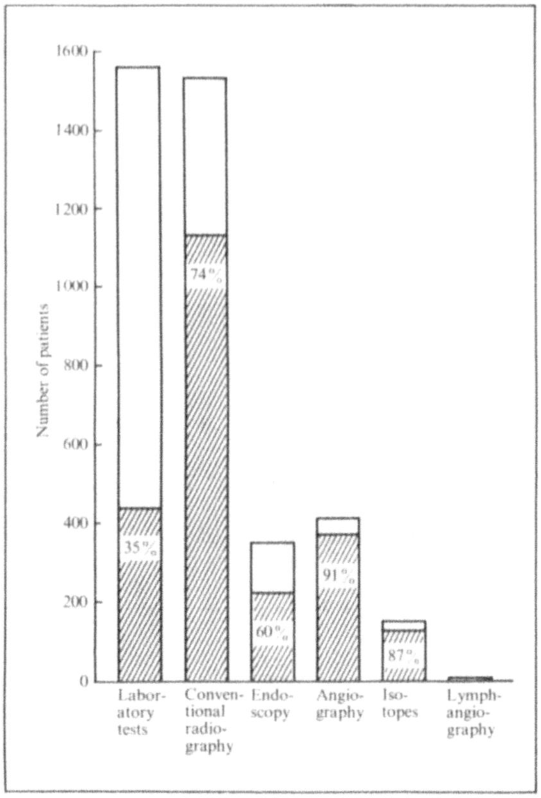

Frequency and productivity ratio of diagnostic procedures in 2784 patients

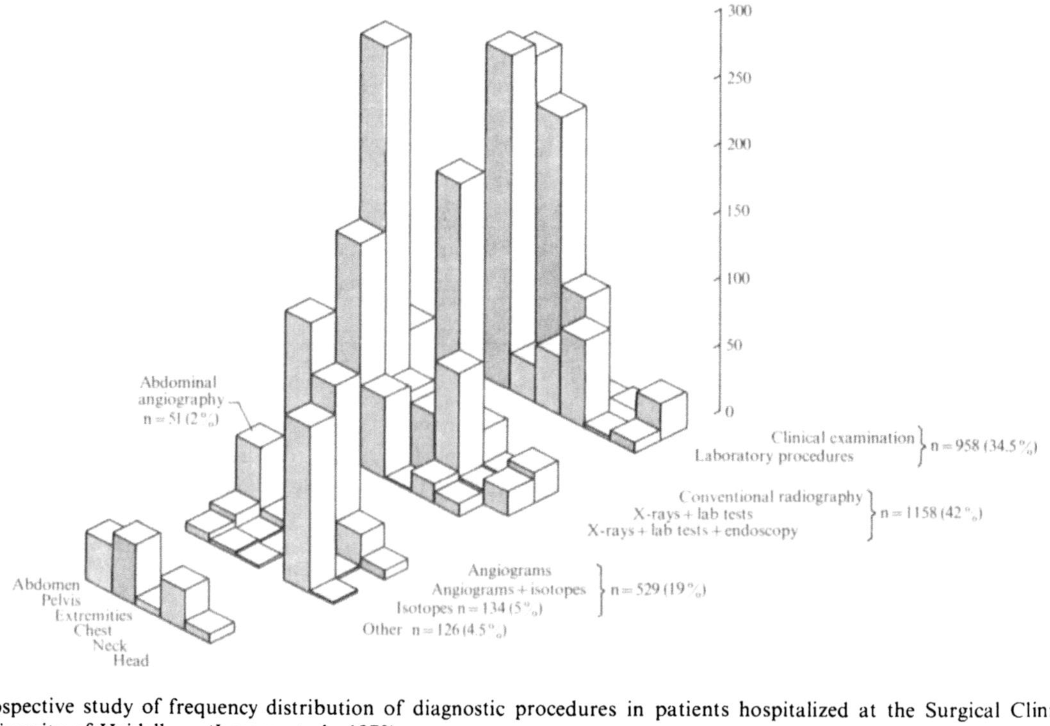

Prospective study of frequency distribution of diagnostic procedures in patients hospitalized at the Surgical Clinic, University of Heidelberg (LINDER et al., 1970)

together since both these vessels have to be visualized in a large number of cases. We should also mention diseases of the pancreas as well as localization of hemorrhages, tumor searches, etc.

Thus, searches for sources of bleeding by means of celiac angiography yielded positive findings in the gastroduodenal region, while the mesenteric route permitted localization in the duodenum and the large and small intestine. "Confirmed" in this case means that verification was obtained either by surgery or autopsy or on the basis of the clinical course. Diagnoses by exclusion were verified by surgery in some cases only. Some later positive findings are undoubtedly concealed in this group. This error was corrected in the statistical analysis following these tables, which presents significant samples.

In all patients who were referred to us for splenoportography, portal hypertension was either clinically confirmed or suspected. Angiographies were undertaken in all cases to determine whether the portal vein was patent and would permit surgical shunting if necessary. In two cases evidence of a functionally effective portocaval shunt was obtained by selective exploration of the inferior vena cava and the anastomosis. Quite often, we were able to localize the source of acute gastrointestinal hemorrhage by the positive demonstration of varicose collateral vessels in the cardia of the stomach and the esophagus.

To minimize the role of random subjective factors in our statistics and our assessment of the diagnostic value of different techniques, Linder et al. (1970) carried out a prospective study at the Surgical Clinic of the University of Heidelberg. Despite a high degree of specialization, the Clinic has a patient population recruited from the University Hospital and Municipal Hospital.

To aid in the understanding of this survey, the following brief sketch is offered to outline the diagnostic decision-making process (Linder et al., 1970).

After history-taking and clinical examination, a presumptive clinical diagnosis is made and further special diagnostic procedures are decided upon. Specifically, during a three-month period in 1969, a total of 40 different diagnostic procedures were carried out in 2784 consecutive inpatients. However, for our pre-

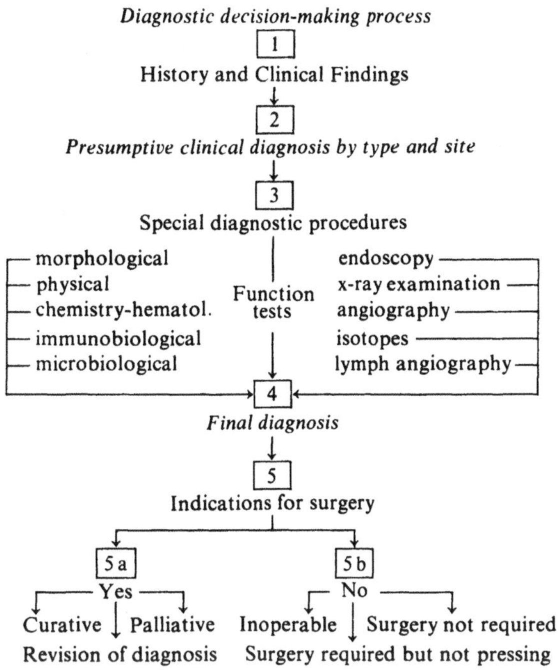

sent purposes, we will concern ourselves only with the roentgenological examinations.

Two-thirds of these 2784 surgical patients underwent conventional radiography. Angiographies accounted for 15% of the diagnostic procedures.

For a critical evaluation of individual diagnostic techniques, the survey was to determine not only the number of procedures employed but also specify those examinations which proved *decisive*.

A kind of "productivity index" was computed on the basis of the frequency of use and the information yield of the various techniques. We should stress that Department physicians and senior physicians were the only ones responsible for evaluating the individual procedures. Seventy-four percent of all x-ray studies provided *important information* for the final diagnosis; the corresponding figure for *angiography* was even higher, about 90%.

But looking at the details of this general picture, we find that the "Frequency Distribution of Diagnostic Procedures," which at first glance is quite bewildering, shows that the Surgical Department of Heidelberg University performed abdominal angiography in only 2% of the total population (51 patients).

Thus, it appears that abdominal angiography was rather infrequently employed as a method of investigation, especially since 1158 conventional x-ray studies with laboratory tests and endoscopies were carried out during the same period. It is precisely this fact, that abdominal angiography was so seldom employed, which makes the question of its effectiveness so interesting (WENZ et al., 1970) (cf. Table).

Angiographic finding	Disease		Total
	Positive	Negative	
Positive	35 (5)	4 (2)	39
Negative	4	8	12
Total	39 (5)	12 (2)	51 (12)

Specificity 0.67; sensitivity 0.90; error I: 0.10; error II: 0.33

Thus, prospective study of a mixed group of patients consisting of tumor, inflammation, and vascular occlusion cases shows that 51 abdominal angiographies yielded correct positive diagnoses 30 times and correct negative diagnoses 8 times. In seven cases the angiographic diagnosis was doubtful; two of the positive diagnoses proved false. Accordingly, the sensitivity amounted to 90%, which means that the probability of detecting an existing disease is relatively high.

Let us now further compare these figures with a larger set of data from a *retrospective analysis* of 2385 abdominal angiographies, 559 of which were done in patients who were examined for a suspected tumor. In 263 of these cases this diagnosis was histologically confirmed.

Angiographic finding	Disease		Total
	Positive	Negative	
Positive	186 (26)	20 (10)	206
Negative	30	27	57
Total	216 (26)	47 (10)	263 (36)

Specificity 0.57; sensitivity 0.86; error I: 0.14; error II: 0.43

Evaluation of the diagnostically verified cases shows that the sensitivity, i.e. the probability of a correct positive finding, is of the same order of magnitude as in the previously mentioned mixed group if the doubtful findings are again interpreted positively. With this stipulation, however, the specificity, that is, the degree of certainty that patients not having the disease will be excluded (error II = 0.43), is low.

Even when questionable findings are invariably given a negative interpretation, the risk of a false positive finding in abdominal tumors is 21%. It follows that visceral angiography is better suited for detecting a tumor when there is sufficient presumptive evidence of it. It is less effective, however, when the clinical evidence is less certain and subjects not having the disease are to be excluded or, in other words, when an abdominal tumor was suspected *in our own case material, we tended to attach an exaggerated importance to angiographic signs among the diagnostic criteria for tumors.*

The conclusions to be drawn from these figures for our own future case material are plain: Even more critical assessment of angiographic findings, even better correlation of angiographic pathomorphology with the evidence at hand, an even more thorough clinical workup on patients to be examined, and discriminating use of all the technical aids afforded us by superselective investigative techniques, pharmacoangiography, electronic picture analysis, and whatever else the future may bring.

We have deliberately chosen abdominal tumors with the problems they so often present in preoperative diagnosis for our critical, statistical evaluation in order also to point out the weaknesses of abdominal angiography and the margin of error to which our analysis of angiograms was subject.

Finally, it should not be forgotten that size and numbers do not necessarily mean quality! The peculiarities of the pathomorphological development of a process, especially its vascularization, extent, and topography, are by and large decisive in determining the "measure" of its angiographic demonstrability. It should be clear, then, that no global appraisal of the diagnostic value of angiography is possible. Knowledge of the capabilities of a diagnostic method is a prerequisite for its intelligent clinical use and evaluation, and this in turn is the only assurance of the continued success of angiography.

VII Plates (Figures 1–183)

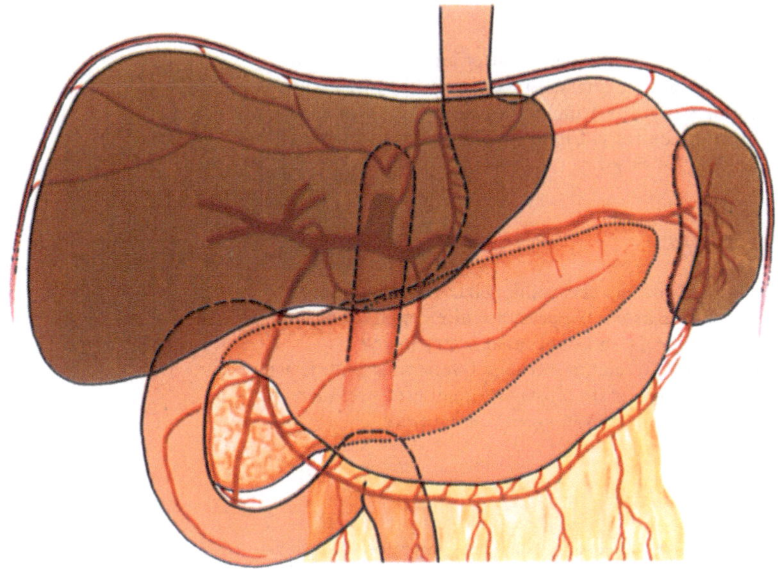

Fig. 1. Distribution of celiac trunk

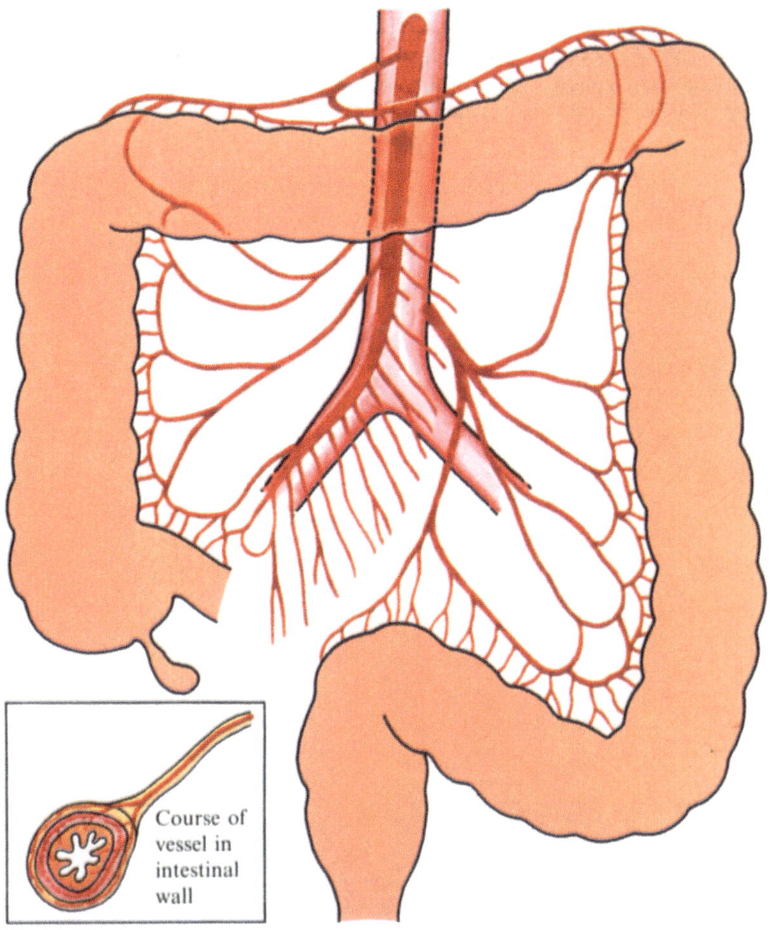

Fig. 2. Distribution of superior mesenteric and inferior mesenteric arteries

Above left and right

Fig. 3a and b. (a) Stenosis at origin of celiac trunk and left gastric artery. Branches of celiac trunk in red. Color x-ray. (b) Annular stenosis of trunk of superior mesenteric artery. Clinical manifestation: intestinal angina. Color x-ray

Center left

Fig. 4. Two-tiers occlusion: celiac trunk and superior mesenteric artery. Appearance after removal of left kidney. Aorta and right renal artery in red. Collateral circulation through inferior mesenteric artery and Riolan's anastomosis into region of occluded abdominal arteries in green. Color x-ray

Center right

Fig. 5. Arteriosclerotic stenosis of superior mesenteric artery. Autopsy specimen (Dr. K. GOERTTLER)

Below left and right

Fig. 6a and b. High, iatrogenic aortic occlusion after ligation of aorta for extirpation of a large tumor in the left kidney at age of 1 year. Six years later extensive network of collateral vessels between proximal aorta and iliac arteries. (a) Early arterial phase. (b) Late arterial phase. Picture of lumbar, vertebral, and spinal collateral vessels. Color x-ray

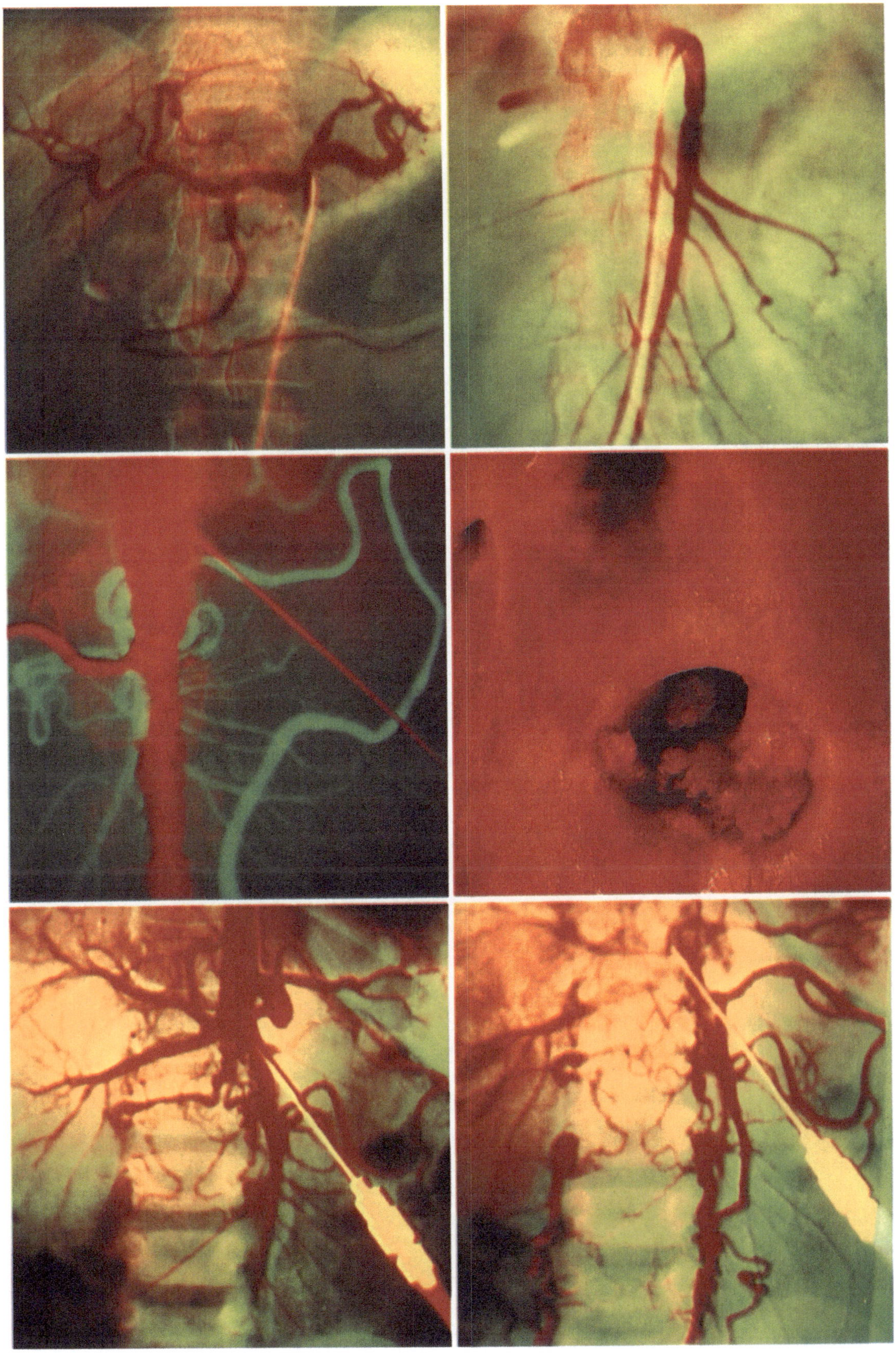

Above left and right, left center

Fig. 7a–c. Familial intestinal polyposis (PEUTZ-JEGHERS). (a) Typical pigmentation in father and daughter. (b) Severe gastrointestinal bleeding. Localization of origin of bleeding in father by selective angiography of superior mesenteric artery. Conspicuously wide afferent jejunal artery in red. Demarcation of richly vascularized tumor in small intestine by basket-weave arrangement of vessels with minute extravasations of contrast agent (arrow). Veins in green. Color x-ray. (c) Bleeding jejunal polyp. Operative photograph. (Dr. F. LINDER)

Right center

Fig. 8. Cecal adenocarcinoma. Tumor stained dark green against red-stained arteries. Afferent vessel: Ileocolic artery. Color x-ray

Below left and right

Fig. 9a and b. Traumatic renal infarct. (a) Detachement of caudal renal vessels with no visualization of parenchyma in lower half of kidney. Color x-ray. (b) Extensive infarct of caudal portion of kidney. Surgical specimen (Dr. L. RÖHL)

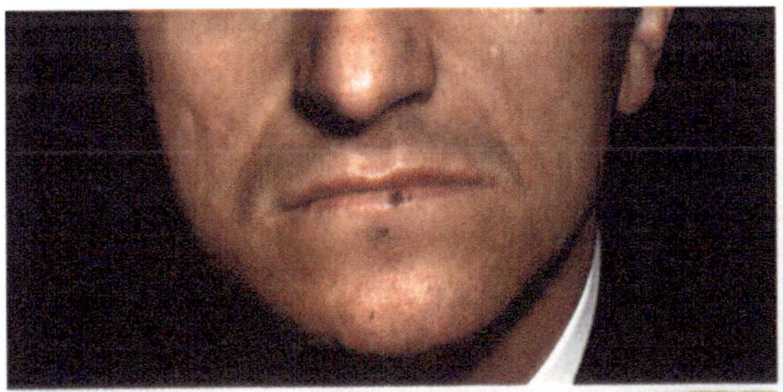

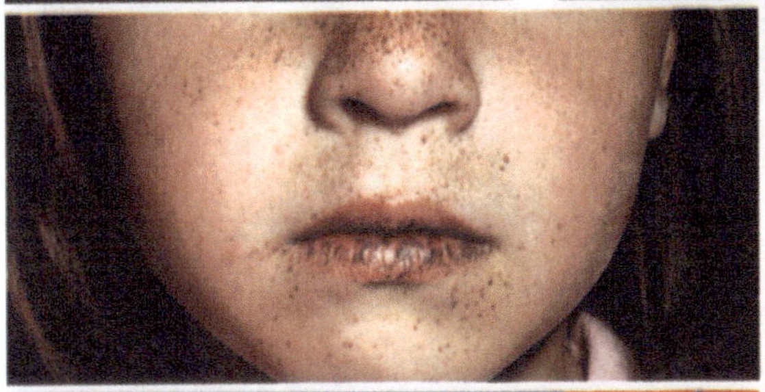

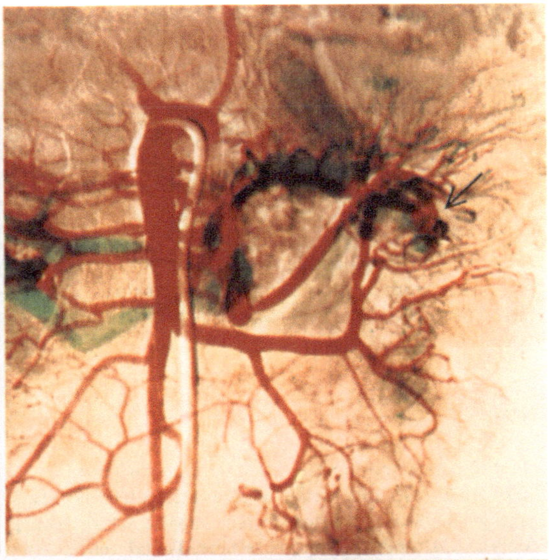

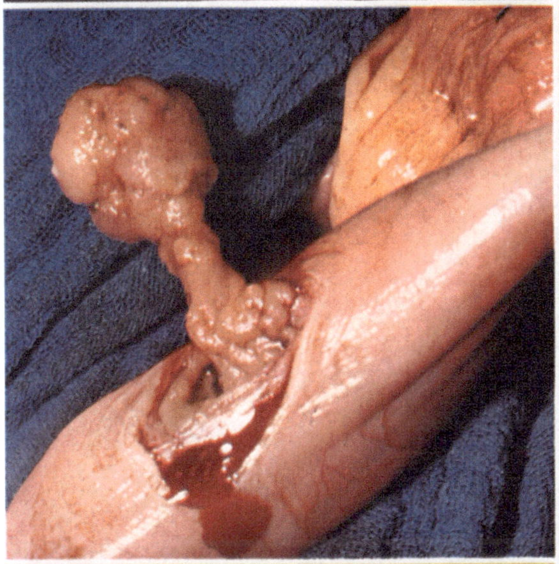

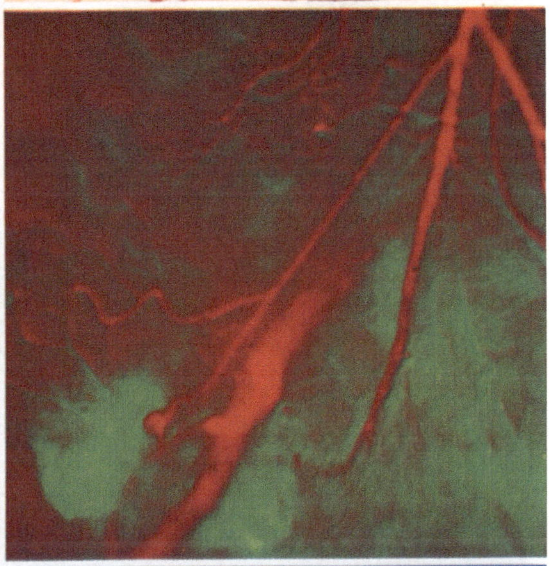

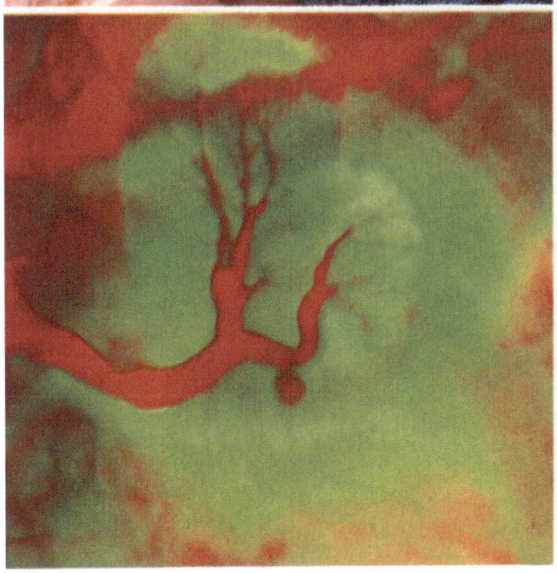

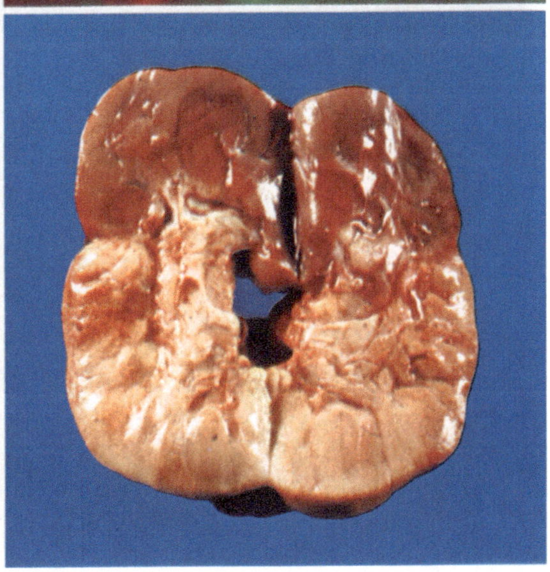

Above left

Fig. 10. Abdominal aortogram showing no pathological alterations. Aorta and its branches in red, venous outflow in green, kidneys in yellow. Color x-ray

Above right

Fig. 11. Aortocaval fistula. Nephrectomy 19 years previously with ligation of the entire pedicle. Aortic side red. Mixing phase blue. Inferior vena cava green. Color x-ray

Center left and right

Fig. 12. (a) Arterioportal fistula. Condition after Billroth II resection. Celiac angiogram: Splenic artery and gastroduodenal artery in red, hepatic artery visible only as a stump. Mixing phase blue. Portal vein light blue. Color x-ray. (b) Arterioportal fistula. Surgical specimen (Dr. J. VOLLMAR)

Below left and right

Fig. 13a and b. (a) Ruptured spleen. Simultaneous visualization of arteries (red) and splenic vein (blue). Extravasations of contrast medium in spleen parenchyma. Broken contour. Color x-ray.
(b) Extensive intra- and subcapsular hematomas in spleen. Surgical specimen

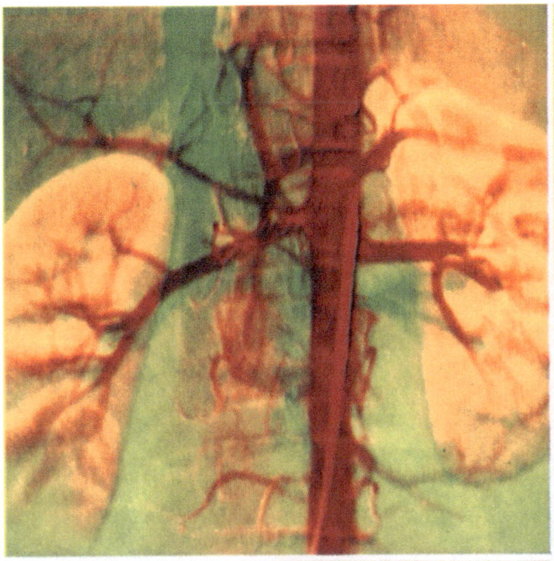
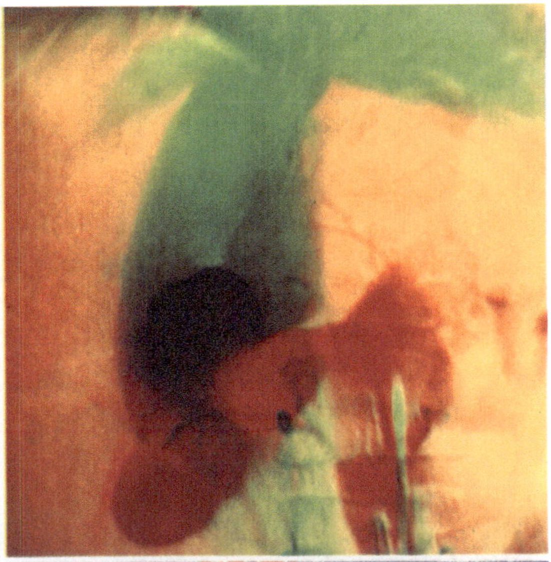
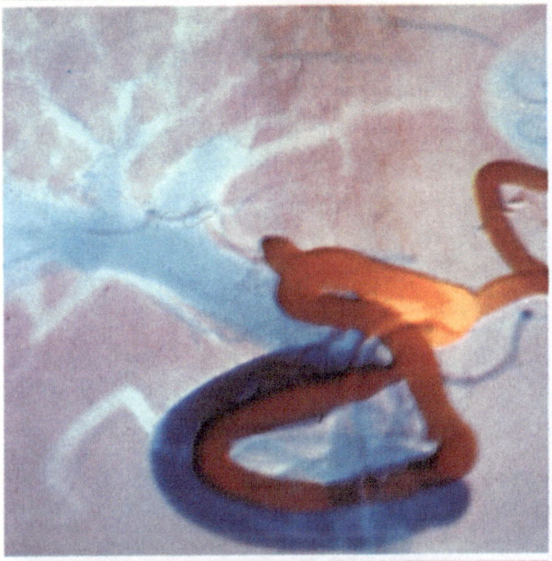
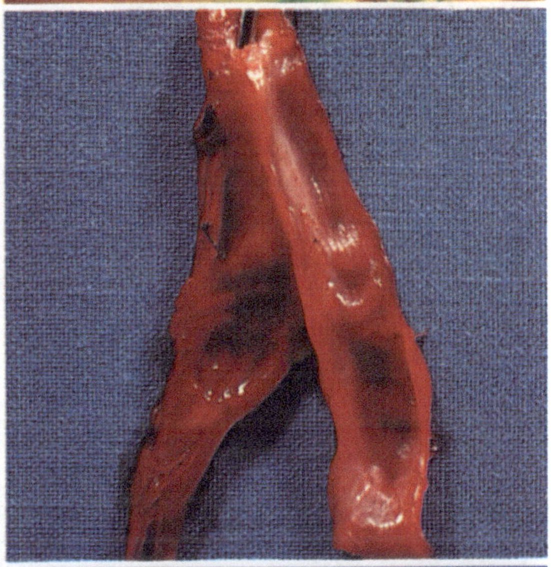
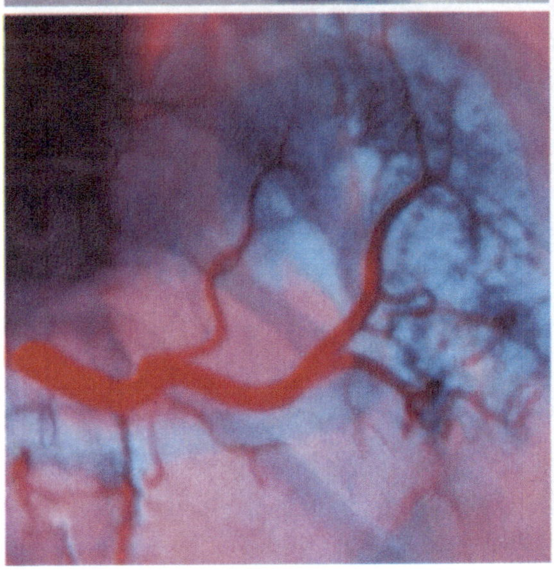
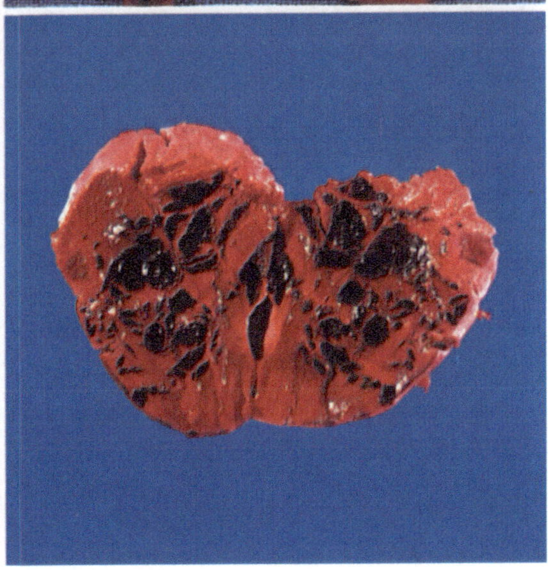

Above left

Fig. 14. Liver trauma. Hepatic artery in red. Liver blue. Right lobe of liver compressed laterally by large hematoma. Color x-ray

Above right, center left and right

Fig. 15a and b. (a) Malignant tumor in Thorotrast liver. Celiac angiogram: Arteries in red, liver in yellow, tumor in right lobe of liver green. Color x-ray. (b) Partial resection of liver. Surgical specimen (Dr. M. TREDE). Bile duct carcinoma with bleeding from tumor as morphological correlate of good angiographic tumor staining. Histological preparation (Dr. K. WEGENER)

Below left

Fig. 16. Portal vein thrombosis. Splenoportogram: Picture of conspicuously wide and tortuous collateral vessel from spleen to porta hepatis; the vessel stained in different colors in the three filling phases. Green – spleen; yellow – splenic veins; red – region of porta hepatis. Color x-ray

Below right

Fig. 17. Cirrhosis of liver. Splenoportogram: Bypass circulation through coronary veins of the stomach with esophageal varices. Color x-ray

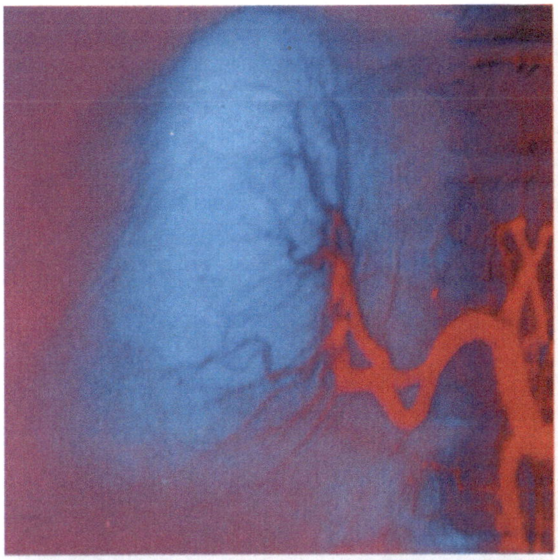

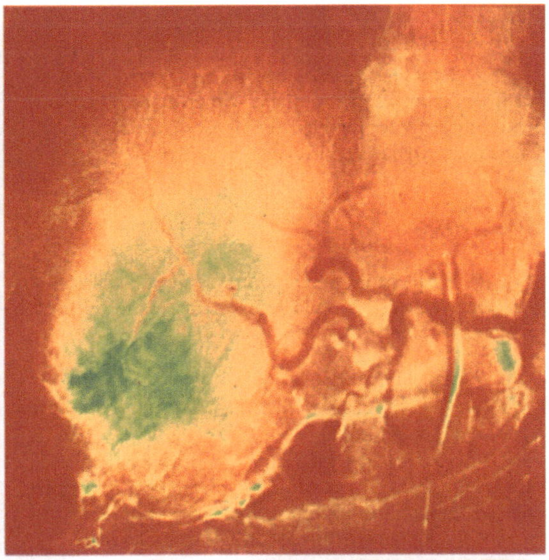

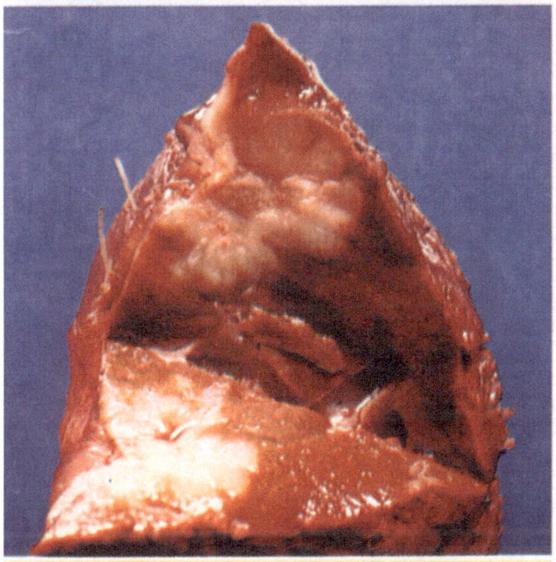

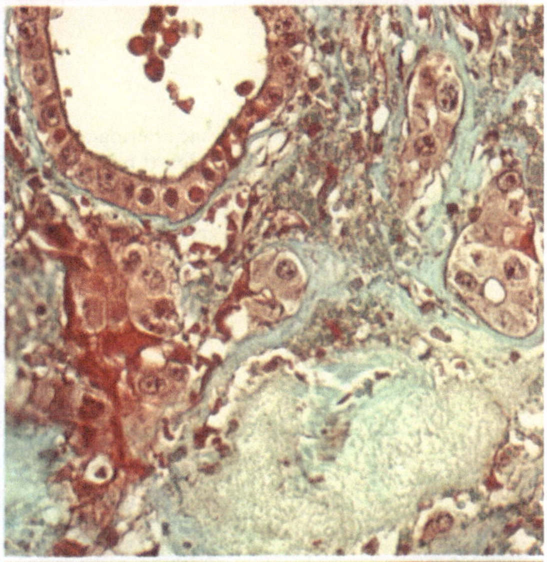

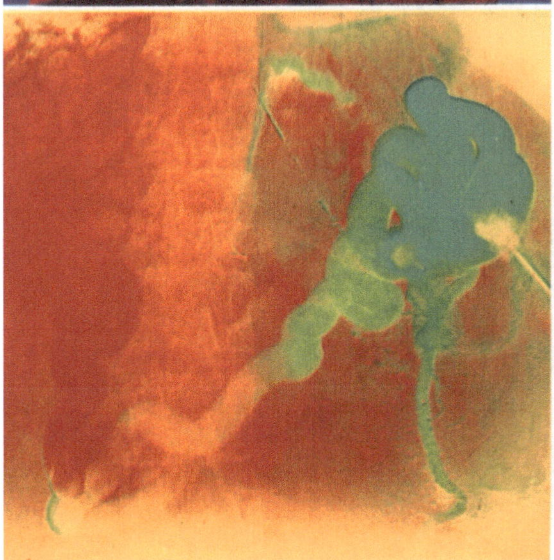

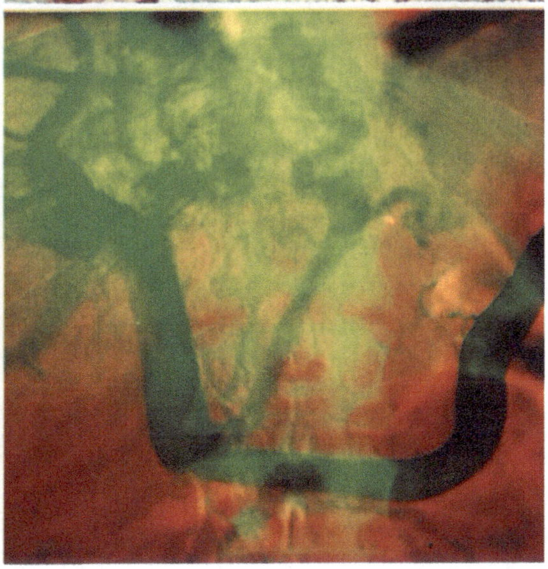

Above left

Fig. 18. Pancreas. Celiac angiogram: Opacification of celiac branches and staining of pancreas in blue. (Balloon catheter for bleeding of esophageal varices in cirrhosis of liver). Color x-ray

Above right

Fig. 19. Purulent inflammation of head of pancreas. Mesenteric arteriogram: Extensive abscess in head of pancreas stained green. Color x-ray

Center

Fig. 20a and b. (a) Cystic tumor in tail of pancreas. Celiac angiogram: Elevation of splenic vein and artery due to tumor (arteries red; veins, spleen and liver green). Color x-ray. (b) Cyst in tail of pancreas, surgical specimen (Dr. F. LINDER)

Below left and right

Fig. 21a and b. (a) Insulinoma. Celiac arteriogram: Opacification of hepatic artery and dorsal pancreatic artery (its origin an anomaly), circumscribed staining of tumor in body of pancreas in red. Color x-ray. (b) Insulinoma, surgical specimen (Dr. F. LINDER)

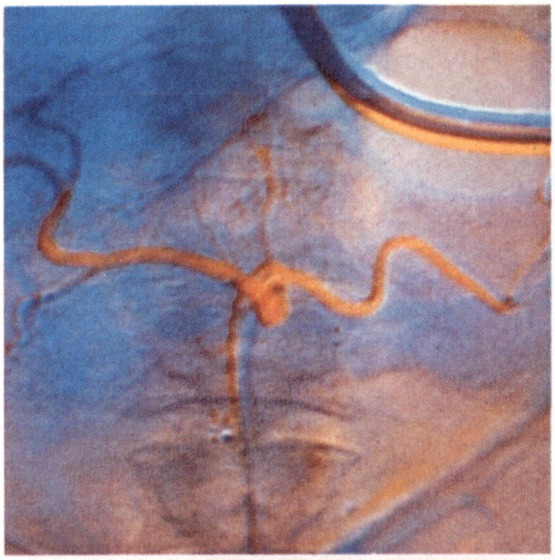

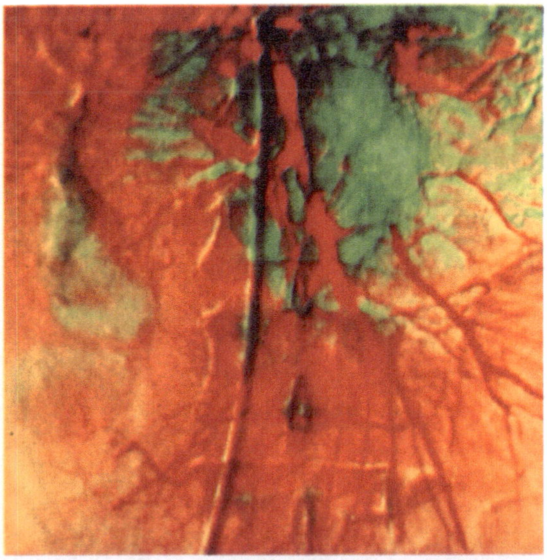

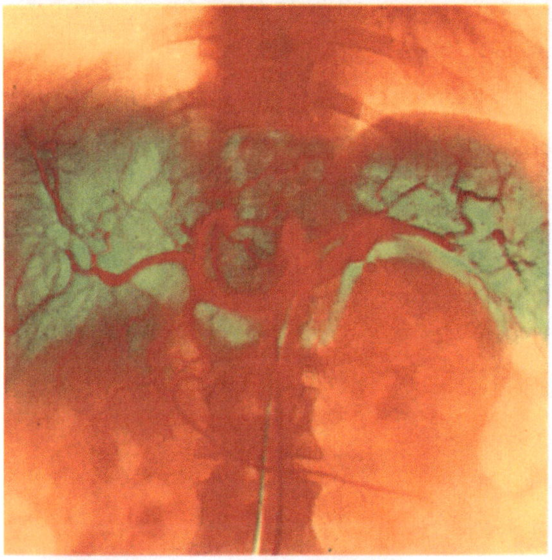

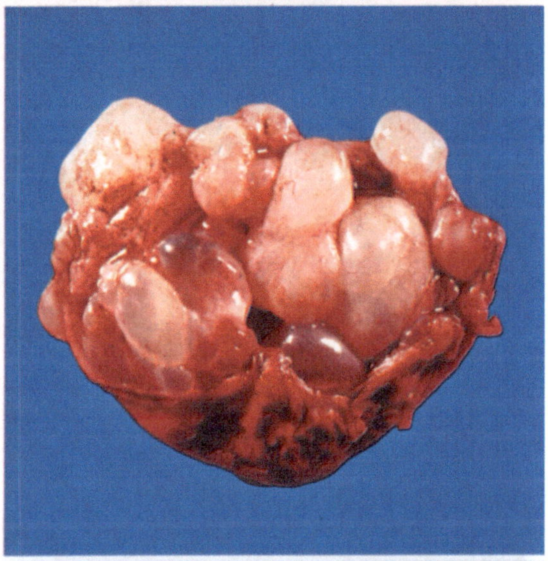

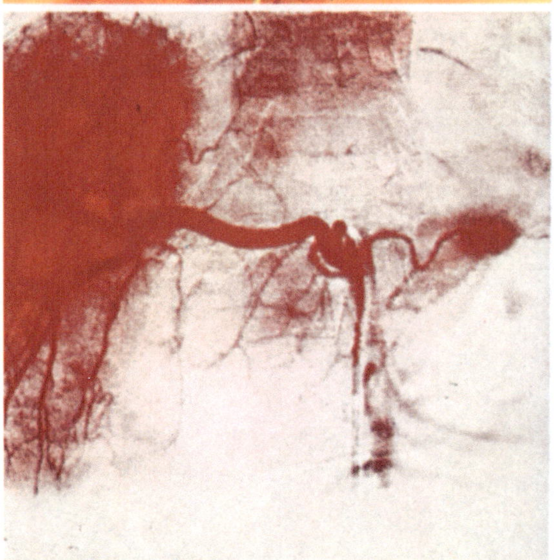

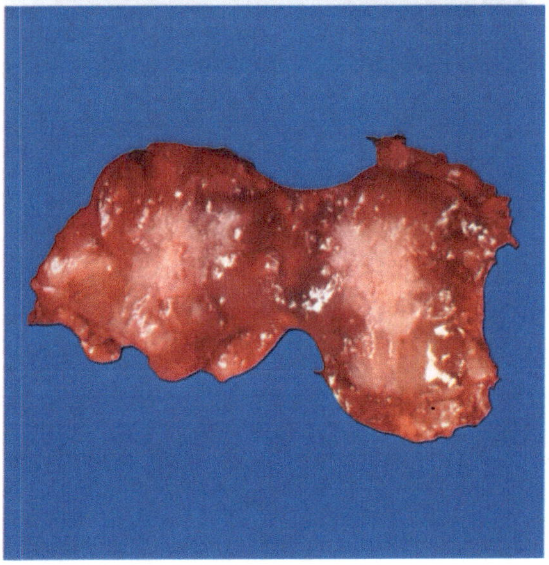

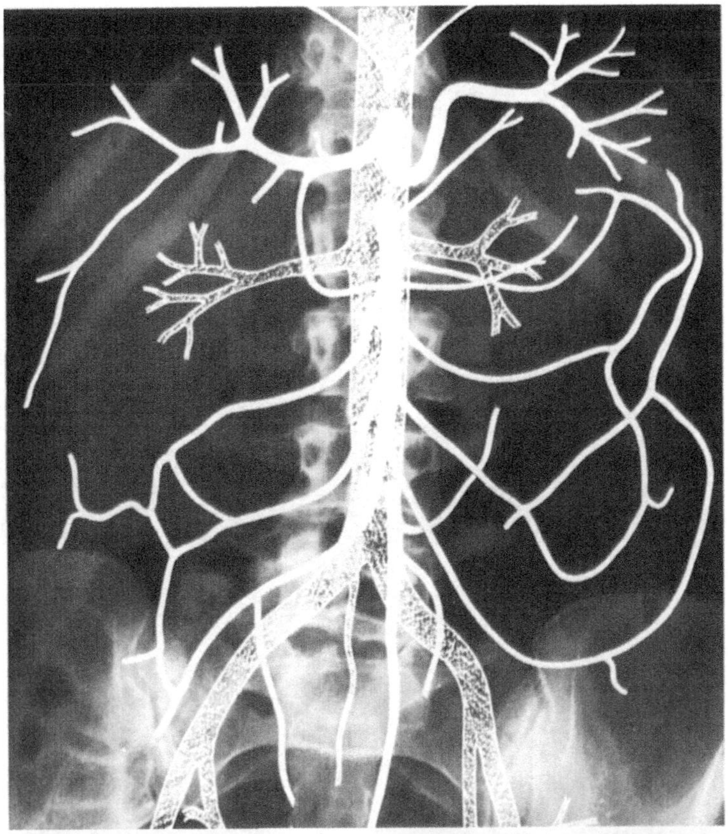

Fig. 22. Full abdominal x-ray with distribution of abdominal aorta and its branches

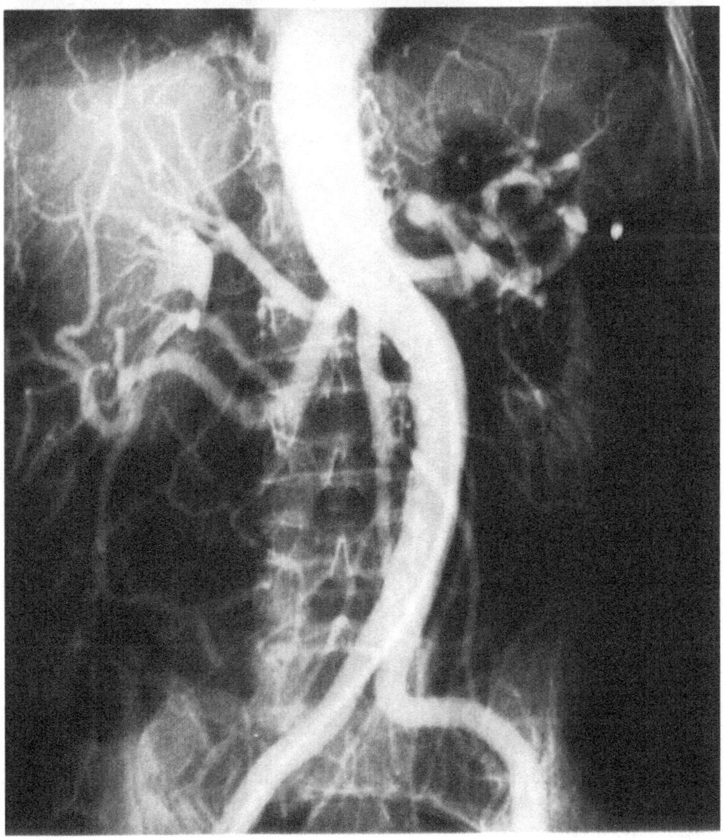

Fig. 23. Kinking of abdominal and iliac arteries secondary to arteriosclerosis. Catheter aortogram

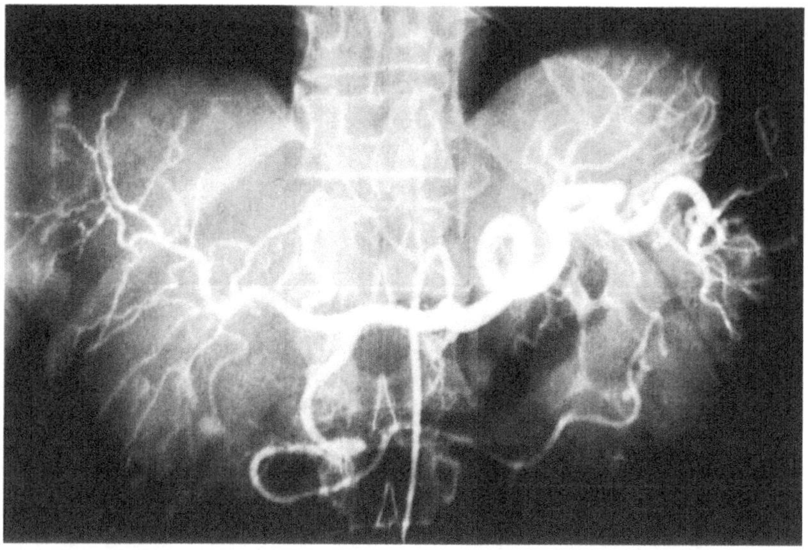

Fig. 24. Normal picture of celiac trunk and its branches.
Celiac angiogram

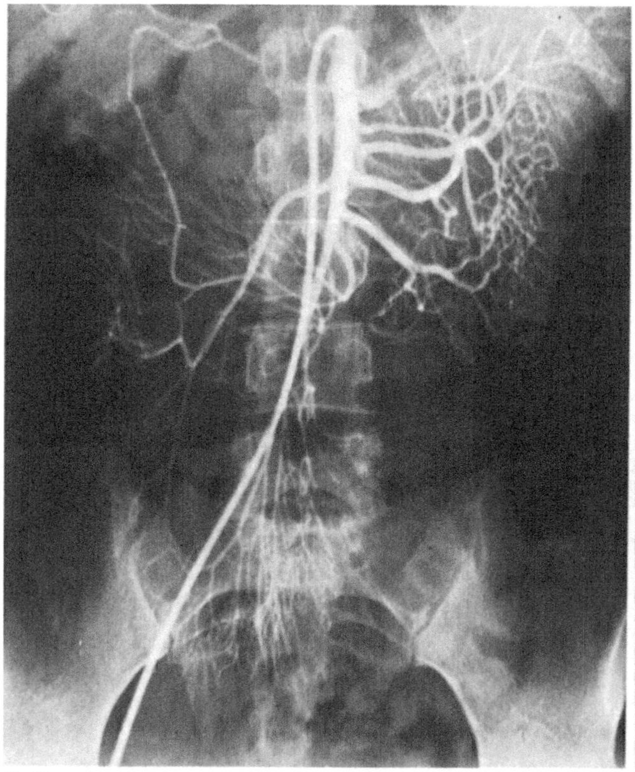

Fig. 25

Fig. 25. Normal picture of superior mesenteric artery and its branches. Selective angiogram of superior mesenteric artery

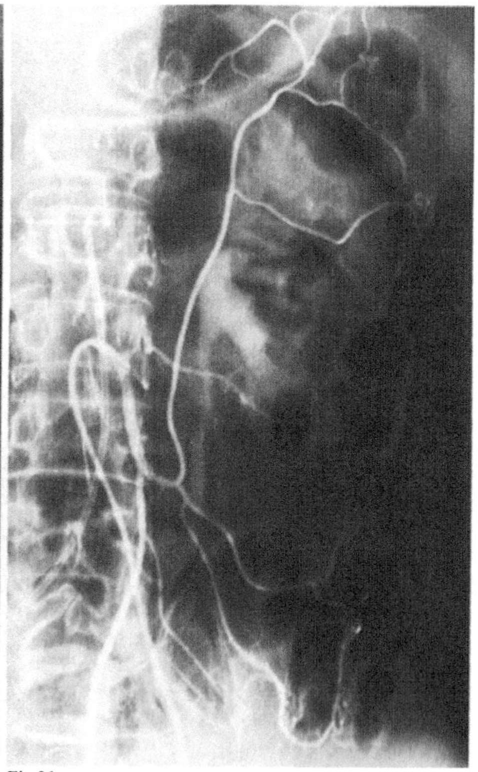

Fig. 26

Fig. 26. Normal picture of inferior mesenteric artery and its branches. Selective angiogram of inferior mesenteric artery

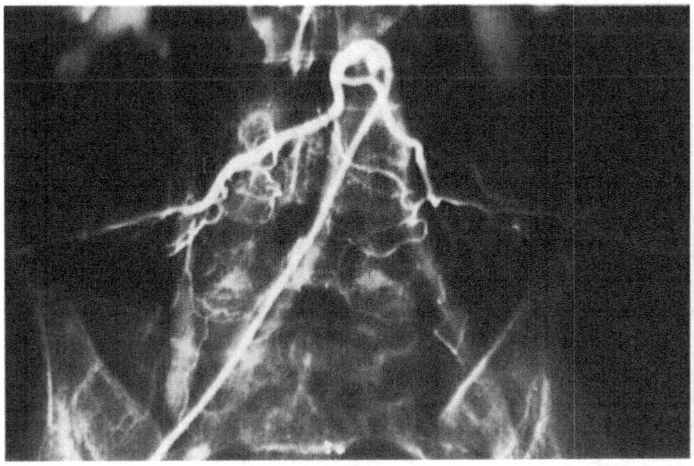

Fig. 27

Fig. 27. Common origin of right and left fourth lumbar arteries at the aorta. Selective angiogram of a lumbar artery

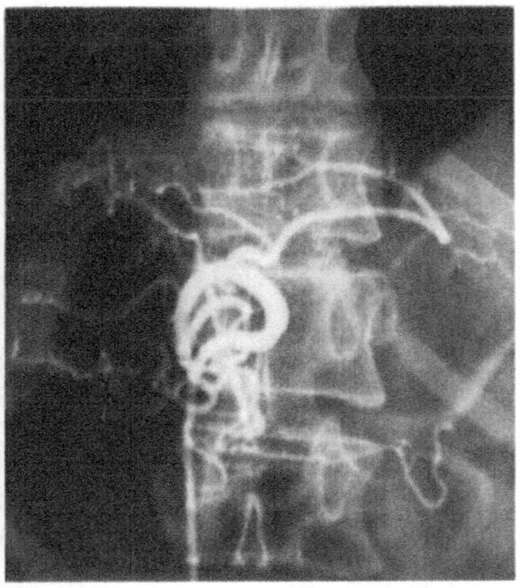

Fig. 28

Fig. 28. Extremely tortuous course of left gastric artery and its branches. Superselective angiogram of left gastric artery

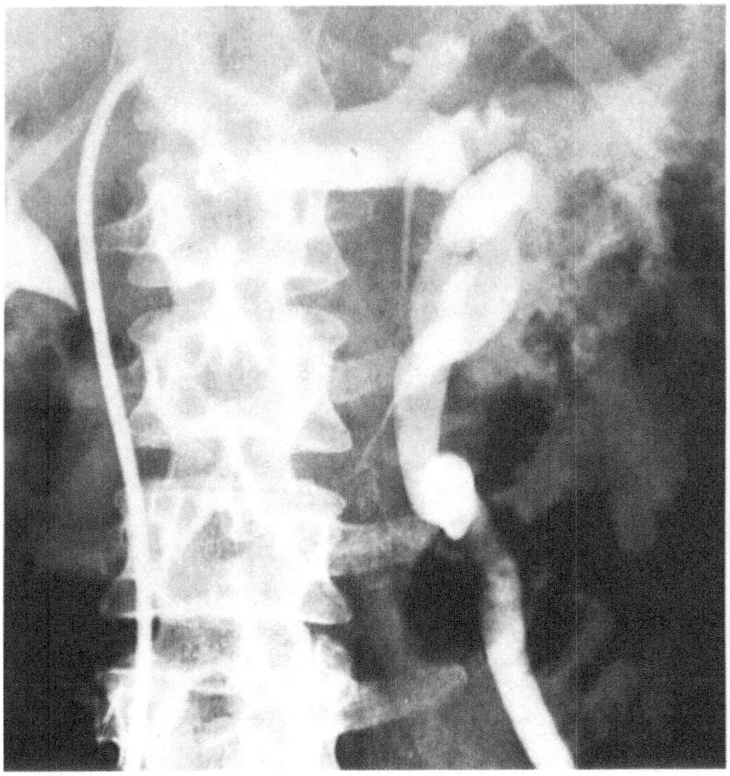

Fig. 29

Fig. 29. Dilated and tortuous left ovarian vein. Selective angiogram of left renal vein with retrograde opacification of left ovarian vein

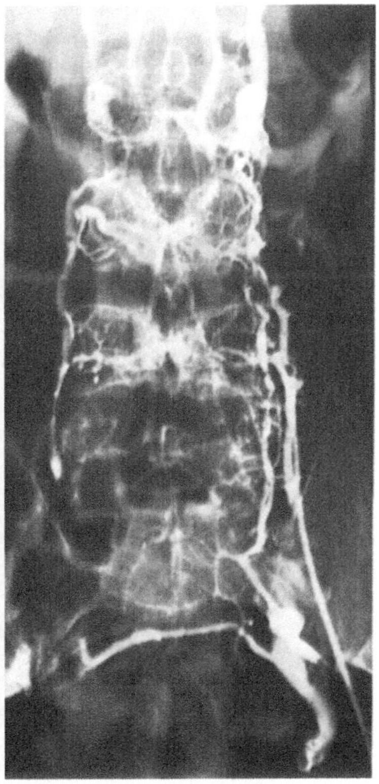

Fig. 30

Fig. 30. Normal picture of left ascending lumbar vein and its tributaries: Vertebral and spinal branches. Superselective angiogram of left ascending lumbar vein

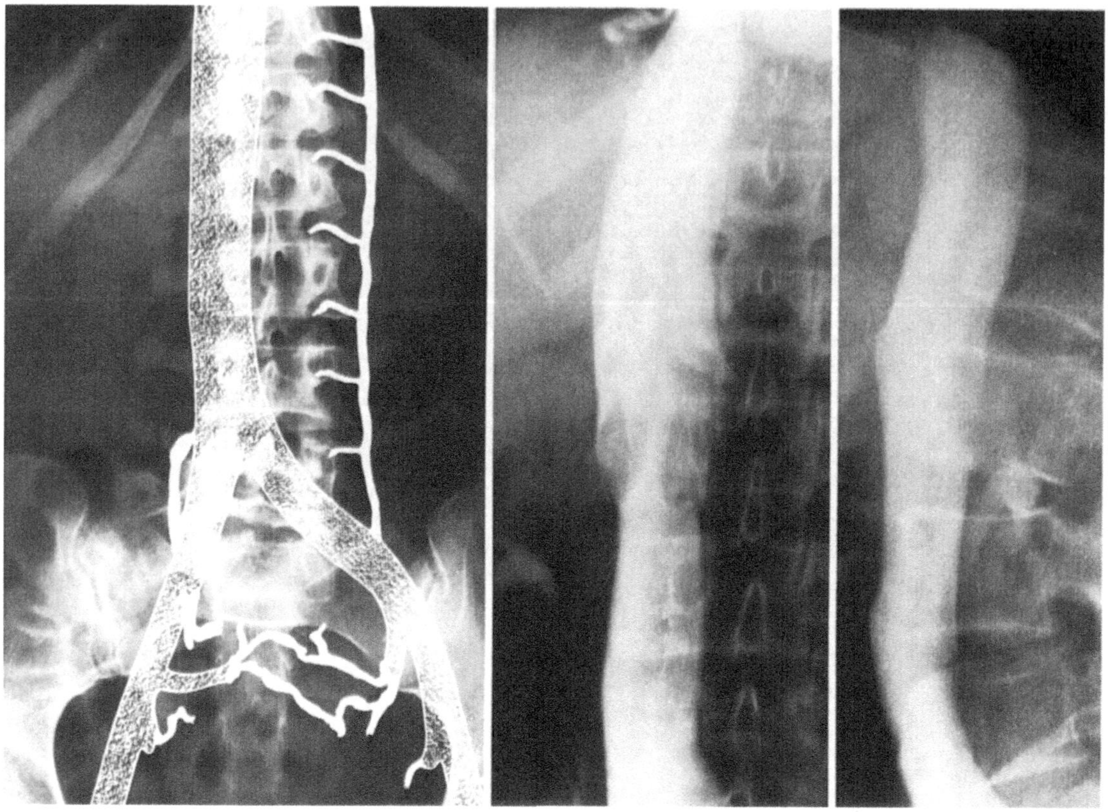

a b c

Fig. 31 a–c. (a) Abdominal x-ray with anatomy of inferior vena cava. (b) Normal course of inferior vena cava in anteroposterior projection. Irregular contours at opening into renal vein. Slight reflux into a hepatic vein. (c) Corresponding lateral view

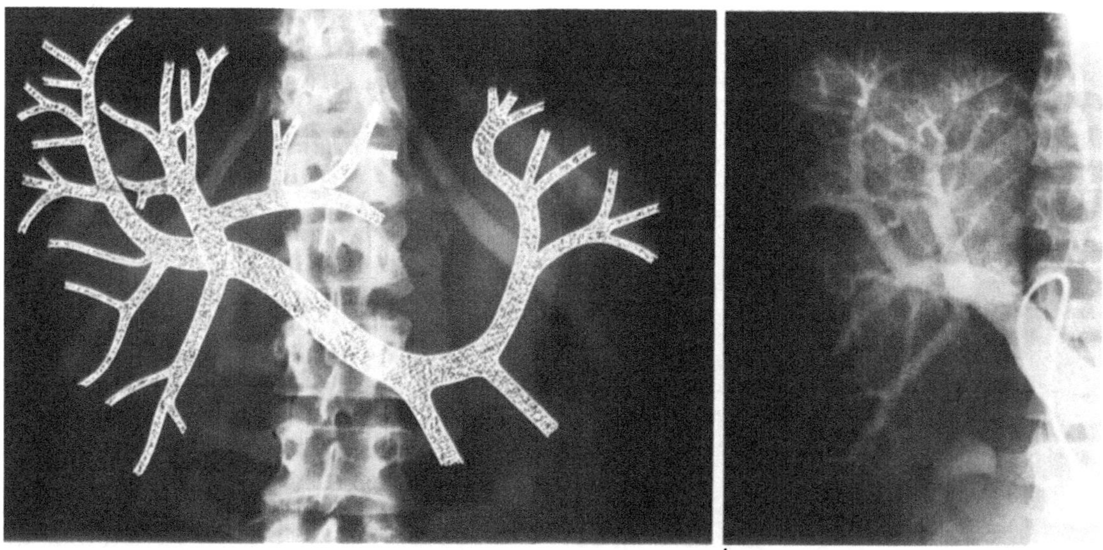

a b

Fig. 32 a and b. (a) Abdominal x-ray with anatomy of portal vein system. (b) Normal ramification of intrahepatic portal vein branches. Omphaloportogram. The catheter is located in the re-opened umbilical vein

Fig. 33a. Normal picture of splenic and superior mesenteric arteries. Simultaneous angiogram of splenic and superior mesenteric arteries taken with the aid of two catheters inserted through right and left femoral arteries

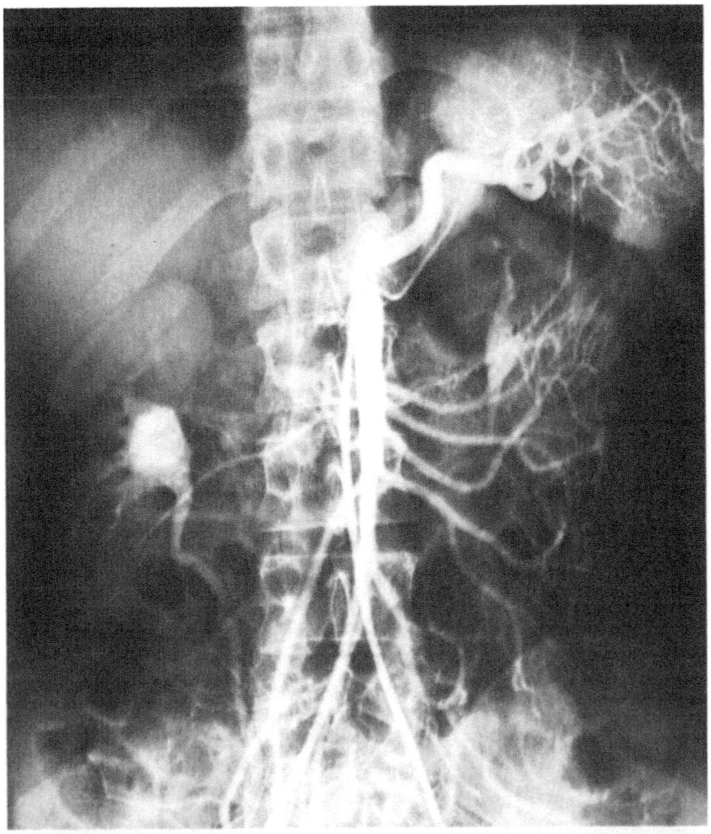

a

Fig. 33b. Venous phase with strong opacification of portal vein system (arterioportogram)

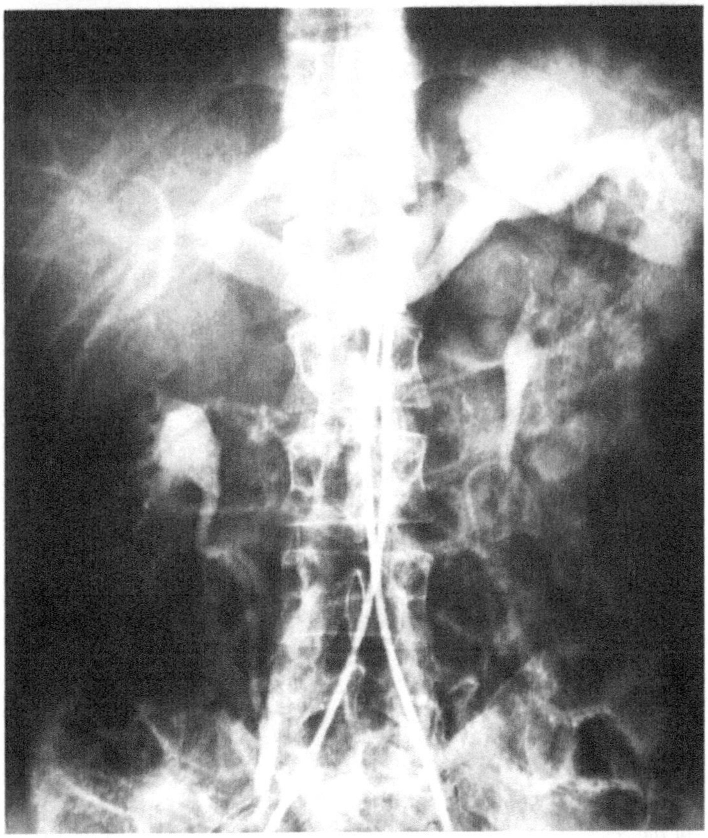

b

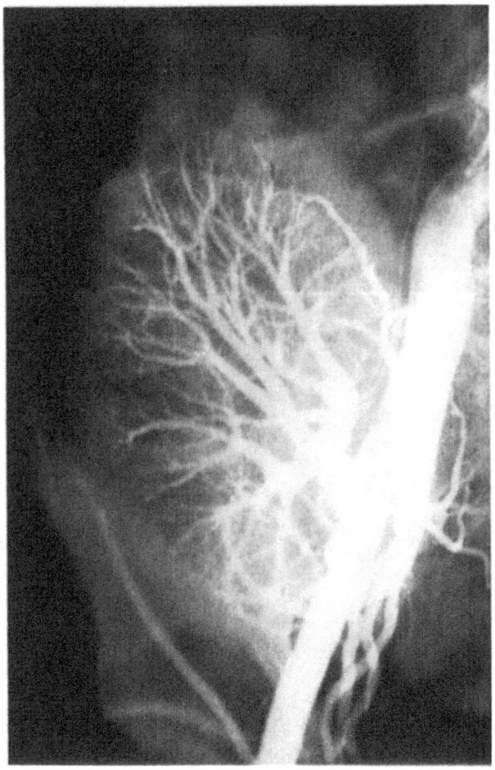

Fig. 34. Normal arteriogram of a transplanted kidney. Retrograde arteriogram taken from right femoral artery with strong opacification of the transplanted organ which is anastomosed to the internal iliac artery and projected onto the right ilium

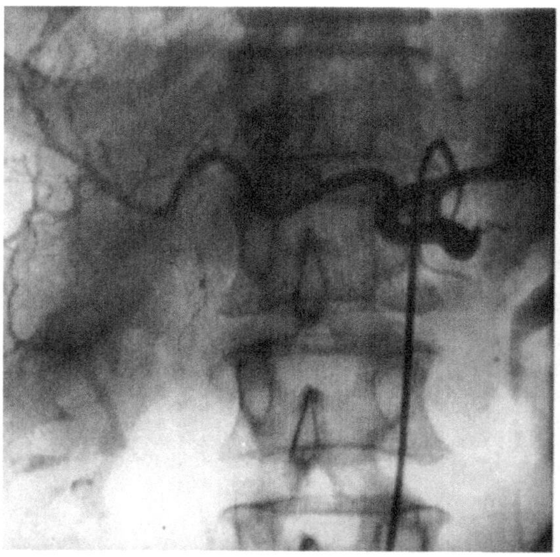

a

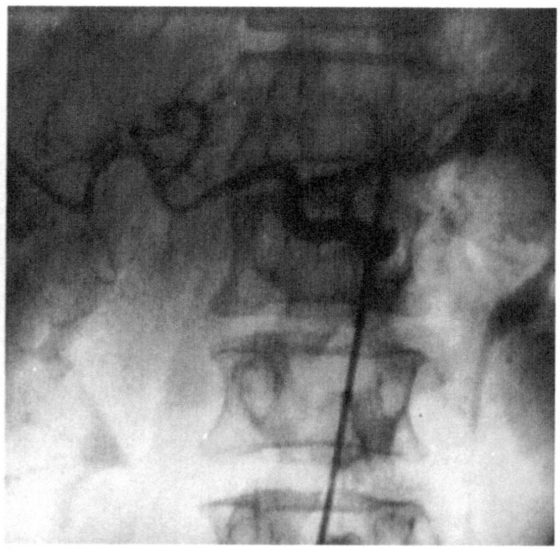

b

Fig. 35a and b. Stereoangiogram: Normal branching of the celiac trunk. Time elapsed between the two pictures 2 seconds. The angles of projection of the two pictures differed by 5°

Fig. 36a and b. Pressure measurement during angiography. (a) Accessory renal arteries in incipient dilating arteriosclerosis. Lumbar aortography with two cannulae, the second cannula used to measure pressure as contrast medium is injected. (b) Pressure curve before, during, and after manual injection of 40 ml Urografin 76%. Brief rise in pressure followed by marked fall

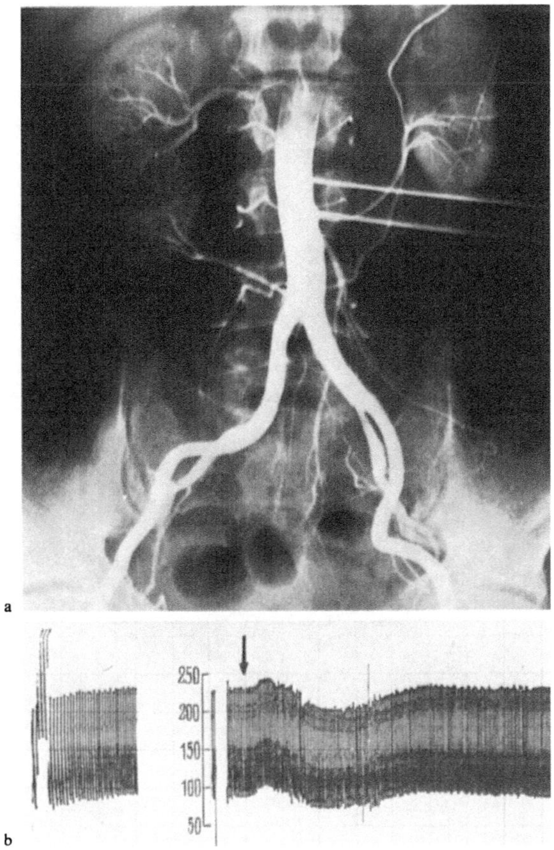

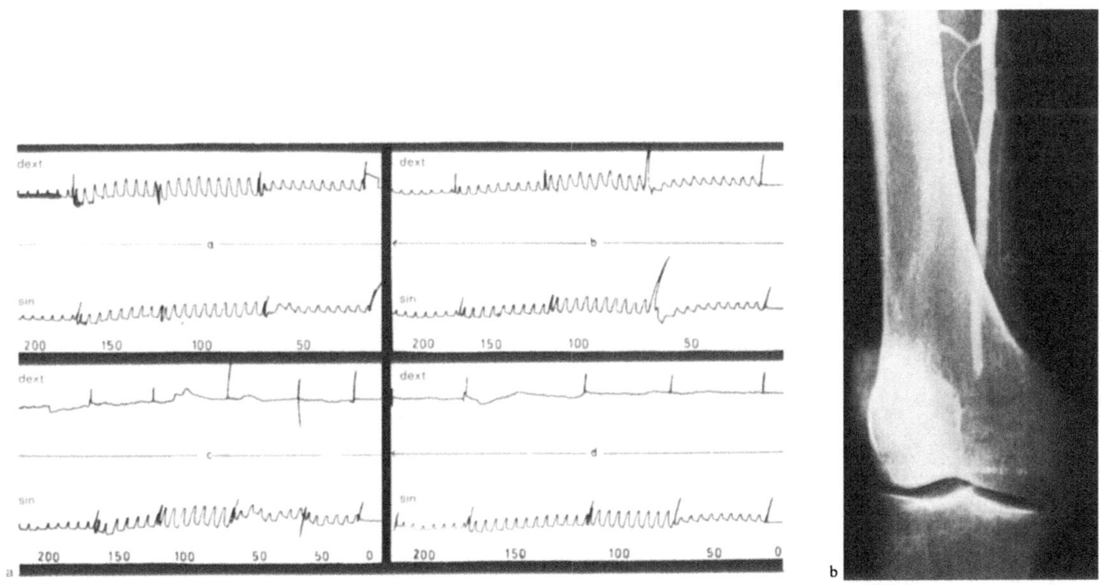

Fig. 37a and b. (a) Postangiographic occlusion of popliteal artery in oscillogram. Measurements made on both lower legs before (above left) and during (above right) injection of contrast medium in catheter aortography. Disappearance of pulse waves after removal of catheter (bottom left); same after two hours (bottom right). (b) Followup arteriogram of right common femoral artery with total occlusion of popliteal artery. Fresh embolism discovered during operation

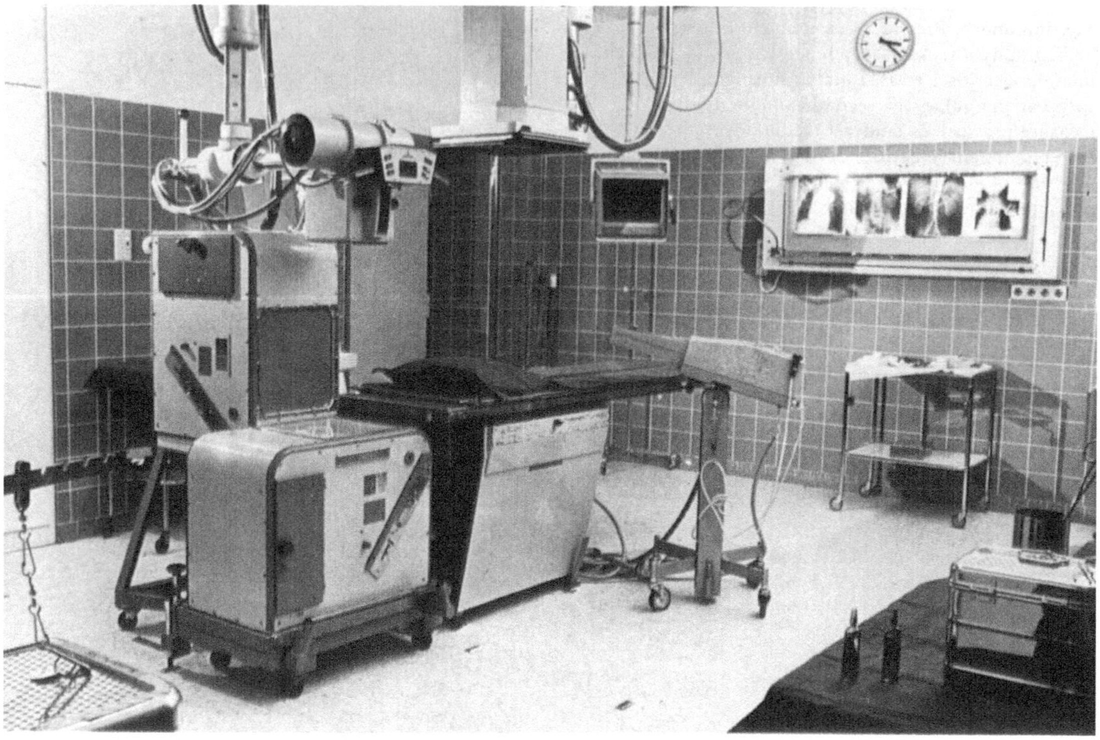

a

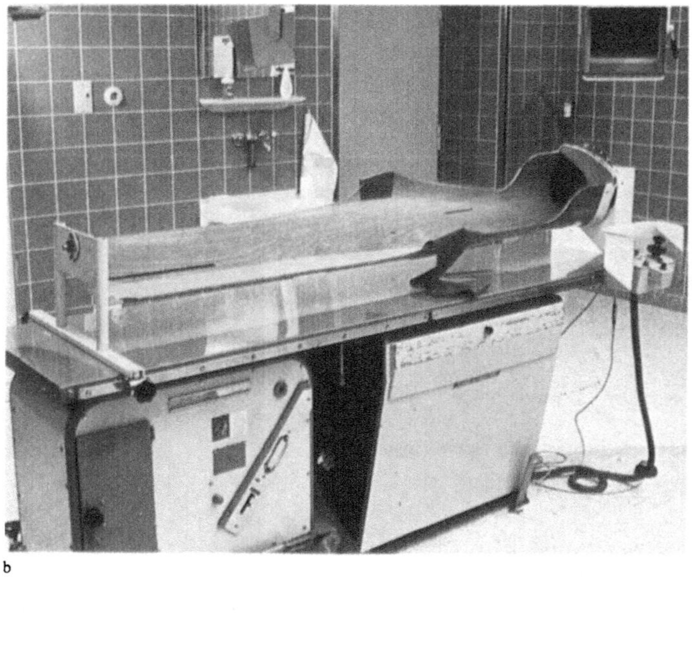

b

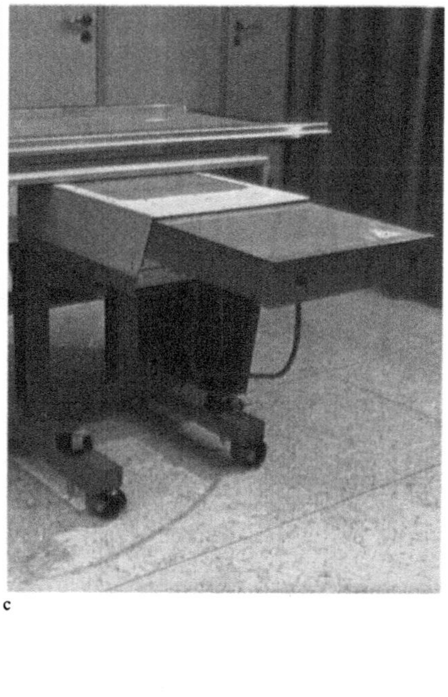

c

Fig. 38a–c. (a) Angiographic equipment for abdominal angiography in the Radiology Department, Surgical Clinic, University of Heidelberg; note the automatic injector "Contrac" (Siemens-Erlangen), (b) Rotating table for abdominal stereoangiography; the table rotates automatically by degrees. (c) Puck film changer for emergency angiography. The device is partially pulled out from under the examination table for display. In foreground, cassette drawer for total of 20 films

Fig. 39a–c. (a) Instruments for direct translumbar and femoral arteriography and venography. (b) Instruments for splenoportography and percutaneous, transhepatic cholangiography.
(c) Equipment for catheter angiography:
1 scalpel;
2 short puncture needle for femoral angiography;
3 long puncture needle for lumbar angiography;
4 syringe with heparinized saline solution;
5 syringe for contrast medium;
6 long needle with teflon sleeve for splenoportography and percutaneous, transhepatic cholangiography;
7 Seldinger needle for catheter angiography;
8 0.5% novocaine;
9 bowl for heparinized saline solution;
10 enameled basin for heparinized saline solution, containing guide wire, and tapered and curved red Ödman catheters;
11 disposable syringe for local anesthesia;
12 pressure syringe for "Contrac" injector;
13 manometer for measuring intrasplenic or intrabiliary pressure;
14 large slit cloth and stellate sheet for draping the patient;
15 swabs and gauze pads;
16 sponge on stick

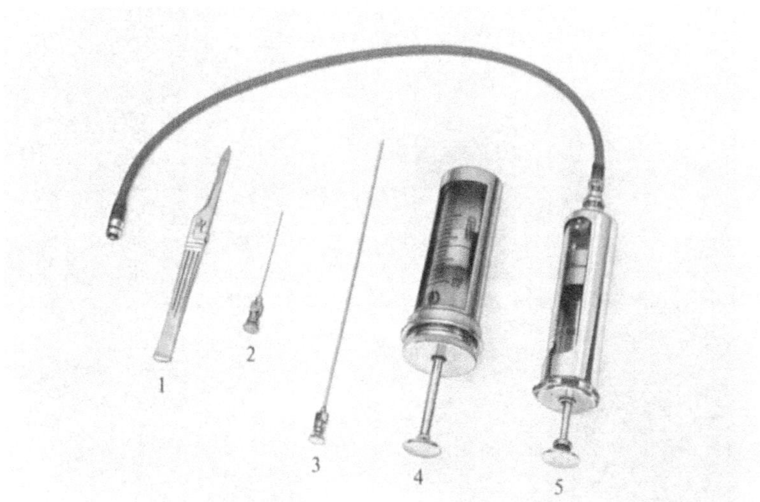

a

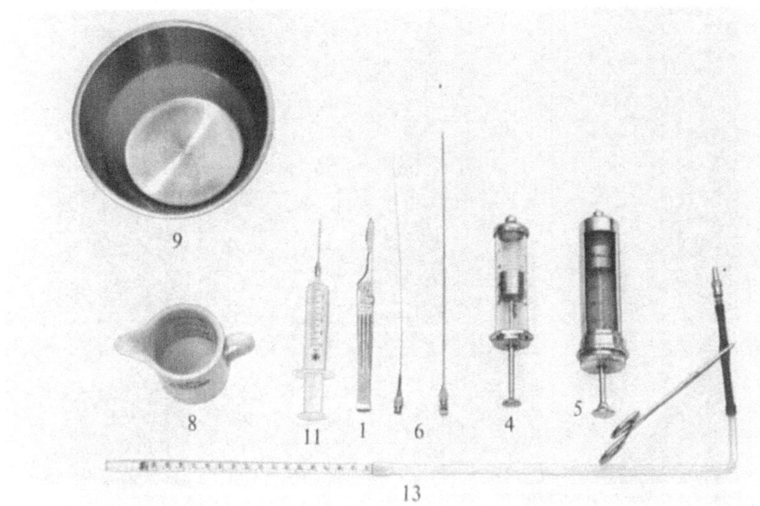

b

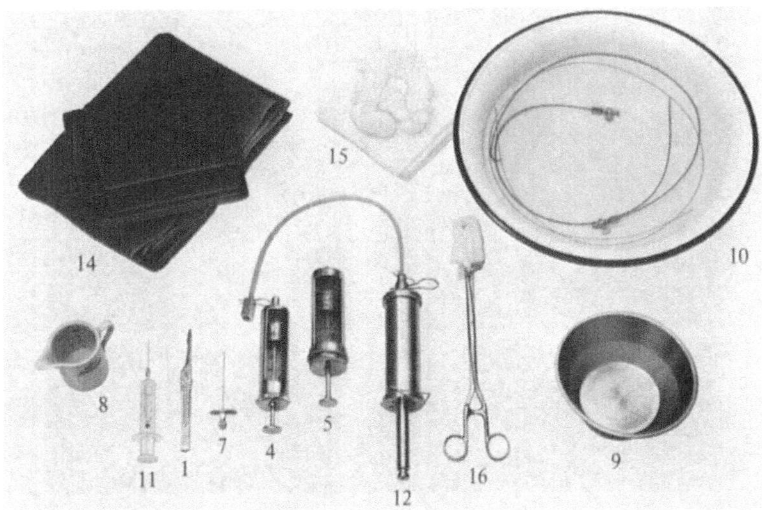

c

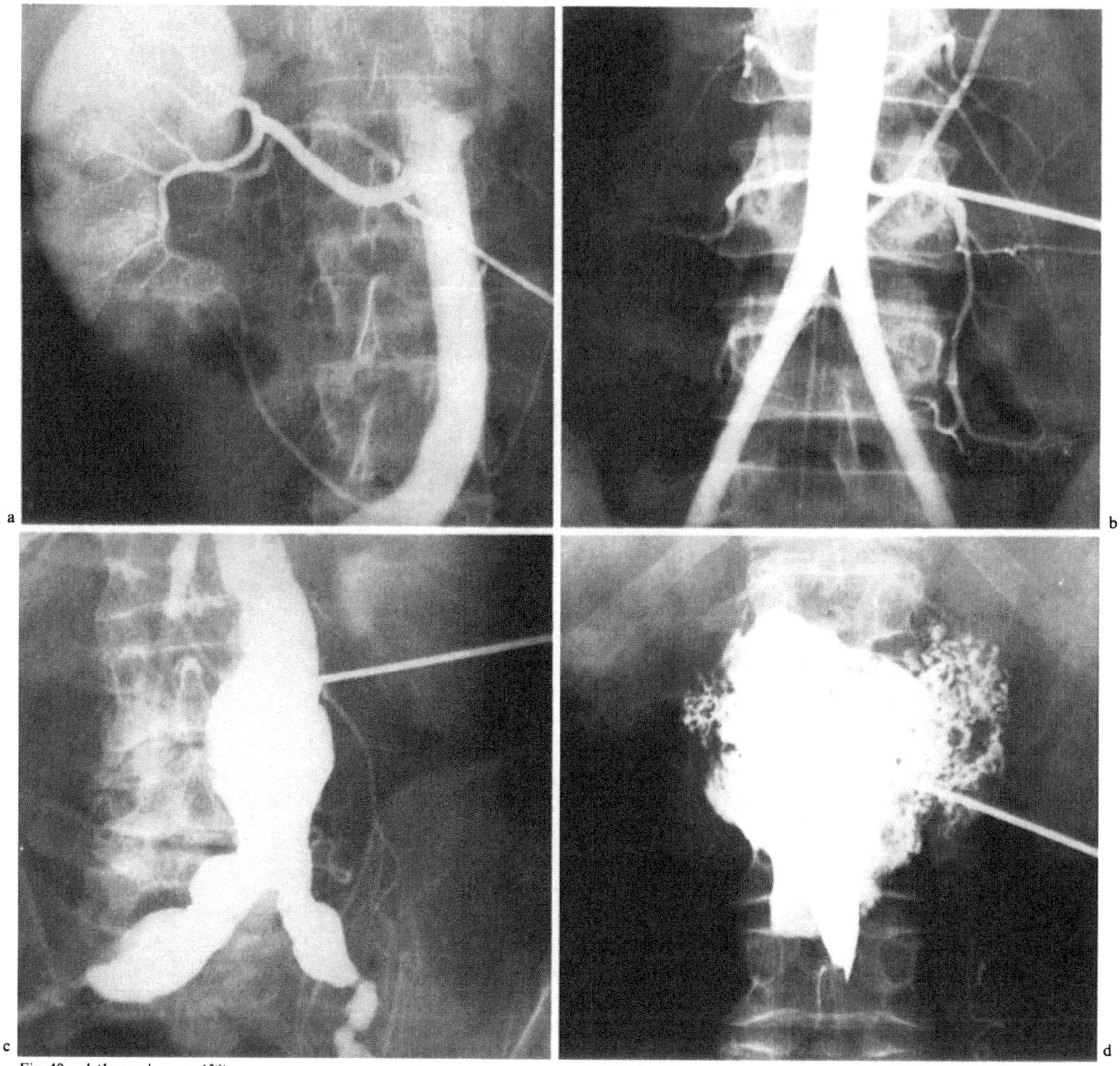

Fig. 40a–d (Legend see p. 139)

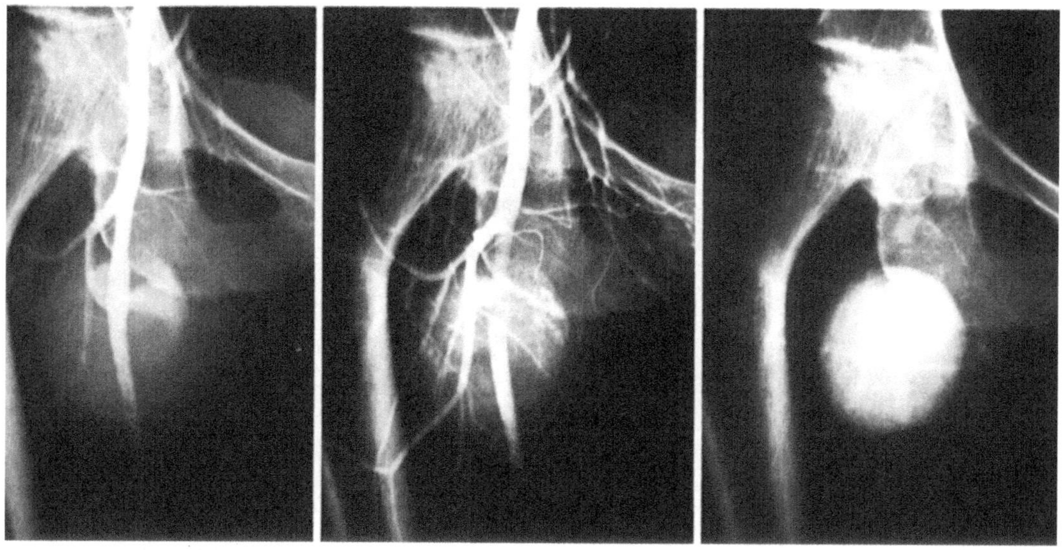

Fig. 41 (Legend see p. 139) a b c

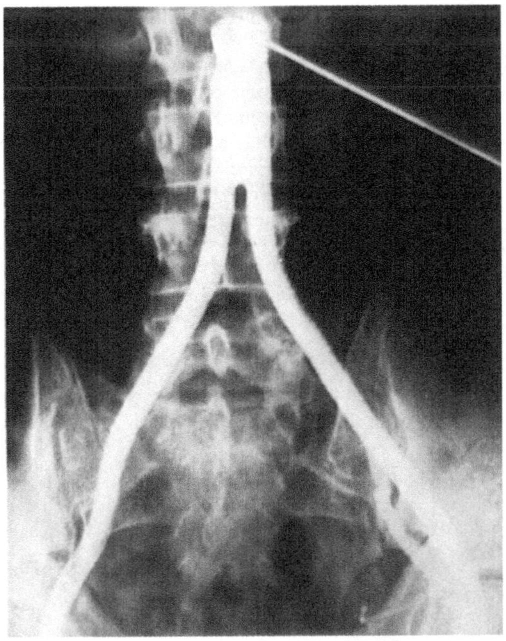

Fig. 42

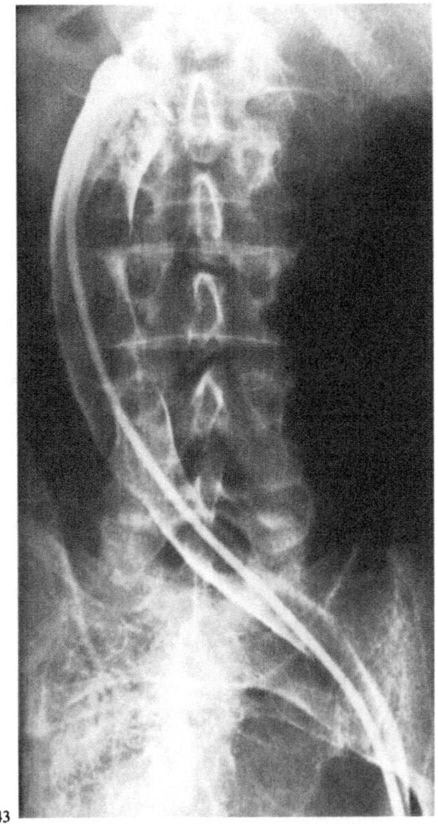

Fig. 43

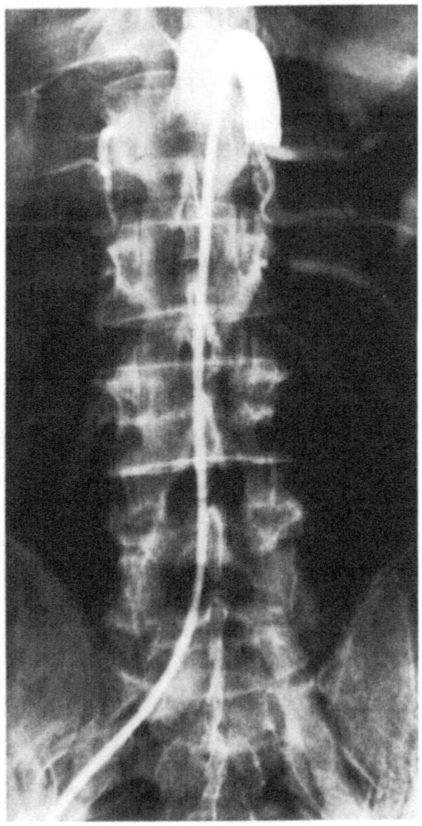

Fig. 44

Fig. 42. Puncture of aortofemoral bifurcation bypass in occlusion of both pelvic arteries. The prosthesis can be recognized by its typical corrugated profile. No branches!

Fig. 43. Dissection of aortic wall by catheter. In this severe case of arteriosclerosis the catheter had worked its way beneath the intima, so that only the aortic wall is visualized after the trial injection.
No subjective or objective sequelae. Angiography later repeated as lumbar aortography

Fig. 44. Intramural injection of contrast agent into proximal section of superior mesenteric artery. Well-defined "stop", while only a small portion of the contrast medium has reached the lumen of the vessel and its branches. No objectively demonstrable consequence

---

Fig. 40a–d. Faulty punctures in lumbar aortography.
(a) Puncture of a right renal artery (note accessory lower polar artery). (b) Puncture of lumbar branch.
(c) Puncture of aortic aneurysm. (d) Extensive extravasation: during injection the needle tip slipped back, spreading contrast medium outside the aorta. One hour after injection, contrast medium could no longer be radiographically detected. Pain in back for two days, otherwise no after-effects. Secondary finding: Selective opacification of left spermatic artery

Fig. 41 a–c. Postangiographic femoral aneurysm (cardiac catheter. (a) Early arterial phase. Extravasations of contrast medium from superficial femoral artery at level of puncture site. (b) Gradual contrast filling of a round tangerine-sized mass.
(c) Persistence of contrast medium beyond venous phase. Secondary finding: Necrosis of head of femur on the right

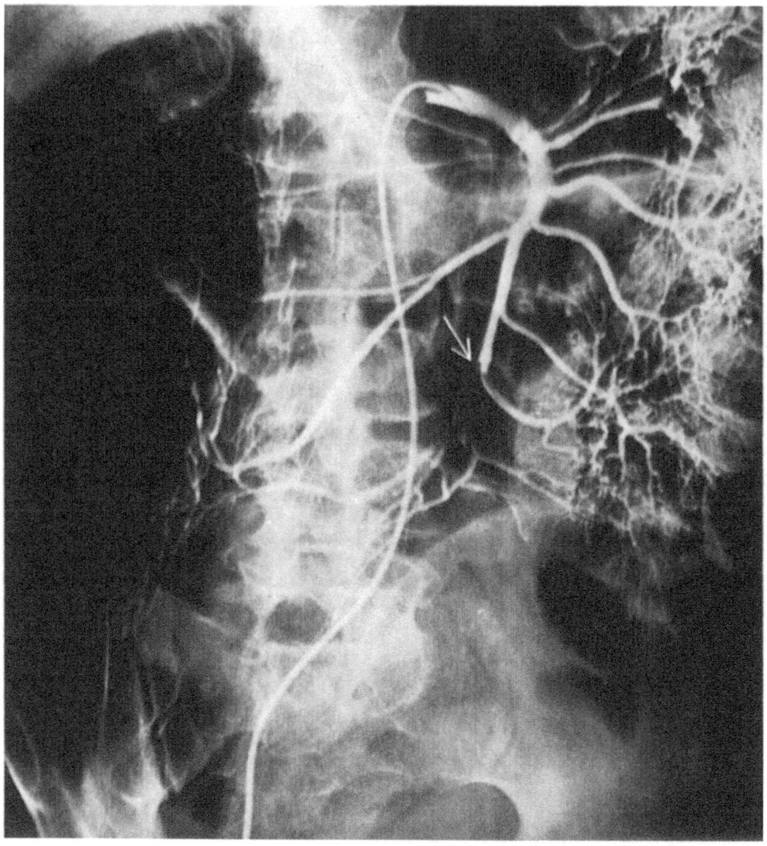

Fig. 45a. Embolic occlusion of the distal portions of trunk of superior mesenteric artery. Some blood is able to flow around the embolism (arrow). The artery is not visible in the region of the ileum. Selective angiography of superior mesenteric artery

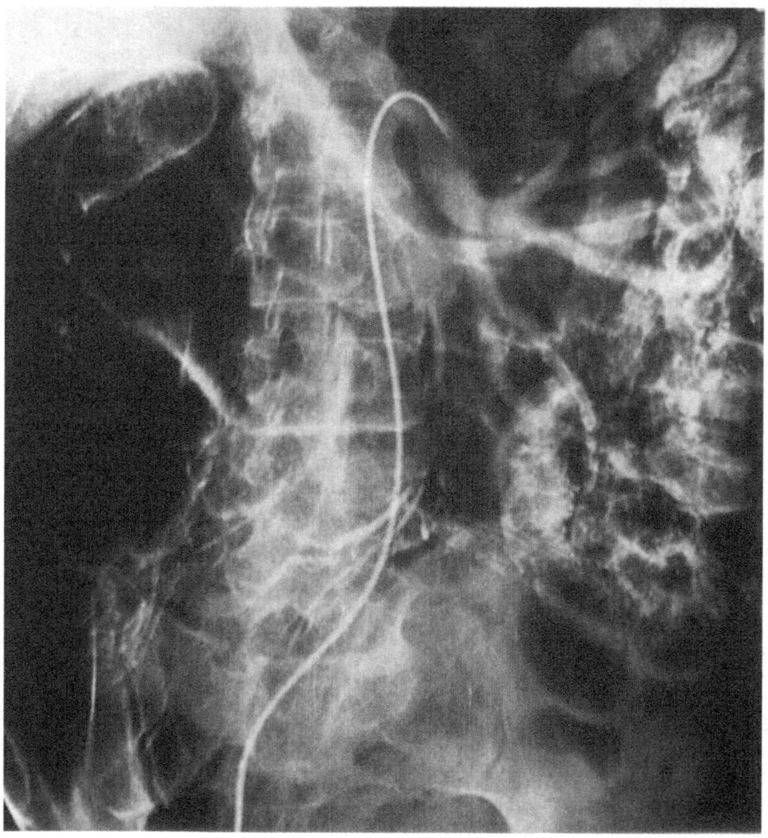

Fig. 45b. Persistence of contrast medium in wide drainage veins in intestinal wall of jejunum and right colon. In addition to the arterial embolism, surgery revealed a venous thrombus at the opening of the superior mesenteric vein into the portal vein

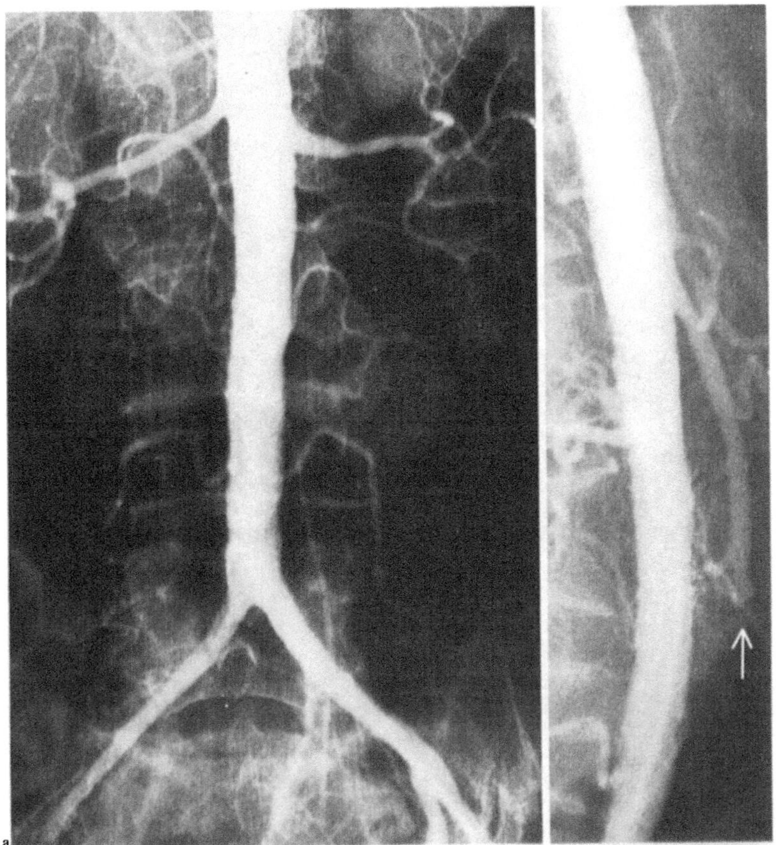

a b

Fig. 46a and b. (a) Embolic occlusion of superior mesenteric artery at the midsection of its trunk. The catheter aortogram shows only branchings of superior mesenteric artery in the proximal third. The vessel is projected onto the aorta and cannot be differentiated. (b) In this side view, the superior mesenteric artery is totally cut off (arrow)

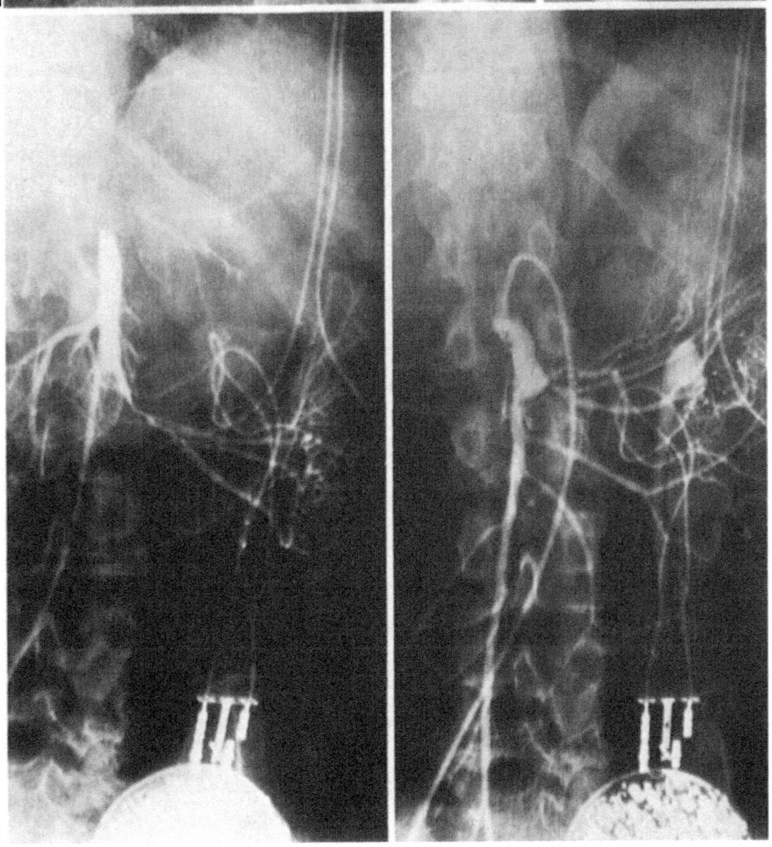

a b

Fig. 47a and b. (a) Embolism in proximal third of main trunk of mesenteric artery in case with implanted pacemaker for continuous arrythmia. Selective angiography of superior mesenteric artery. (b) Postoperative followup arteriogram. The main trunk of the artery is patent again

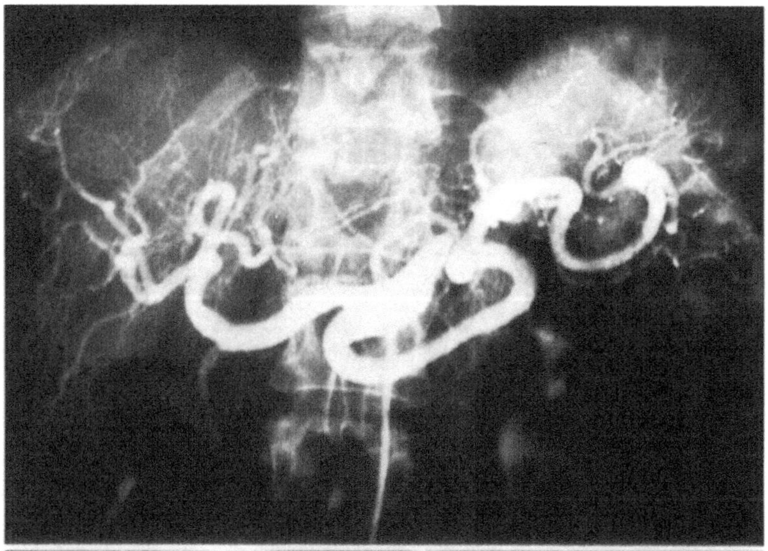

Fig. 48. Stenosis of celiac artery at origin. Poststenotic dilatation of the trunk. Clinical diagnosis: Abdominal angina. Concomitant partial occlusion of gastroduodenal artery. Celiac angiogram

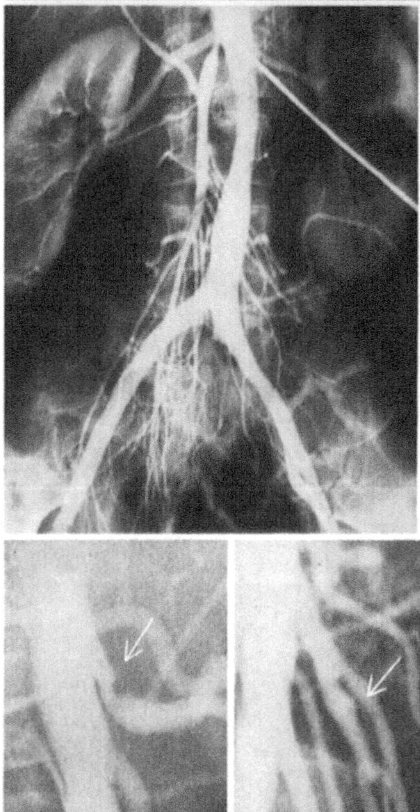

Fig. 49

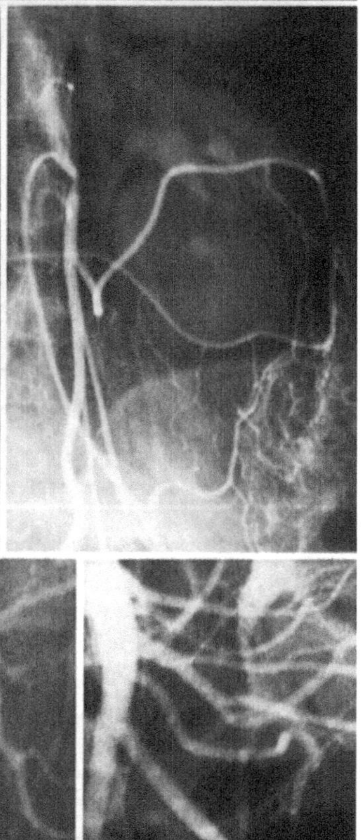

Fig. 50

Fig. 49. Circumscribed stenosis of superior mesenteric artery at origin as a secondary finding in layer aortography occasioned by occlusion of both femoral arteries. Lumbar aortogram

Fig. 50. Stenosis of inferior mesenteric artery at origin with no clinical symptoms. Selective angiogram of inferior mesenteric artery

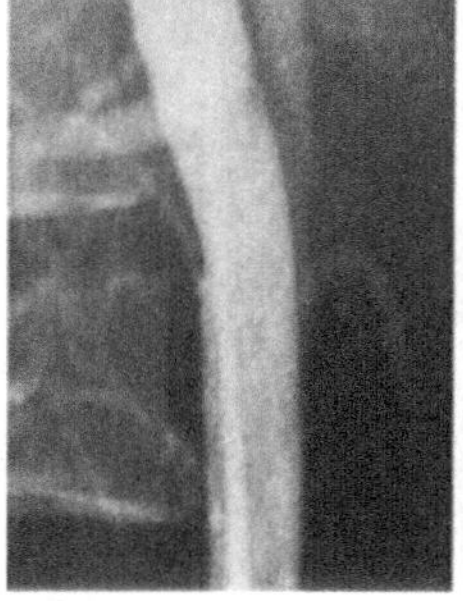

Fig. 51

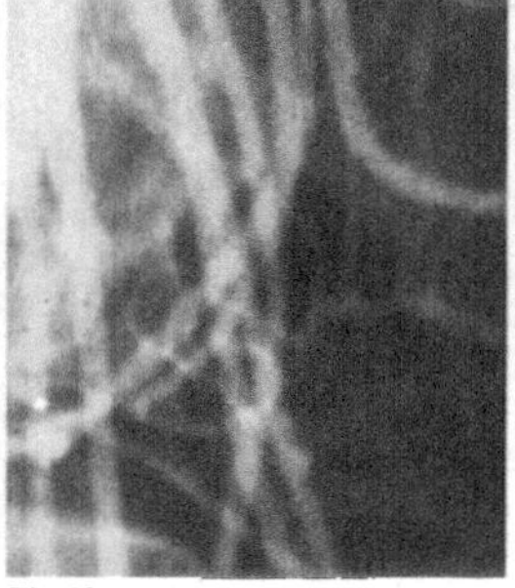

Fig. 52

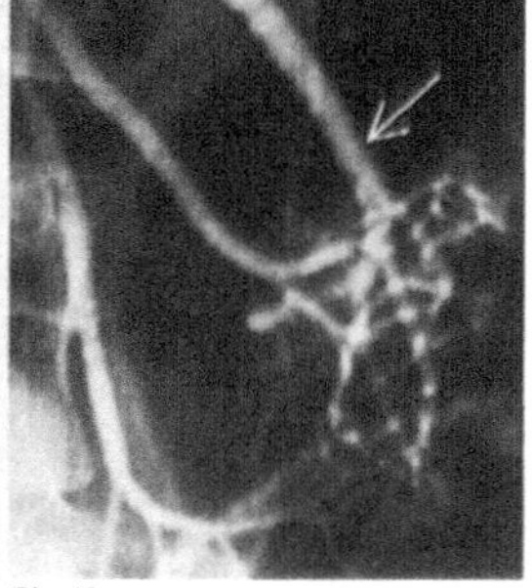

Fig. 53

Fig. 51. Celiac artery stenosis: Median arcuate ligament compression syndrome (arrow). Catheter aortography in lateral view

Fig. 52. Polyarteritis nodosa. Multiple aneurysms barely perceptible in the region of the aortic branches, here at the superior mesenteric artery (arrow). The diagnosis was histologically confirmed. Catheter aortogram

Fig. 53. So-called "string-of-pearls phenomenon" (arrow). Secondary finding in search for tumor. Selective angiography of superior mesenteric artery

Fig. 54. Diagram of visceral collateral vessels: Pancreatic arcade (1) between the celiac trunk and superior mesenteric artery; Riolan's anastomosis (2) between superior and inferior mesenteric arteries; superior hemorrhoidal artery (3) between inferior mesenteric artery and left internal iliac artery

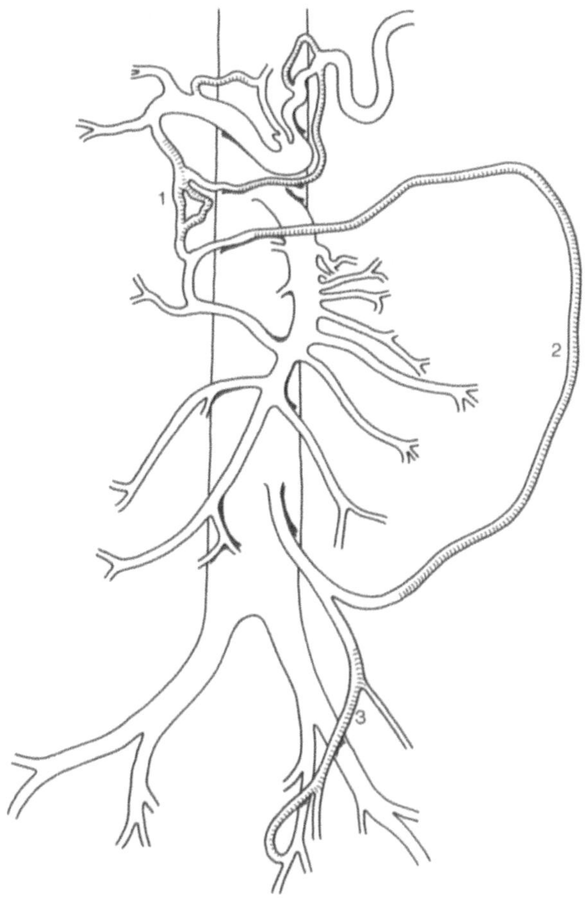

Fig. 55. Celiac occlusion. Picture of celiac artery filled retrograde above superior mesenteric artery through dilated vessels of pancreatic arcade (arrow)

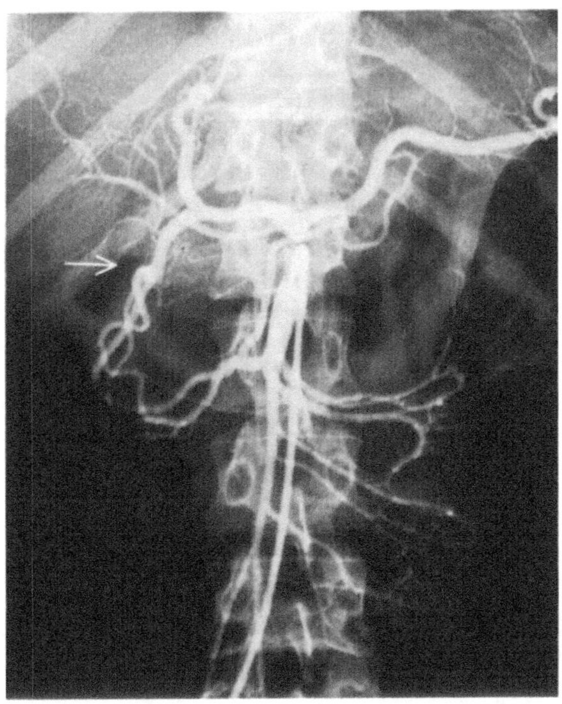

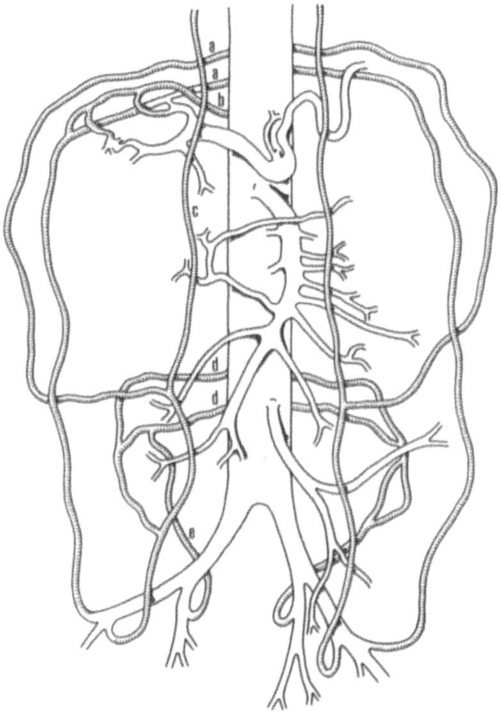

Fig. 56. Diagram of collateral vessels from systemic circulation in occlusions of abdominal aorta and its branches, the intercostal [a], phrenic [b], epigastric [c] and [e], and lumbar [d] arteries

Fig. 58. Aortic occlusion just above the bifurcation (Leriche syndrome). Extensive collateralization via inferior mesenteric artery, lumbar arteries dilated by way of compensation, and the caudal aorta

Fig. 59. Infrarenal aortic occlusion. Riolan's anastomosis (arrow), which has taken over supply distally

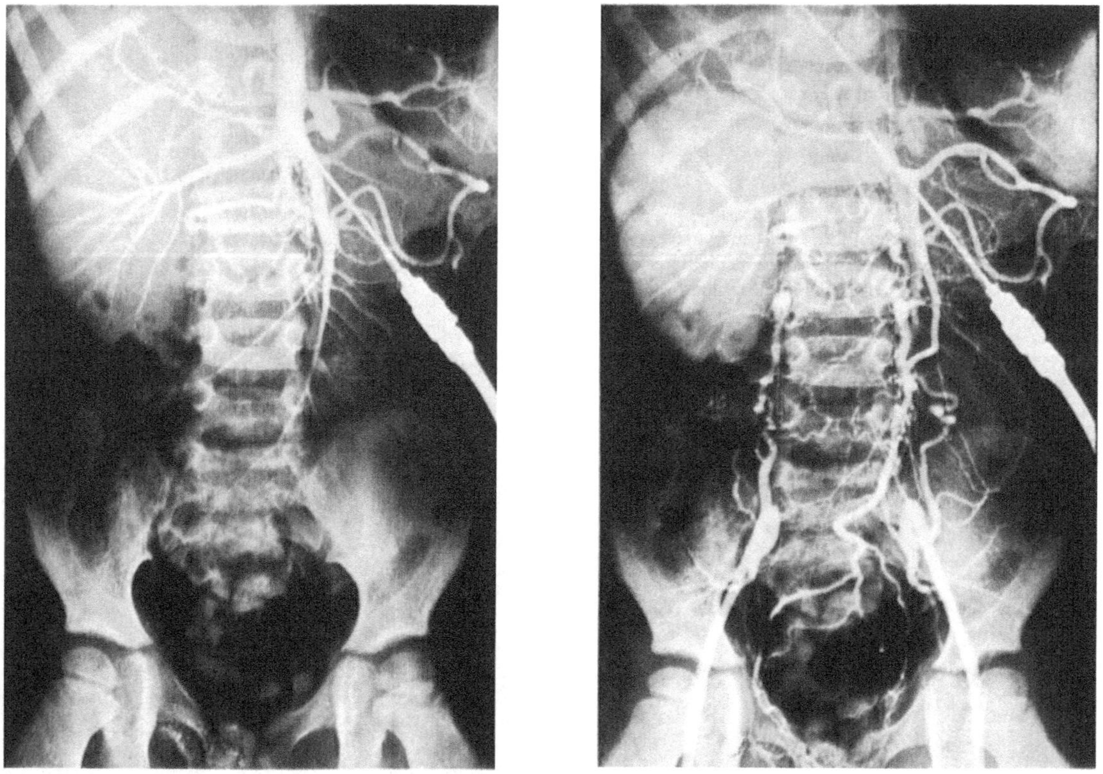

a

b

Fig. 57a and b. (a) Iatrogenic aortic occlusion. Ligation of aorta when patient was 13 months old for extirpation of tumor in left kidney. Total occlusion of aorta at level of right renal artery. Translumbar aortogram. (b) Picture of collateral system with complete refilling of iliac arteries in late arterial phase, when the boy was seven years old

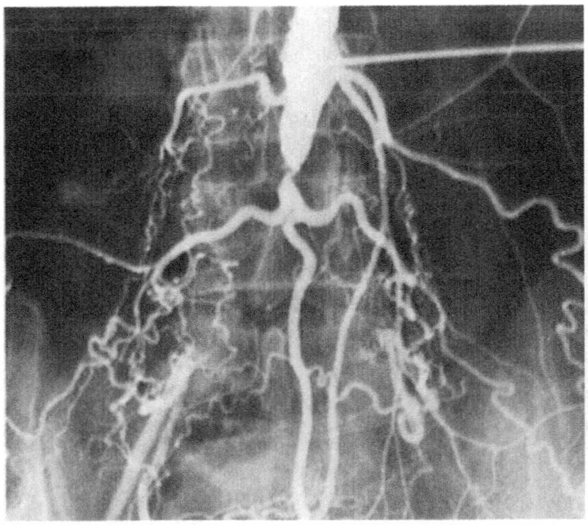

Fig. 58 (Legend see p. 144)

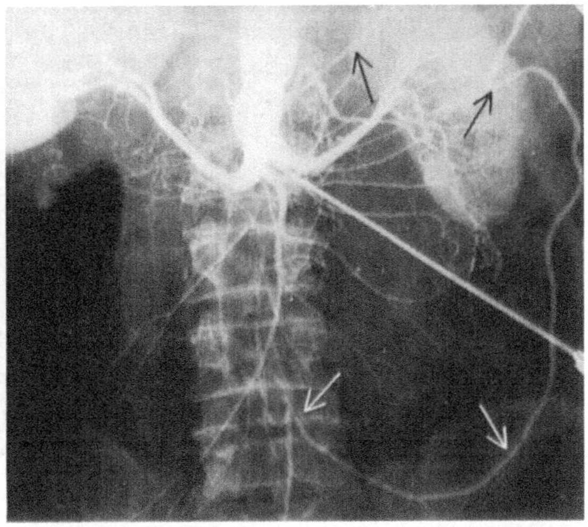

Fig. 59 (Legend see p. 144)

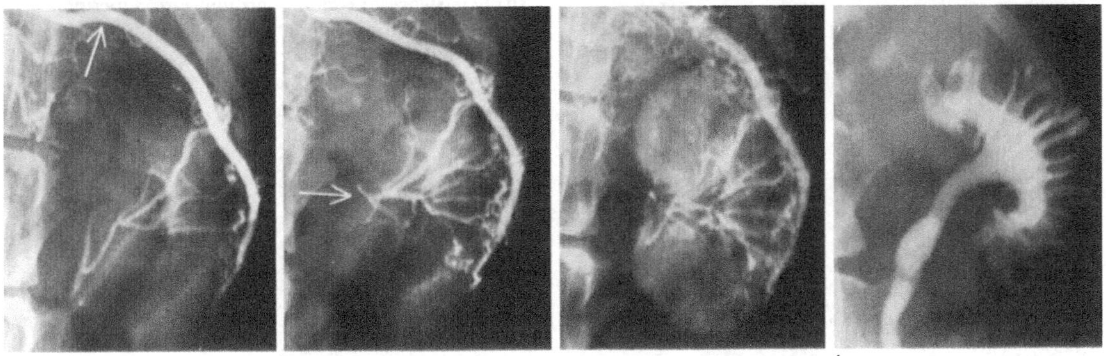

a b c d

Fig. 60a–d. Arterial supply of left kidney via splenic artery. Experiment on dog after removal of right kidney; severance of left renal artery and implantation of splenic artery and vein in parenchyma of left kidney. (a) Early arterial phase of a celiac angiogram in dog, with visualization of splenic artery (arrow) which passes through the renal parenchyma and fills intrarenal branches of renal artery from the periphery through anastomoses. (b) Good staining of intrarenal vessels (arrow). (c) Picture of homogeneous parenchyma throughout the kidney in late phase. (d) Final excretory urogram with cavity system and ureter

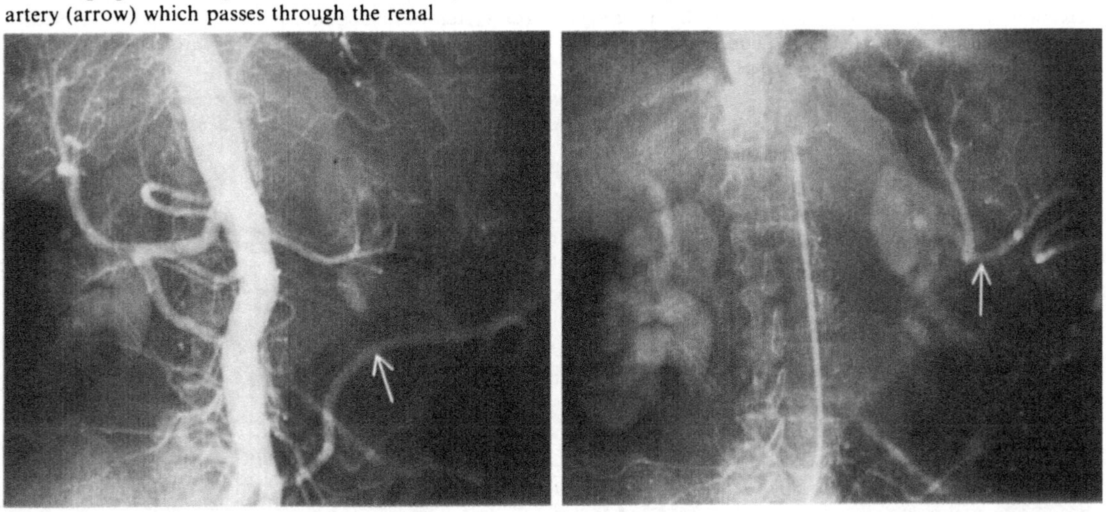

a b

Fig. 61a and b. (a) Splenic artery occlusion of uncertain origin. Arterial phase: Early visualization of strong collateral vessel extending in a wide arc from superior mesenteric artery caudad and then left into upper abdomen (arrow). The splenic artery is absent. (b) Four seconds after injection, good contrast filling of splenic artery through this collateral vessel (arrow)

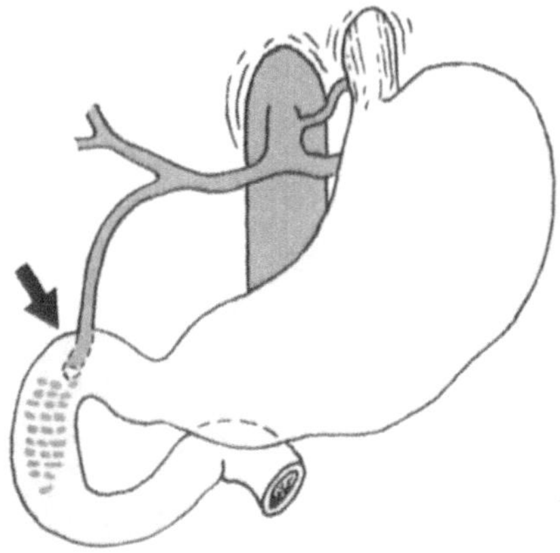

Fig. 62

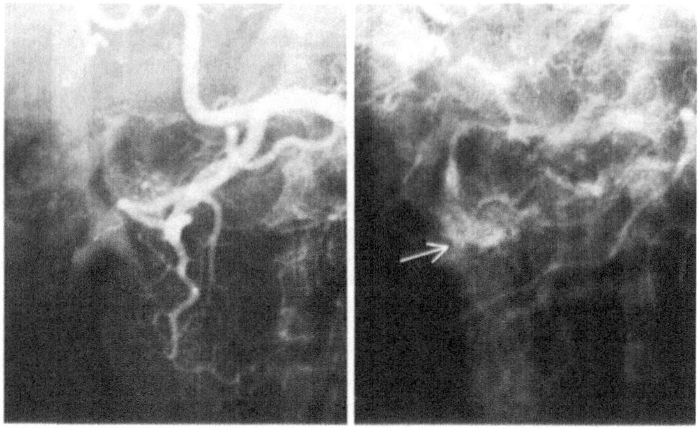

Fig. 63a

Fig. 63b

Fig. 62. Schematic of angiographic localization of bleeding in duodenum

Fig. 63a and b. (a) Bleeding duodenal ulcer. Unremarkable ramification of hepatic artery. Prolific vascular network from gastroduodenal artery. Selective angiography of common hepatic artery. (b) Persistence of contrast medium near superior duodenal flexure and faint contrast coating within duodenal lumen (arrow)

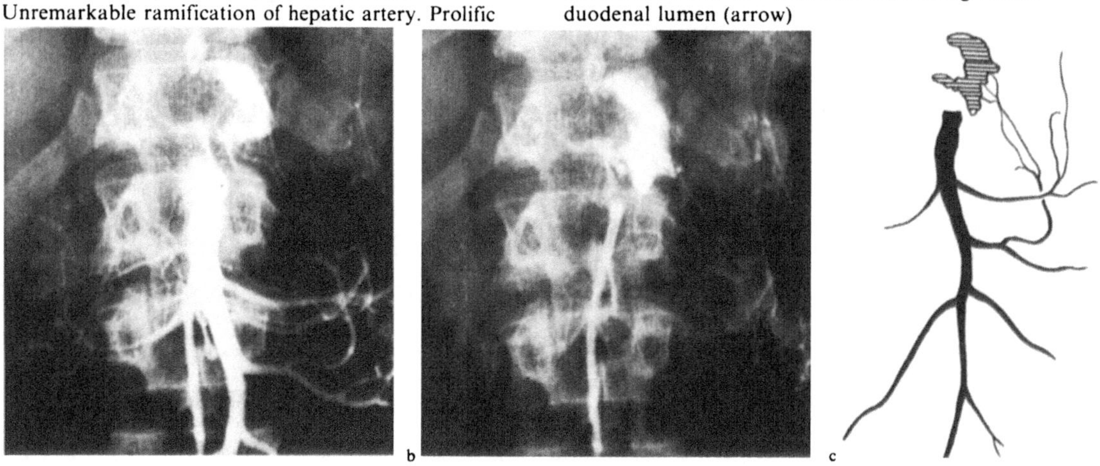

a b c

Fig. 64a–c. Gastric hemorrhage two days after Billroth II resection. (a) Extravasation of contrast medium through small jejunal branches. Selective angiography of superior mesenteric artery. (b) Enlargement of contrast material extravasate in late arterial phase. (c) Sketch of angiogram. Purse-string suture of bleeding vessel in anastomosis at relaparotomy

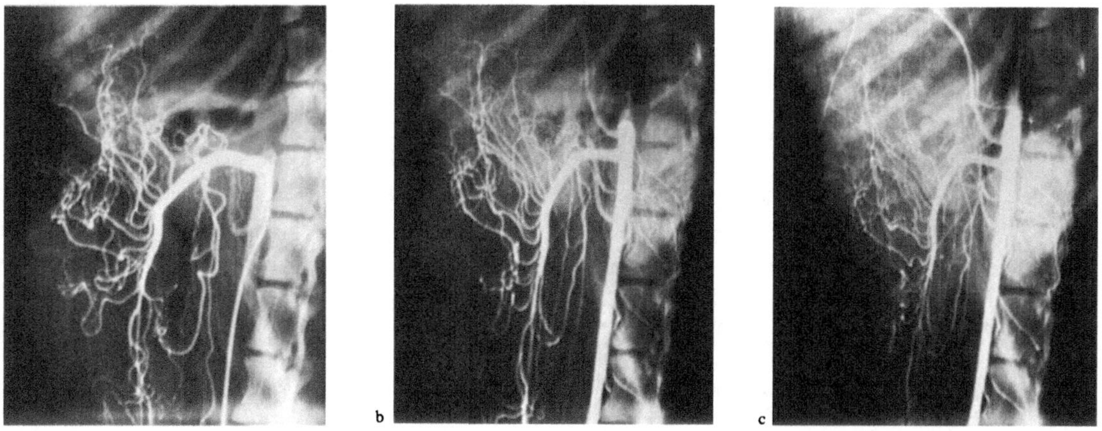

a b c

Fig. 65a–c. Experimental hemorrhagic shock. Angiographic picture of superior mesenteric artery in dog. (a) Beginning of experiment. (b) During hemorrhage. (c) In state of severe hemorrhagic shock. Reduction of vessel caliber, rarefaction of peripheral vessels with relatively large parenchymal areas blocked off, apparently through arteriovenous shunts; premature filling of efferent veins

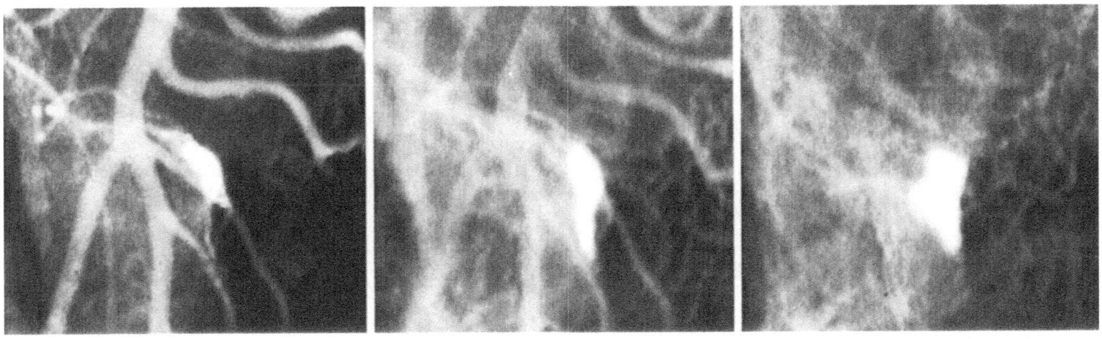

a b c

Fig. 66a–c. Bleeding neurinoma of small intestine. Postlaparotomy condition without detection of source of bleeding. (a) Crescent-shaped extravasate of contrast medium from a jejunal branch. Selective angiography of superior mesenteric artery. (b) Enlargement of contrast extravasate and mild contrast filling of a round tumor in late arterial phase. (c) Further change in contrast distribution. The tumor is more prominent. Relaparotomy revealed a bleeding neurinoma in the jejunum about 3 cm in diameter

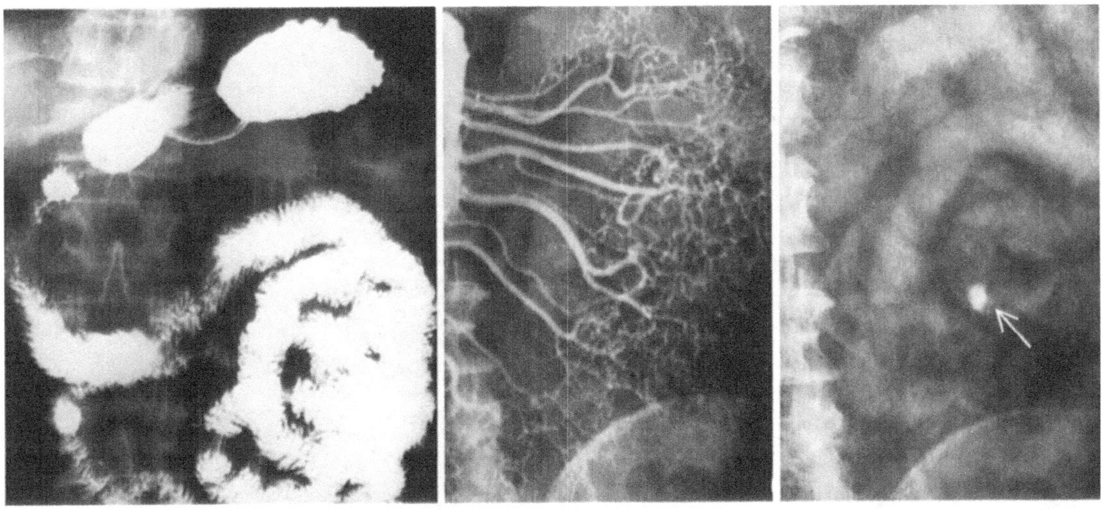

a b c

Fig. 67a–c. Bleeding jejunal polyp. (a) Unremarkable gastrointestinal series. (b) No pathological alterations in arterial phase of selective angiography of superior mesenteric artery. (c) Persisting spot of contrast medium in the middle jejunum in late phase (arrow)

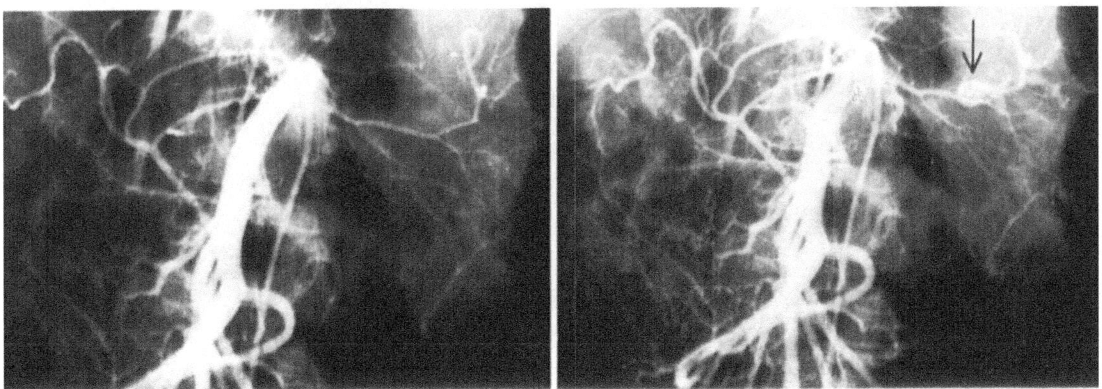

a b

Fig. 68a and b. Bleeding peptic ulcer in jejunum. (a) No pathological findings in early phase of selective angiography of superior mesenteric artery. (b) Three seconds after injection of contrast medium into the upper jejunal branch, there is a round density (arrow) at about the level of the anastomosis after a Billroth II resection, which upon repeat laparotomy proved to be the floor of a peptic ulcer in a typical spot. Neither a gastrointestinal series nor endoscopy detected the ulcer

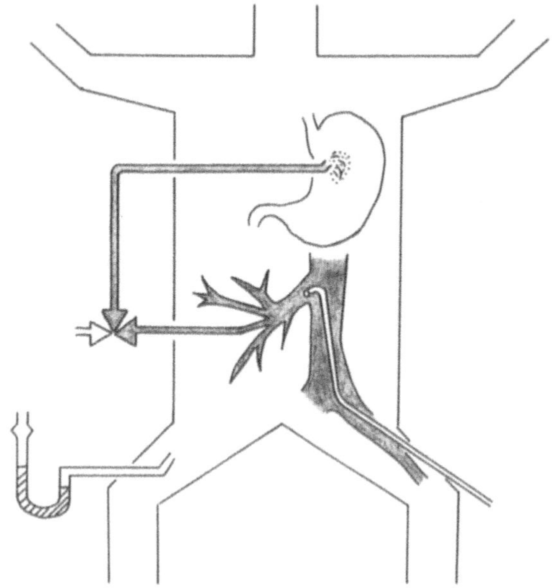

Fig. 69. Experimental angiographic detection of bleeding. Experimental setup for quantitative determination of the minimum quantity of contrast medium required for localization in a dog. The blood flow rate was measured extracorporeally through a catheter one end positioned in the superior mesenteric artery and the other inserted into the stomach

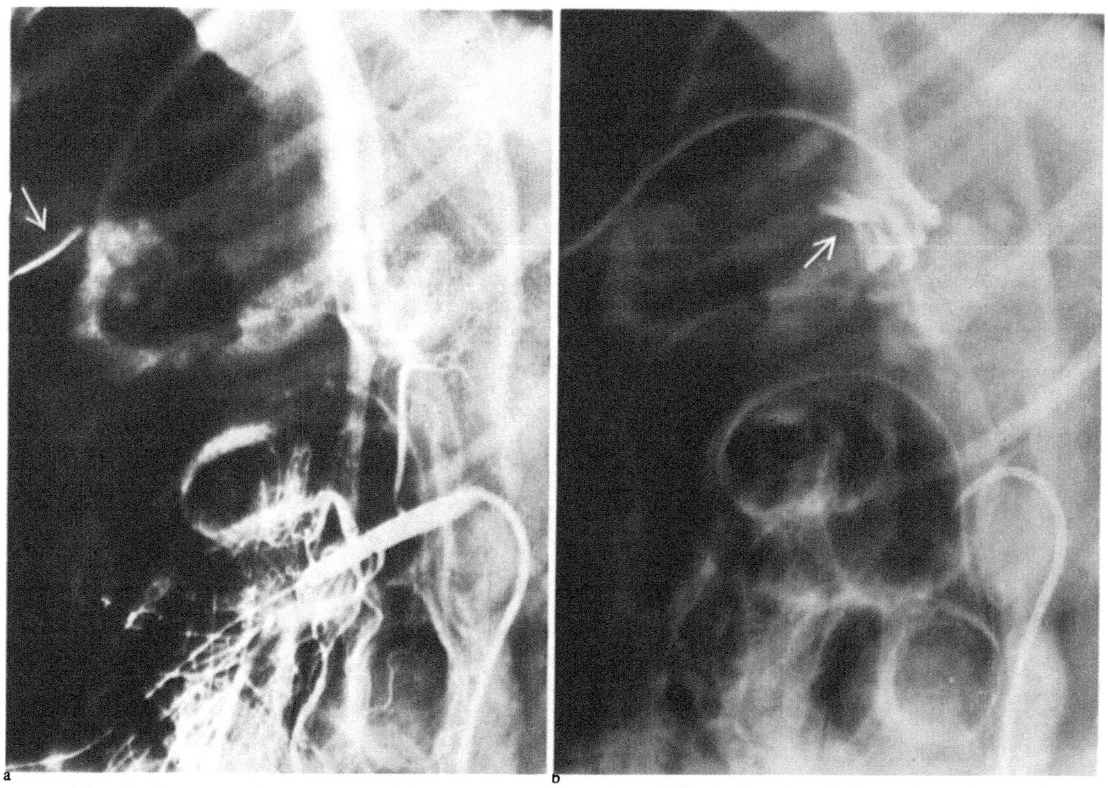

a

b

Fig. 70a and b. Experimental angiographic detection of bleeding into stomach. (a) Curved red Oedman catheter in superior mesenteric artery. Contrast medium in arterial branches as well as in the fixed catheter which has one end situated extracorporeally, visible in the upper left of the picture (arrow). (b) Three seconds after start of injection the contrast medium drained into visualizing an area of mucosa (arrow)

Fig. 71 a–c. Congenital aneurysmal dilatation of intra- and extrahepatic portal vein (portomegaly, LEGER). A six-year-old boy with gastrointestinal bleeding from esophageal varices and portal hypertension. Liver tissue histologically normal. (a) Picture of splenic and portal veins with aneurysmal dilatations in region of porta hepatis. Splenoportography. (b) Marked reflux of contrast medium into both the mesenteric vein and vena coronaria ventriculi. (c) Strong opacification of intrahepatic portal vein system with concomitant visualization of extensive varicose veins at level of cardia of stomach and esophagus

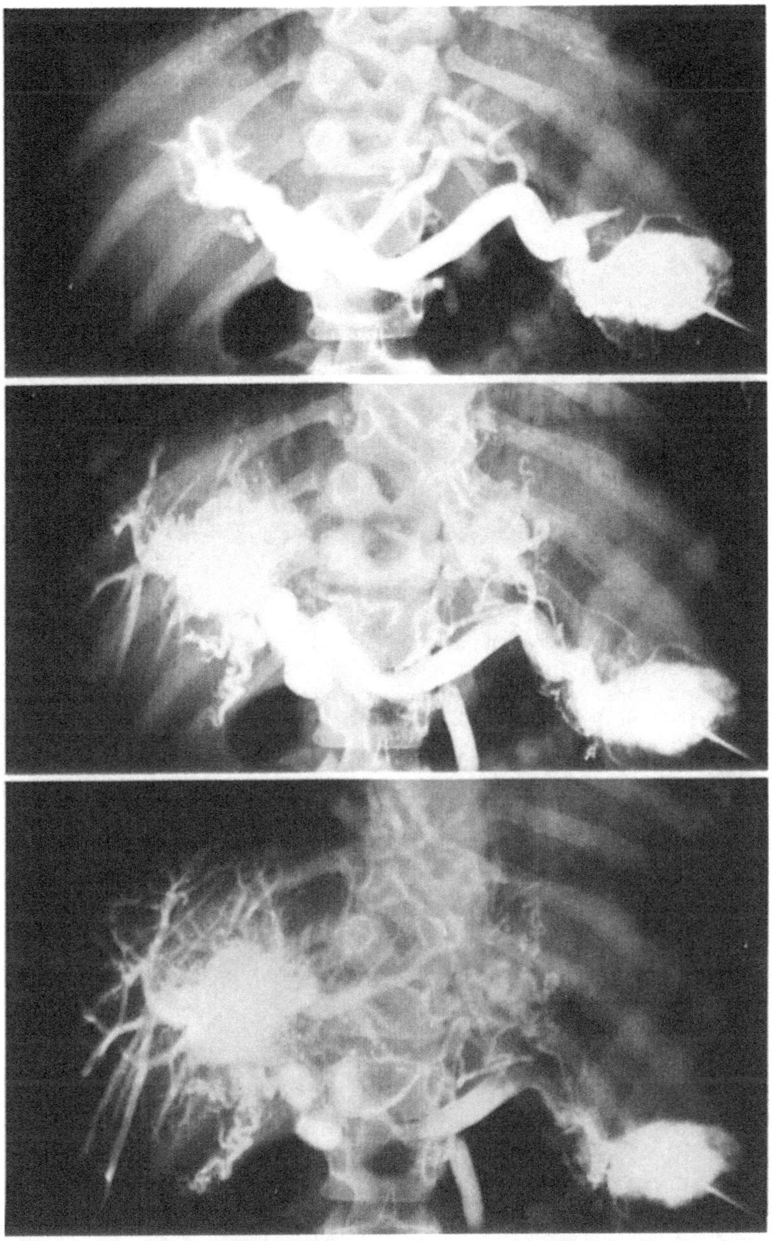

a b c

Fig. 72 a and b. (a) Cirrhosis of liver. Dilated splenic vein and portal vein. Sparse intrahepatic portal vein system. Vena coronaria ventriculi dilated to width of thumb. Intrasplenic pressure considerably elevated at 40 cm H_2O. Splenoportogram. (b) Late phase; picture of extremely dilated collateral vessels extending towards the esophagus

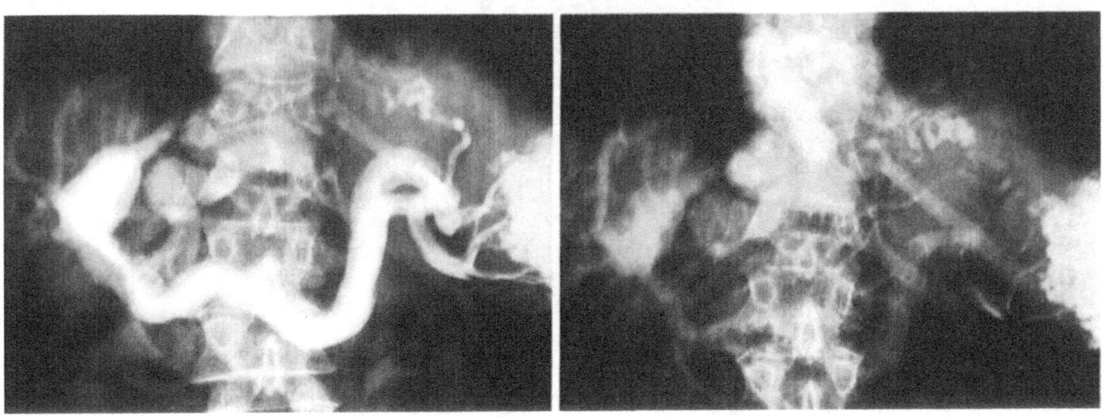

a b

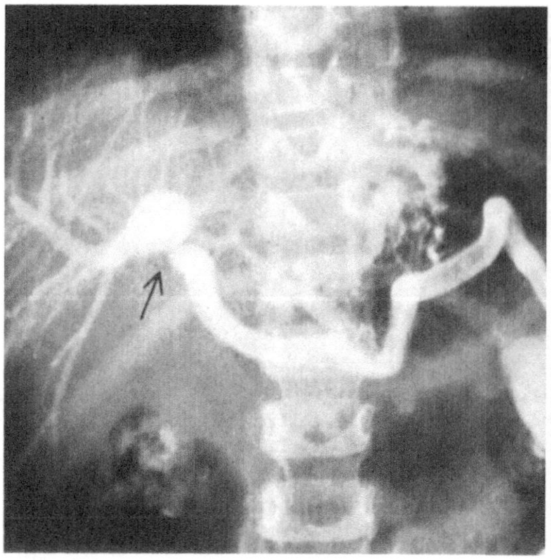

Fig. 73

Fig. 73. Congenital portal vein stenosis. At porta hepatis marked narrowing of trunk of portal vein with poststenotic aneurysmal dilatation (arrow). Bypass circulation through vena coronaria ventriculi. Portal hypertension (intrasplenic pressure 32 cm H_2O) in 10-year-old child. Splenoportogram

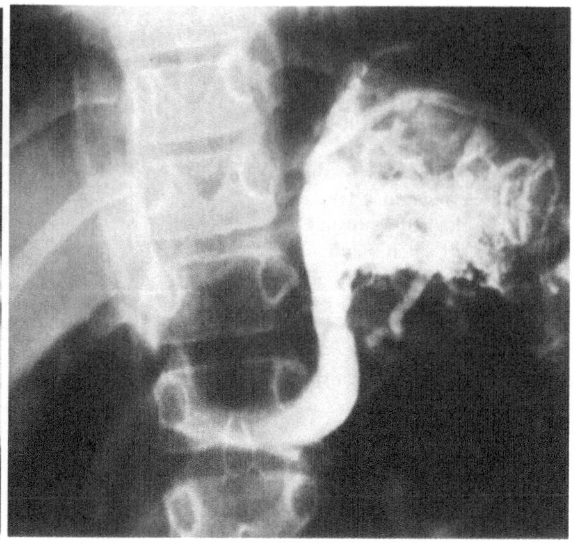

Fig. 74

Fig. 74. Thrombosis of portal vein after sepsis of umbilical cord. Spontaneous portocaval anastomosis in 8-year-old child with portal hypertension (intrasplenic pressure 20 cm H_2O). Splenoportogram with outline of numerous collateral veins, the splenic vein trunk, and direct outflow of contrast medium into inferior vena cava

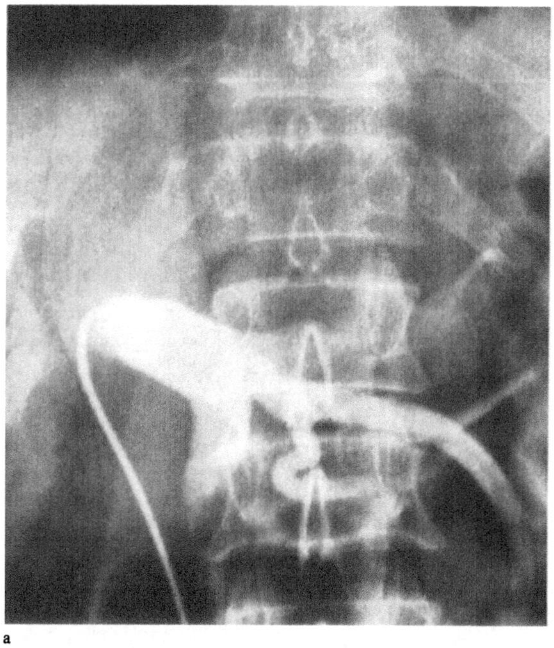

a

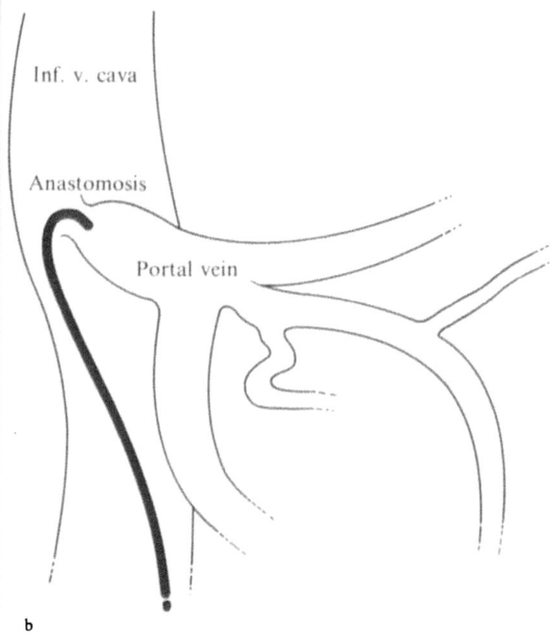

b

Fig. 75a and b. Portocaval anastomosis in cirrhosis of liver. (a) Angiographic picture of anastomosis; the contrast medium was injected through a catheter threaded into inferior vena cava and then inserted easily into the portal vein positioned end-to-side. (b) Explanatory diagram

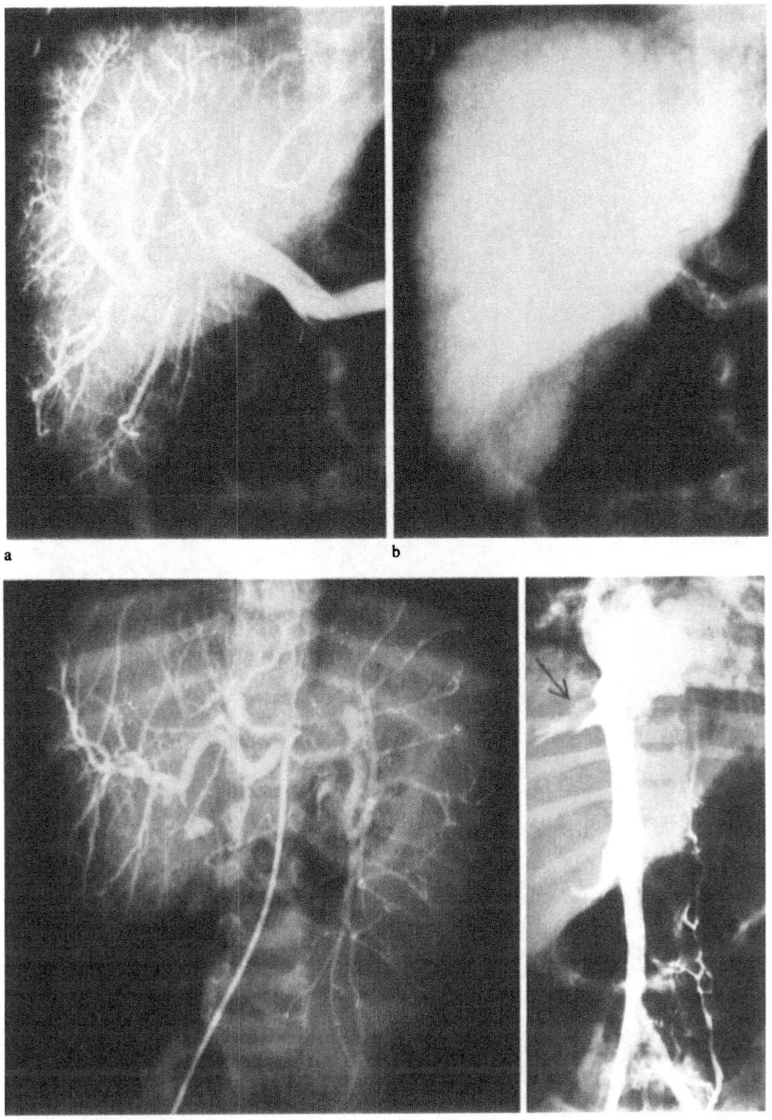

Fig. 76a–d. Budd-Chiari syndrome in four-year-old child. (a) Unremarkable distribution of portal vein branches in enlarged liver. Splenoportogram (intrasplenic pressure 30 cm H_2O). (b) Ivory-like opacification of liver in late phase of splenoportography as result of obstruction of outflow from hepatic veins. (c) Hepatosplenomegaly with widely splayed arterial branches. Selective angiography of celiac artery. (d) Thrombosis of hepatic veins at opening into inferior vena cava (arrow). Cavogram

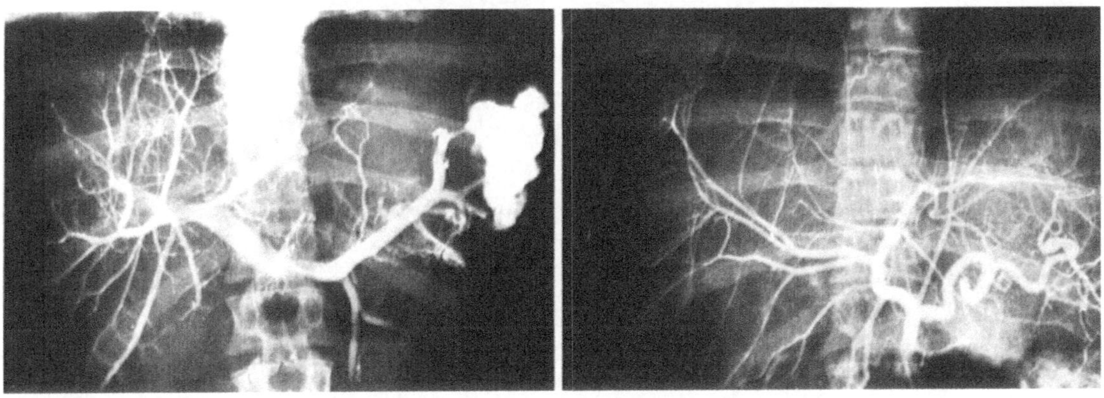

Fig. 77a and b. Budd-Chiari syndrome. (a) Unremarkable portal vein system with persisting contrast medium in enlarged liver. Portal hypertension (intrasplenic pressure 40 cm H_2O). Liver displaced from lateral stomach wall by ascites. Splenoportogram. (b) Arterial branches extremely splayed; hepatosplenomegaly. Selective angiography of celiac trunk

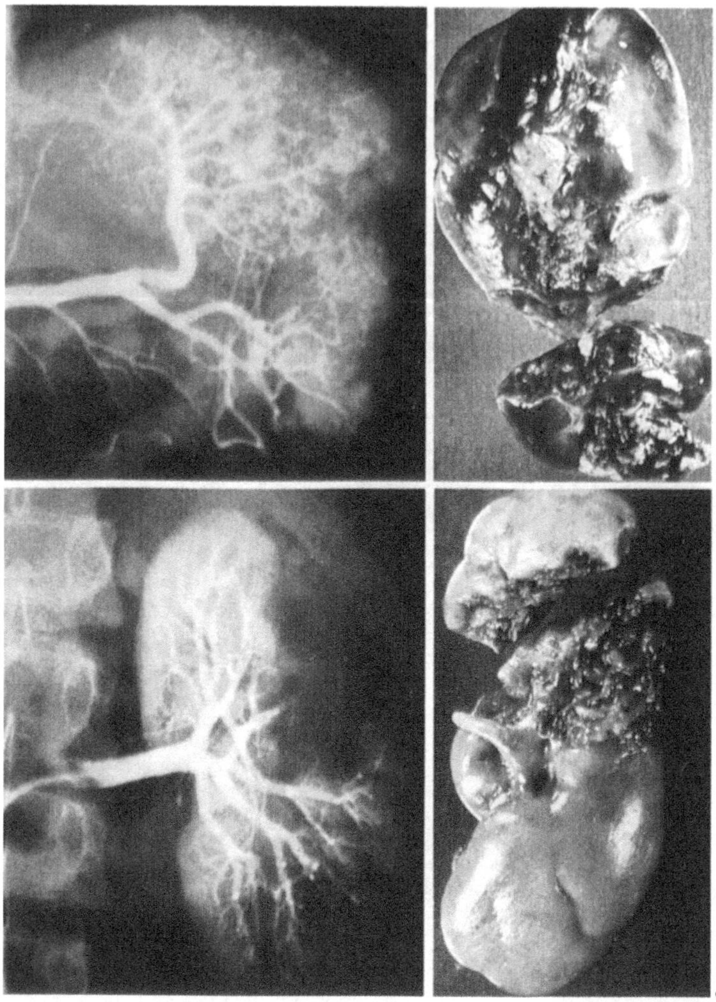

a b c d

Fig. 78 a–d. Compound rupture of spleen and kidney. (a) Transverse rupture of spleen (middle and lower thirds). Extravasation of contrast medium. Early contrast filling of splenic vein. Superselective angiography of splenic artery. (b) Surgical specimen. (c) Oblique rupture of left kidney. Vascular lacerations; cuneiform filling defect. Selective arteriography of left kidney. (d) Surgical specimen

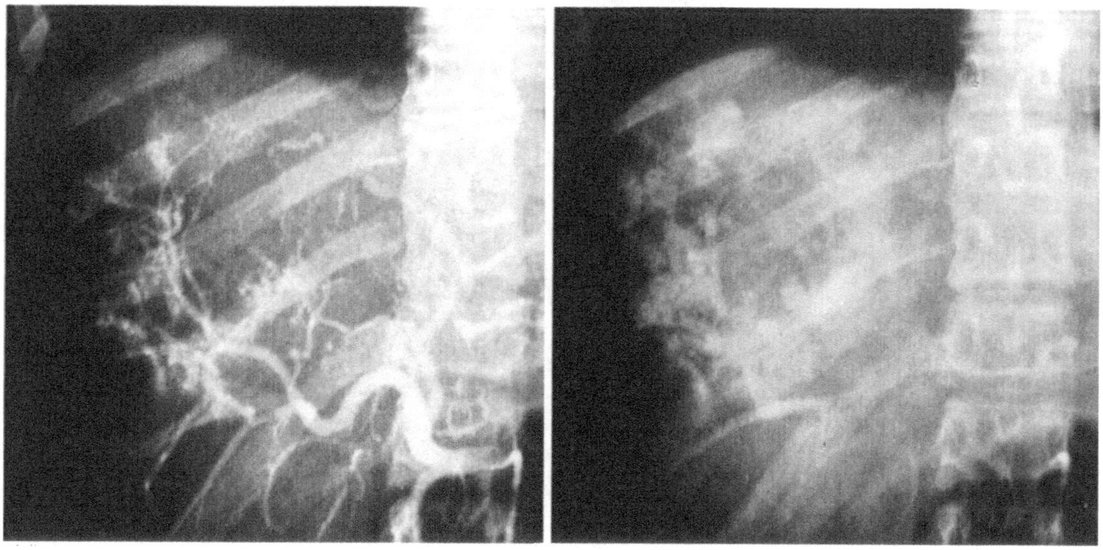

a b

Fig. 79 a and b. Ruptured liver in 17-year-old girl, traffic accident 3 days previously. Pains in upper right abdomen. No abdominal rigidity. (a) Multiple contrast medium extravasates in center of right lobe of liver with vascular avulsions. Angiogram of celiac artery. (b) Enlargement of contrast medium extravasates and parenchymal filling defects in late phase (surgically extensive rupture of right liver lobe)

Fig. 80a–c. Blunt abdominal injury with damage to spleen and pancreas in 15-year-old school girl kicked by a horse.

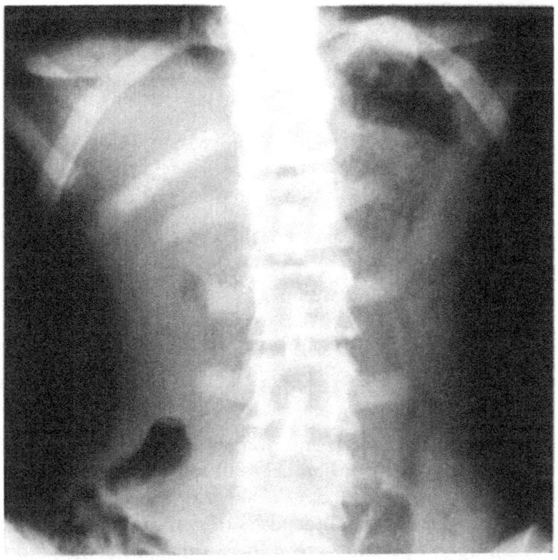

(a) Abdominal x-ray without contrast medium. Liver shadow poorly outlined.
Right psoas muscle effaced, spleen shadow enlarged, large stomach bubble. Convex scoliosis of lumbar vertebral column on left.

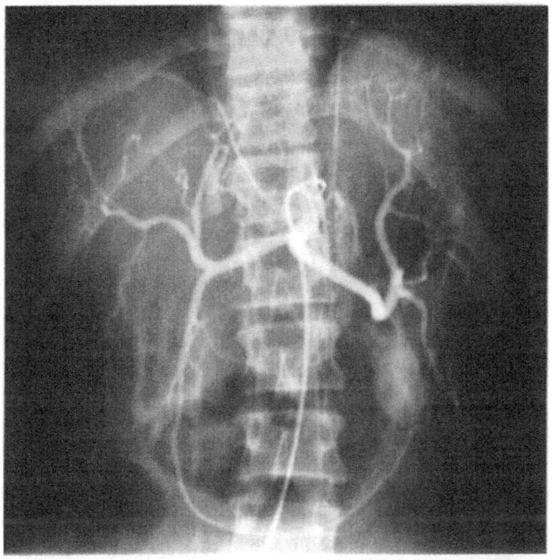

(b) Stretched common hepatic artery and marked extension of gastroduodenal and right gastroepiploic arteries. "String-of-pearls" on extended splenic artery. Selective angiogram of celiac trunk.

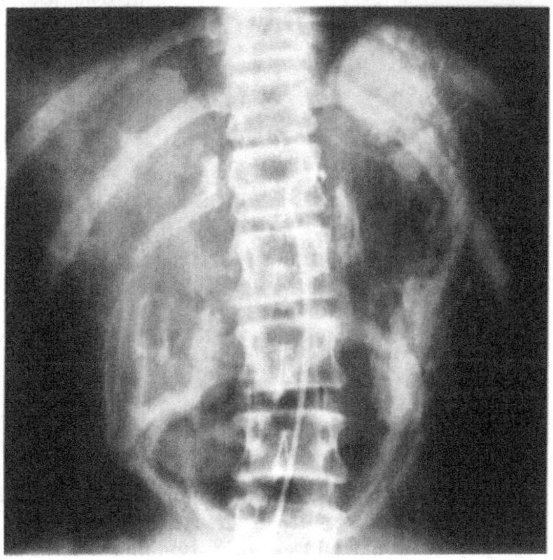

(c) Break in middle third of splenic parenchyma in the form of a transverse rupture. Accumulation of contrast medium further distally on greater curvature of stomach and near duodenum. The operation (Dr. Linder) confirmed the finding of a ruptured spleen, multiple hematomas, and involvement of the pancreas in the form of edematous swelling

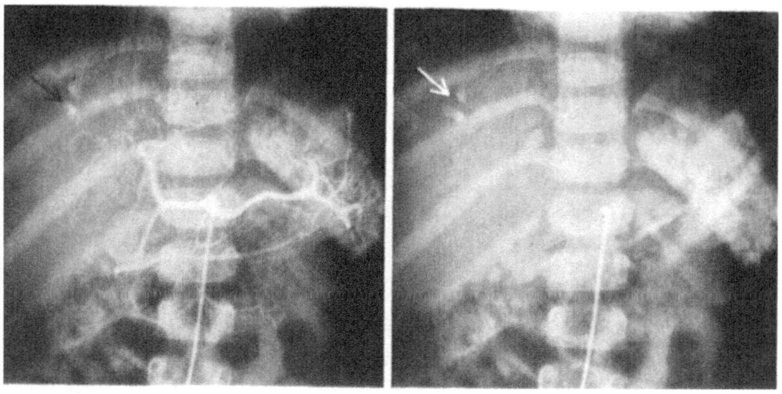

a b

Fig. 81 a and b. Spleen and liver injury. (a) Contrast medium extravasation in center of liver from branches of left hepatic artery (arrow). The right hepatic artery arises from the superior mesenteric artery. Celiac angiogram. (b) Persistence of small deposits of contrast medium in center of liver (arrow) which upon operation prove to be subcapsular hematomas due to torn liver capsule. Contours of spleen irregular; subcapsular hematomas also in this organ

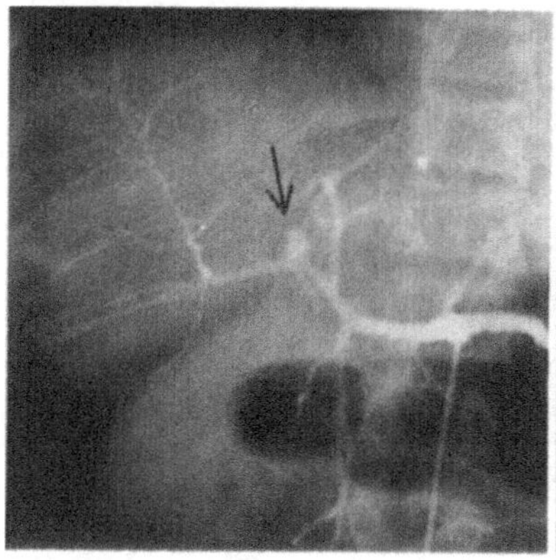

Fig. 82. Ruptured liver with traumatic aneurysm. Right hepatic artery with interrupted contour near porta hepatis. Visualization of small false aneurysm (arrow). Laceration of capsule at the same level confirmed on laparotomy. Celiac angiogram

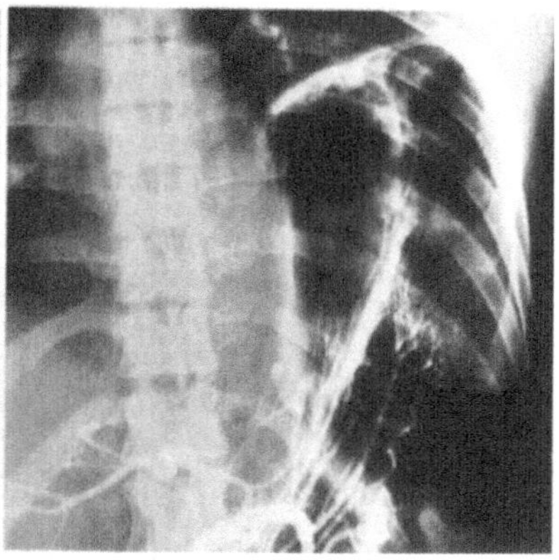

Fig. 83. Ruptured diaphragm on left with prolapse of several small bowel loops. Intrathoracic displacement of extremely taut jejunal arteries in selective angiography of superior mesenteric artery. Splenic rupture ruled out by angiography

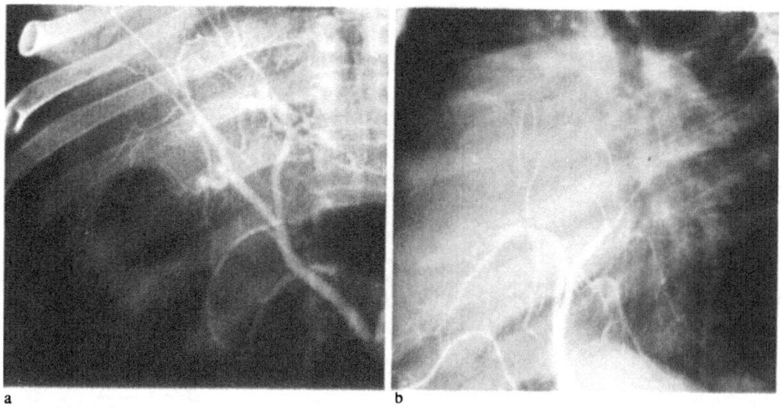

a b

Fig. 84a and b. Ruptured diaphragm on right with intrathoracic displacement of liver. (a) Detection of hepatic arteries extending into thorax by celiac angiography. (b) Lateral view. Liver rupture ruled out

a b c

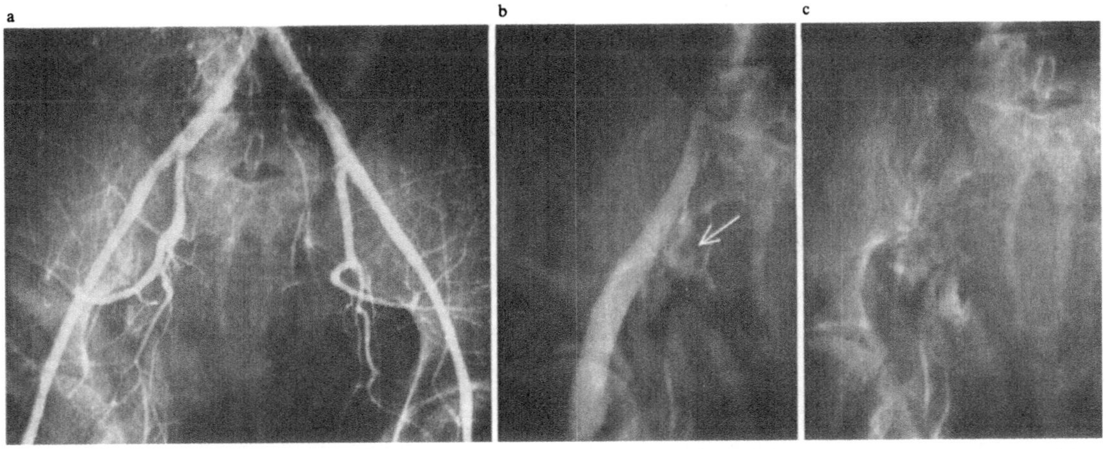

Fig. 85a–c. Blunt abdominal injury with venous rupture. (a) The arterial network in the pelvic region is unremarkable. Catheter aortogram. (b) Direct visualization of the right iliac vein reveals constriction at level of right lateral wing of sacrum, showing a fracture. Incipient contrast medium extravasation with rapid distribution caudad (arrow). (c) Persistence of contrast medium extravasates in a case of iliac vein rupture

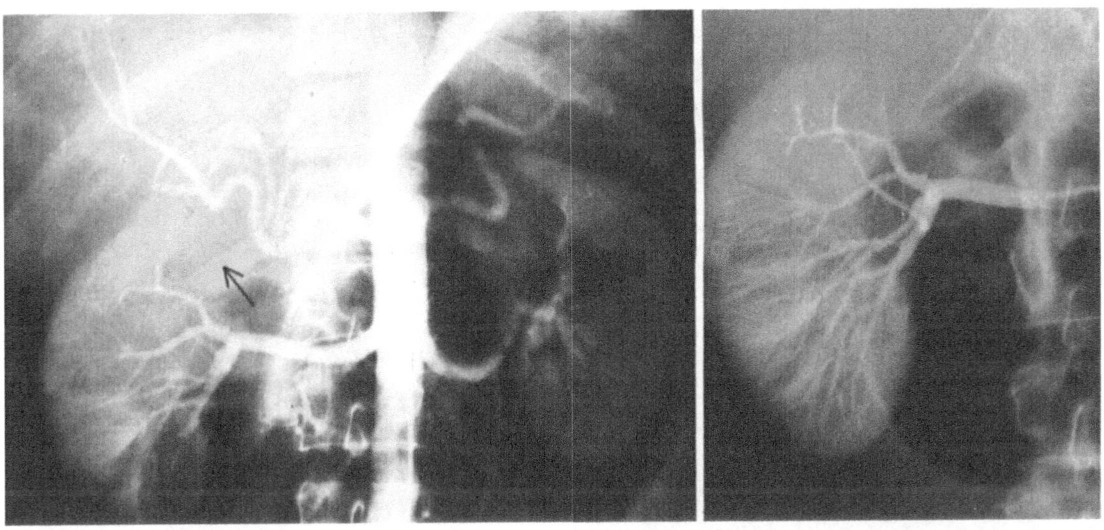

a b

Fig. 86a and b. Blunt abdominal injury – retroperitoneal hematoma. (a) Unremarkable distribution of aortic branches with extremely tympanous stomach. The upper medial portion of right kidney is not visualized (arrow). Catheter aortogram. (b) Identical findings in right kidney on selective angiogram of that organ. Surgery disclosed extensive retroperitoneal hematoma on the right with compression of upper part of right kidney

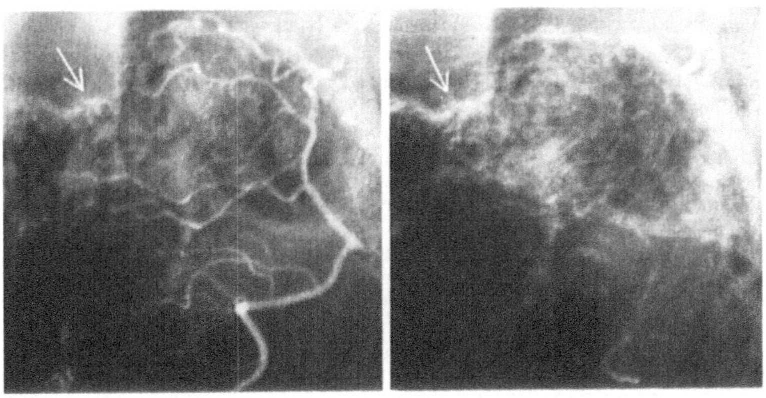

Fig. 87a Fig. 87b

Fig. 87a and b. Rupture of right colic flexure. Blunt abdominal injury with ambiguous symptoms in right upper abdomen. No clear signs of free perforation. (a) Irregular outline of large-intestine wall at level of hepatic flexure, adjacent vessels exhibiting a corkscrew course (arrow). Selective angiography of superior mesenteric artery. (b) Interrupted contour more distinct in parenchymal phase (arrow). Extensive hematoma in vicinity of right colic flexure, with sealed perforation. revealed on laparotomy

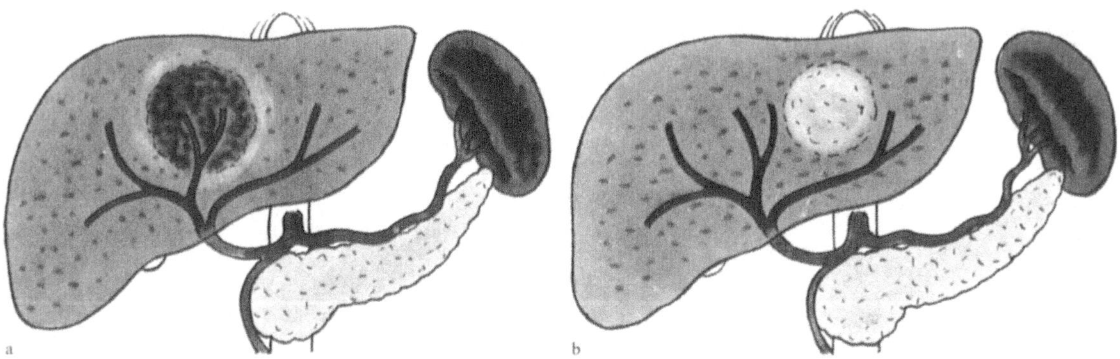

Fig. 88a and b. (a) Angiographic tumor opacification. (b) Angiographic tumor radiolucency

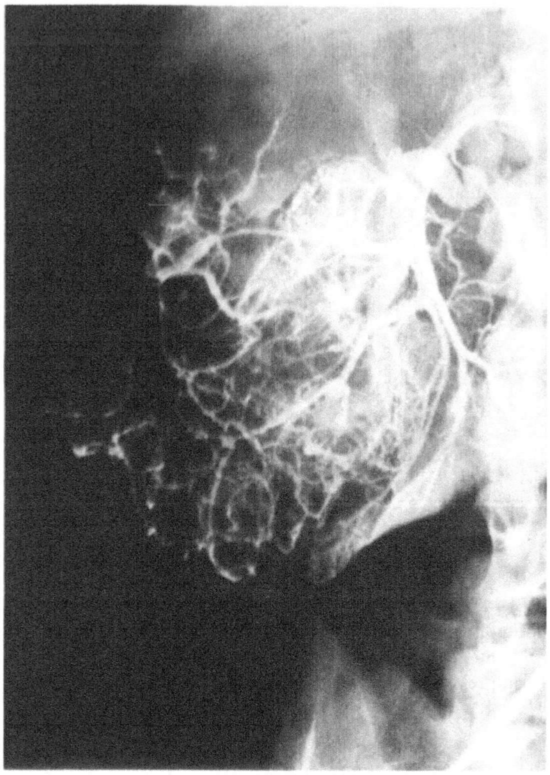

Fig. 89

Fig. 89. Hypernephroma: Highly vascularized tumor with pathological vessels. Pools of blood, arteriovenous shunt connections, destruction of parenchyma, and infiltration of surrounding tissue. Selective angiography of right renal artery

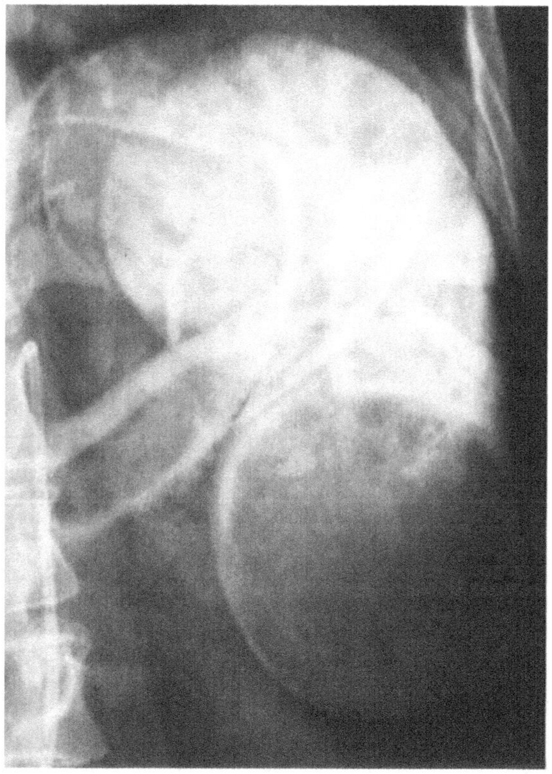

Fig. 90

Fig. 90. Splenic cyst. Tennis ball-sized radiolucency in parenchymal phase of superselective angiogram of splenic artery. Surgery: Isolated cyst at lower pole of spleen

---

Fig. 91. Cylindromatous metastasis of left liver lobe. Condition after extirpation of cylindroma on left lower jaw. Palpable tumor in left upper abdomen. Celiac angiography disclosed an atypical leftward deflection of left hepatic artery supplying a richly vascularized tumor the size of a child's head, with pathological vessels and unclear outline in the caudal portions. Surgery (Dr. E. GOGLER) disclosed a cylindromatous metastasis pervading the left liver lobe, which was extirpated

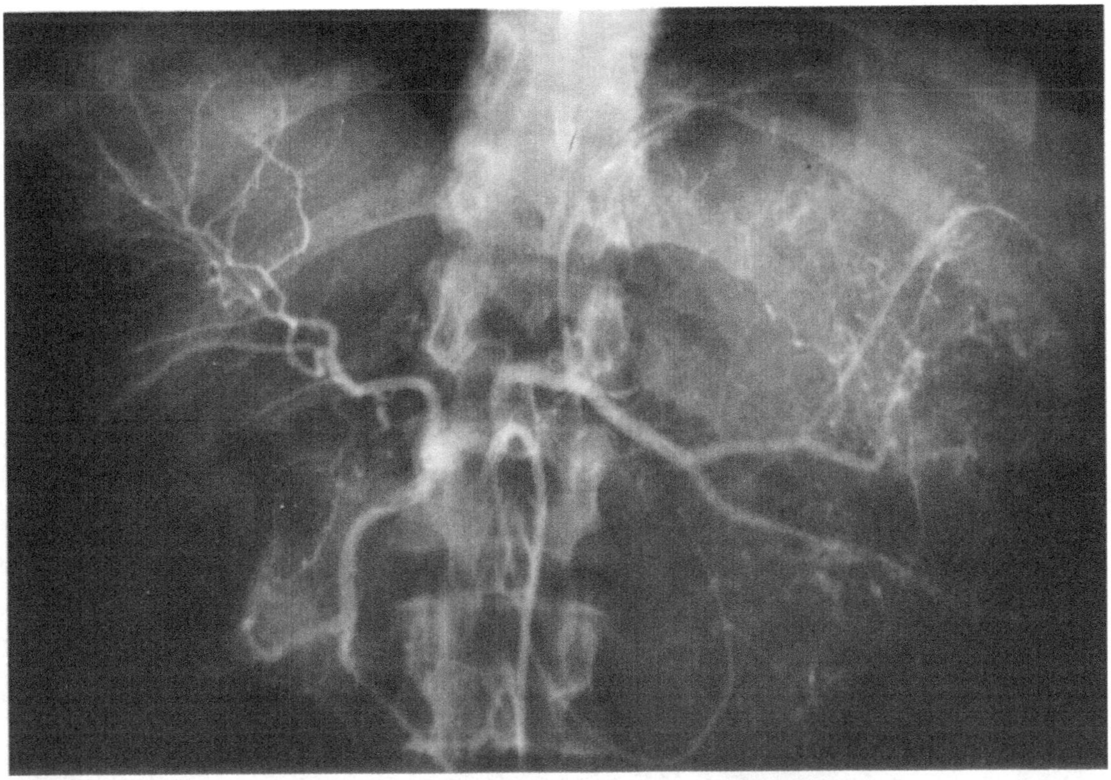

Fig. 91 (Legend see p. 156)

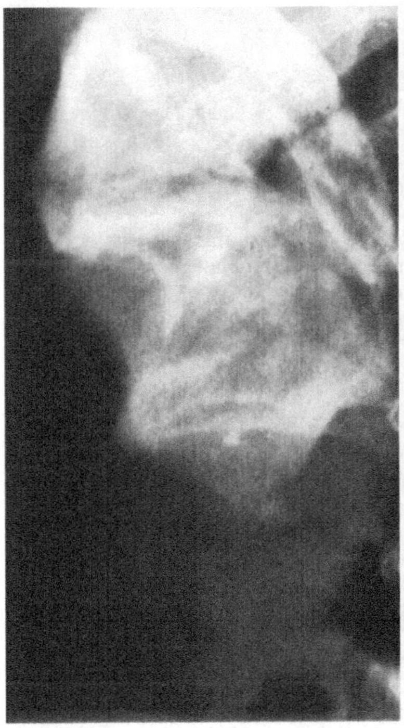

Fig. 92

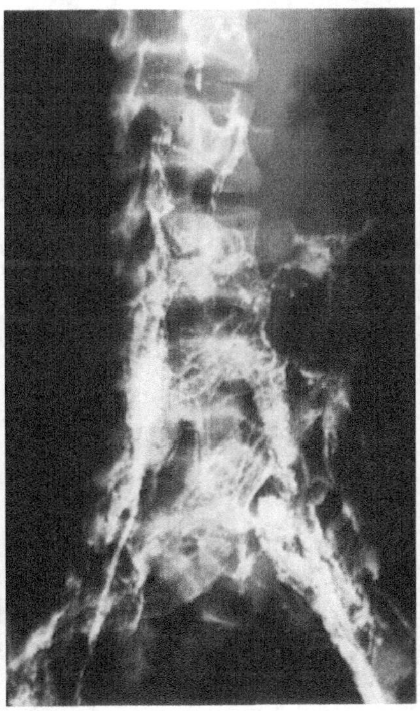

Fig. 93

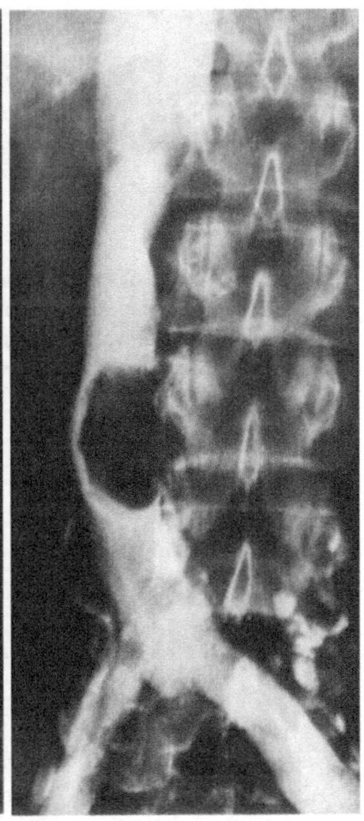

Fig. 94

Fig. 92. Subcapsular filling defects of right kidney owing to multiple hematomas after injury during anticoagulant therapy. Parenchymal phase of selective renal arteriogram

Fig. 93. Para-aortic seminomatous metastases. Filling defects and signs of displacement in lymphangiogram

Fig. 94. Metastasis of teratoid scrotol carcinoma. Clearly outlined egg-sized filling defect in inferior vena cava. Cavogram

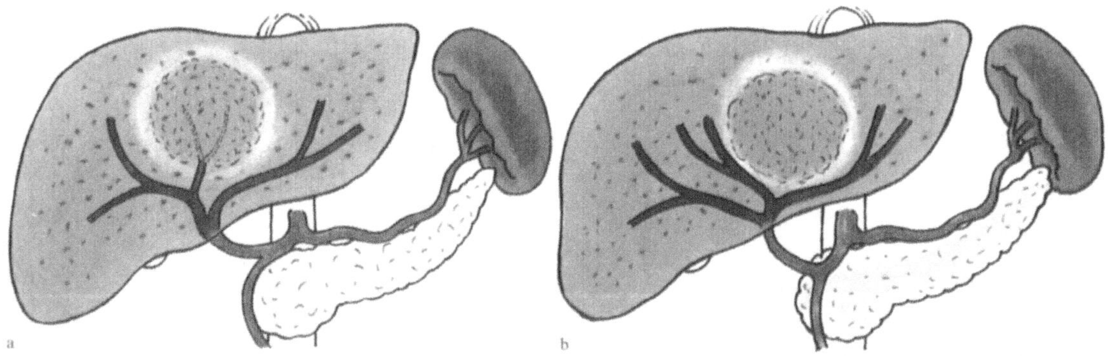

Fig. 95 a and b. (a) Vascular stenoses or occlusions due to tumor growth in angiogram. (b) Vascular displacements due to tumor growth in angiogram

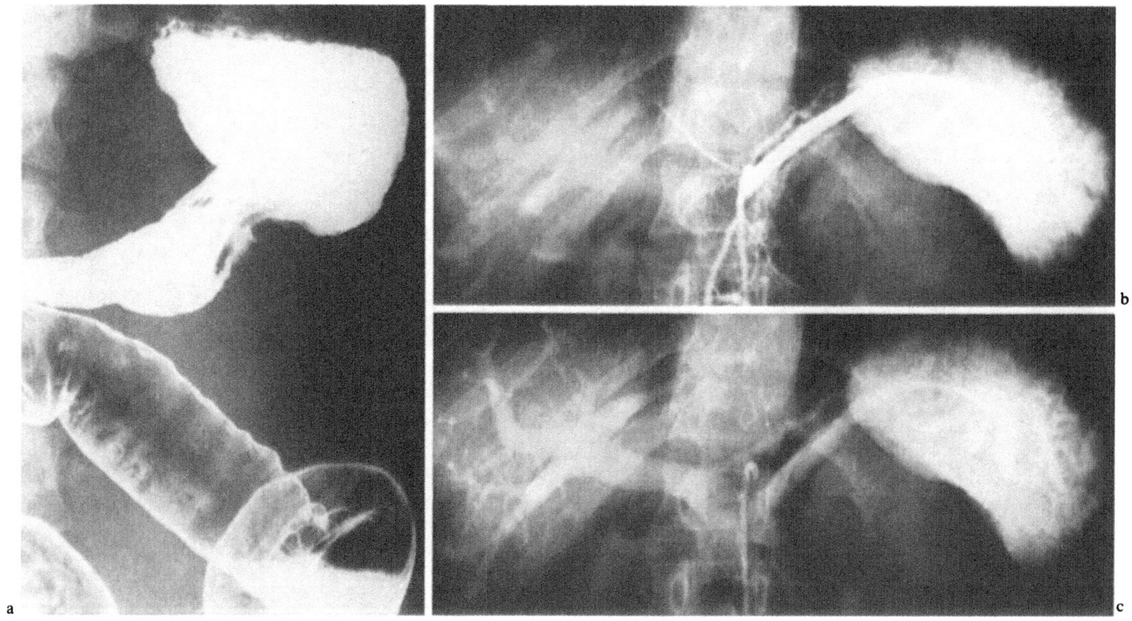

Fig. 96 a–c. Tumor of tail of pancreas. (a) Simultaneous visualization of stomach and colon. (b) Splenic artery elevated. Spleen not enlarged. Selective angiography of splenic artery. (c) Elevation and compression of splenic vein in arterioportogram

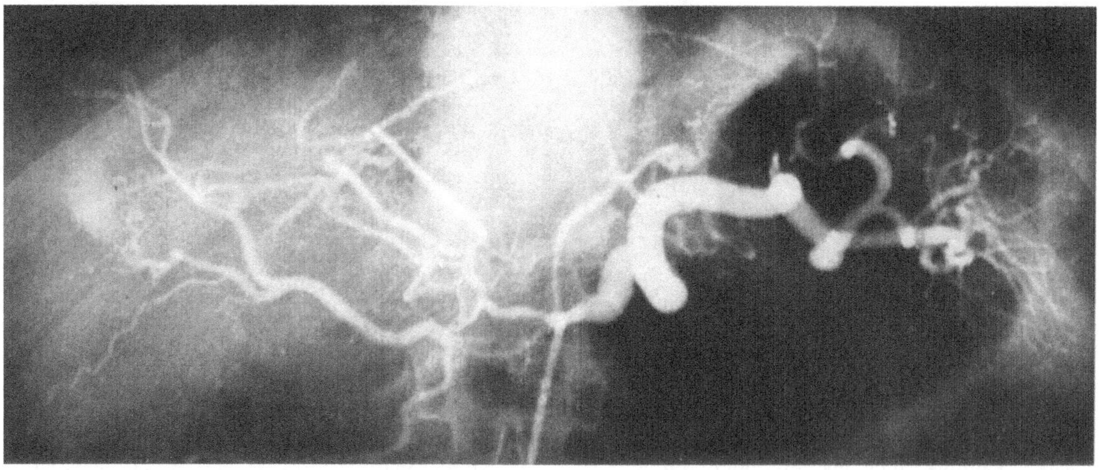

Fig. 97. Pancreatic carcinoma. Severe stenosis of common hepatic artery and origin of splenic artery. Celiac angiogram

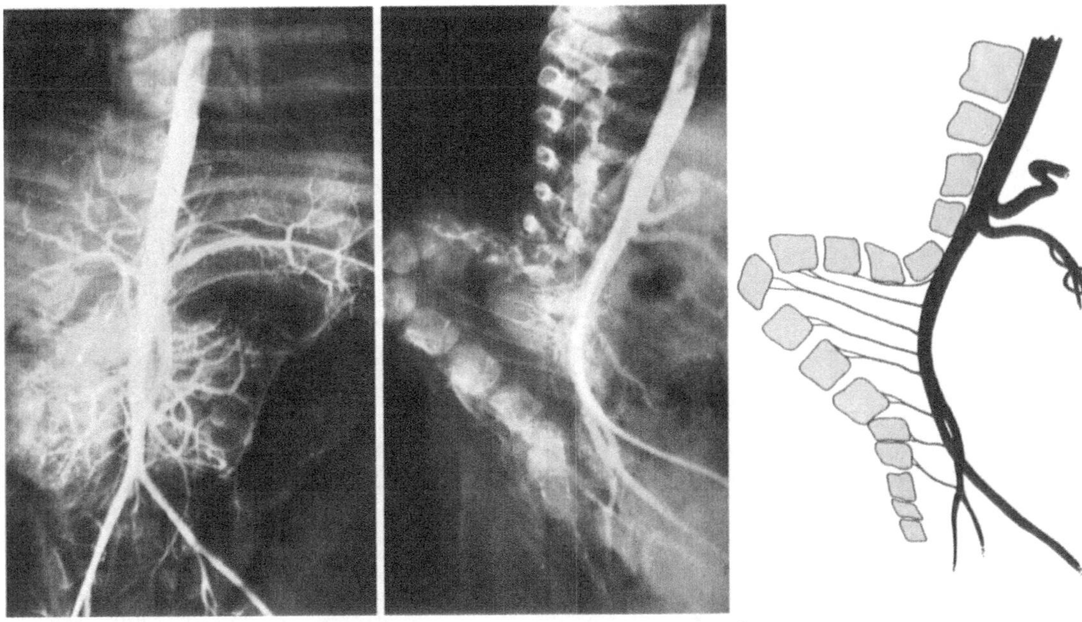

a b c

Fig. 98 a–c. Severe lumbar kyphoscoliosis with myelomeningocele. A four-year-old child scheduled for corrective surgery. (a) Catheter aortogram in anteroposterior view. (b) Anatomic relation between aorta and spinal column with greatly stretched lumbar branches. (c) Diagram

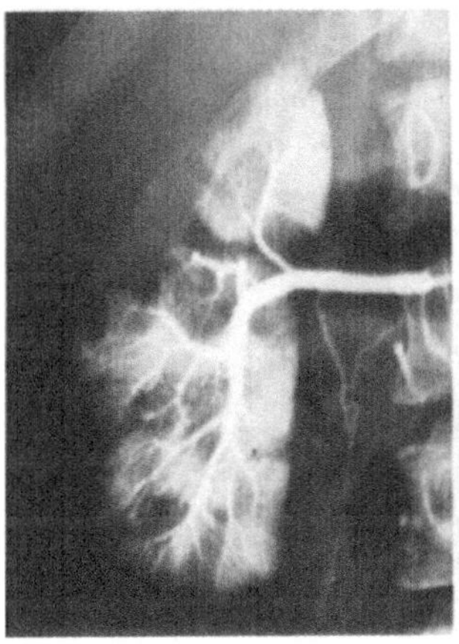

Fig. 99

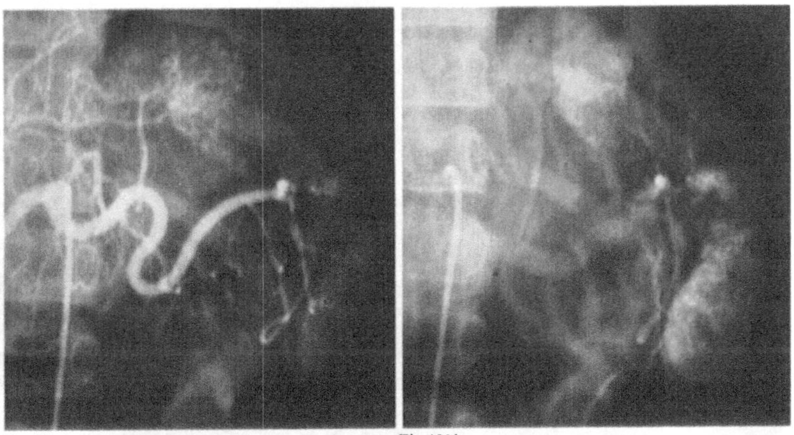

Fig. 100a Fig. 100b

Fig. 99. Ruptured right kidney. Transverse rupture of upper pole of kidney. Avulsions of renal arteries and parenchymal lesions. Selective angiogram of right renal artery. Picture of arteries of the renal pelvis and the ureteral artery

Fig. 100a and b. Ruptured spleen. (a) Avulsions of several arterial branches in early phase of celiac angiography. (b) Parenchymal phase with visualization of separated or disrupted fragments of spleen and marked filling of splenic vein

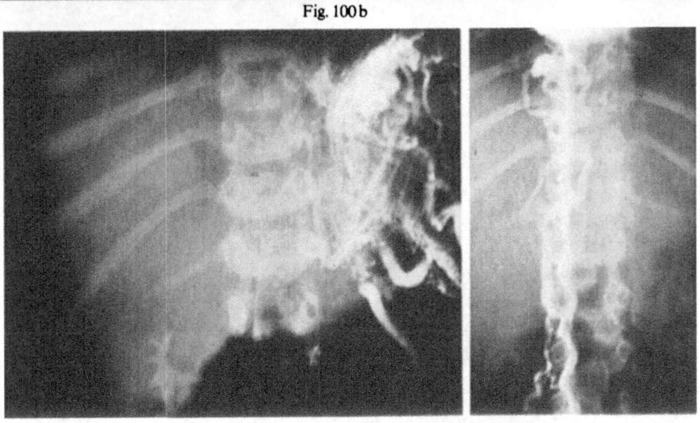

Fig. 101a Fig. 101b

Fig. 101 a and b. Primary liver carcinoma. (a) Total occlusion of portal vein with visualization of numerous collateral veins; liver shadow enlarged. Splenoportogram. (b) Total occlusion of inferior vena cava by liver tumor. Ladder-like collaterals of predominantly vertebral branches

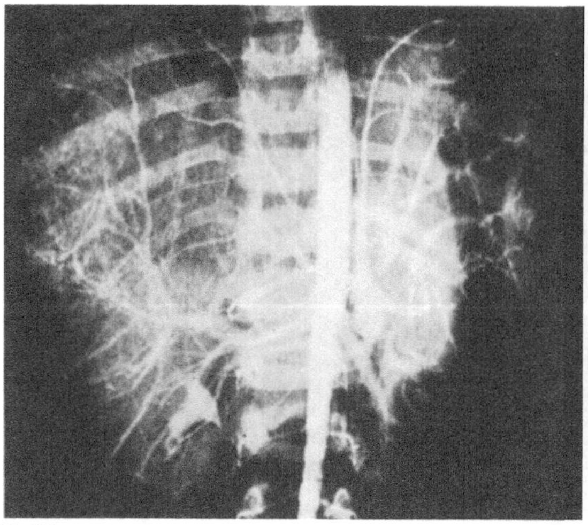

Fig. 102a

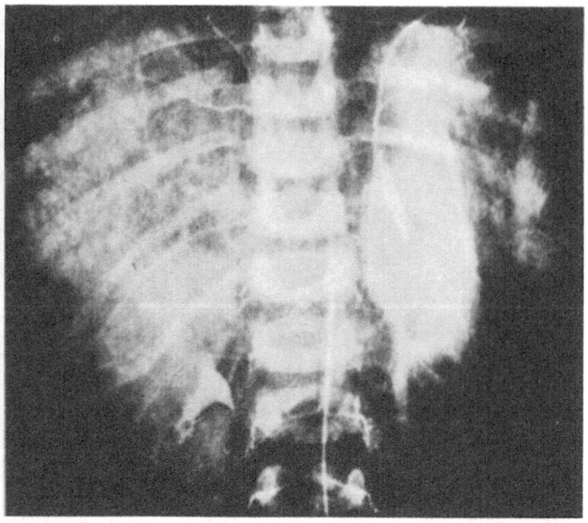

Fig. 102b

Fig. 102a and b. Malignant teratoma metastases of liver. (a) Flush aortography. Arcuate caudalward displacement of common hepatic artery. Pathological vessels visualized via hepatic artery in distinctly enlarged liver.
(b) Uneven opacification of liver parenchyma; pools of blood and radiolucencies in venous phase

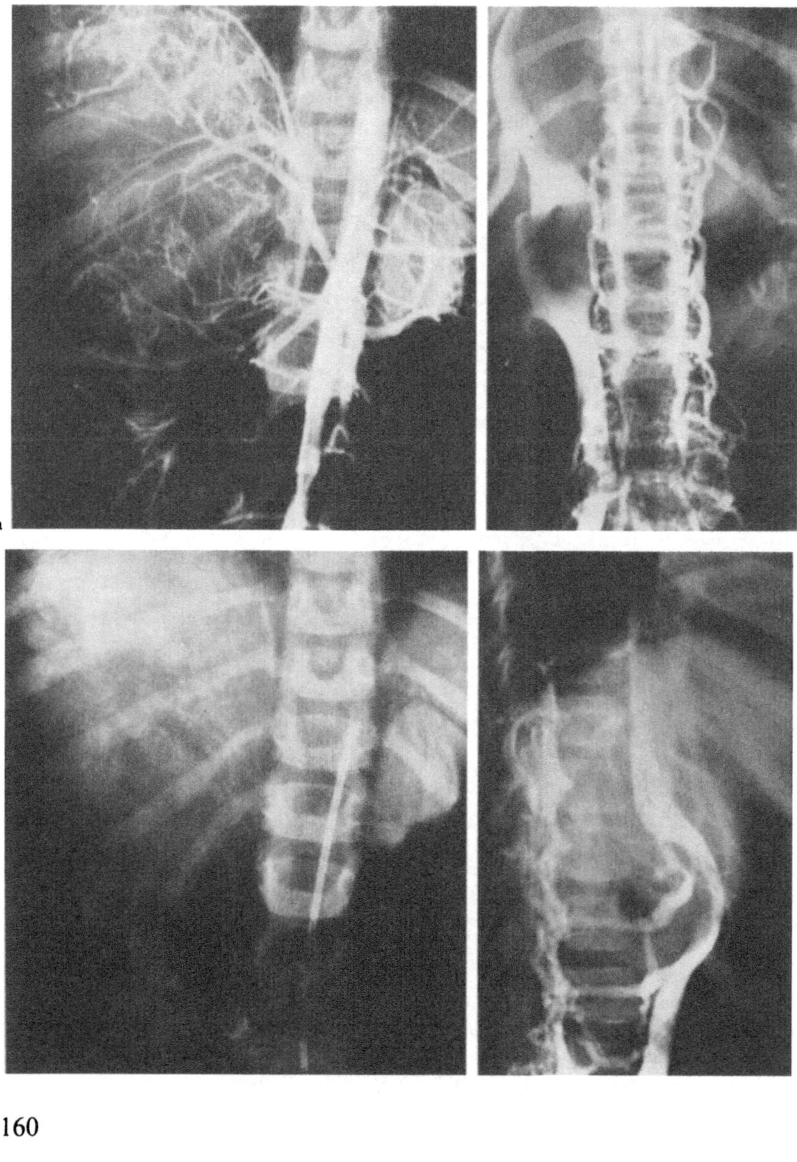

a c b d

Fig. 103a–d. Adrenal carcinoma. (a) Richly vascularized tumor the size of a child's head projected on to right hypochondrium and supplied by adrenal arteries with the diameter of a finger. Catheter aortogram.
(b) Irregular tumor staining with plaque-like calcific deposits. Parenchymal phase. (c) Three years after extirpation of tumor, para-aortic lymph node metastases with impression upon inferior vena cava. Clearly outlined egg-sized displacement area at level of first and second lumbar vertebrae in cavogram.
(d) Displacement of inferior vena cava with compression from dorsal side in lateral view

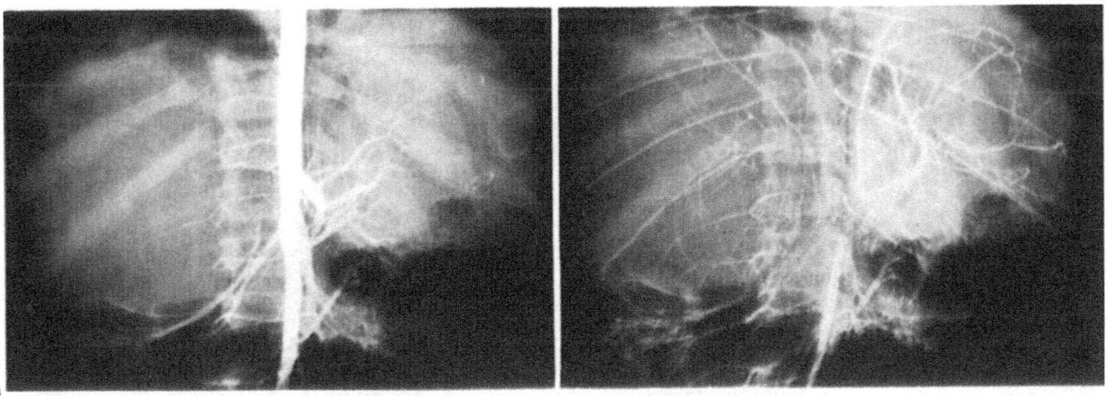

a b

Fig. 104a and b. Sympathicoblastoma on the right. (a) Tumor the size of a child's head displacing renal and hepatic vessels caudad. Catheter aortography. (b) Tumor supplied mainly through intercostal, lumbar, and suprarenal arteries

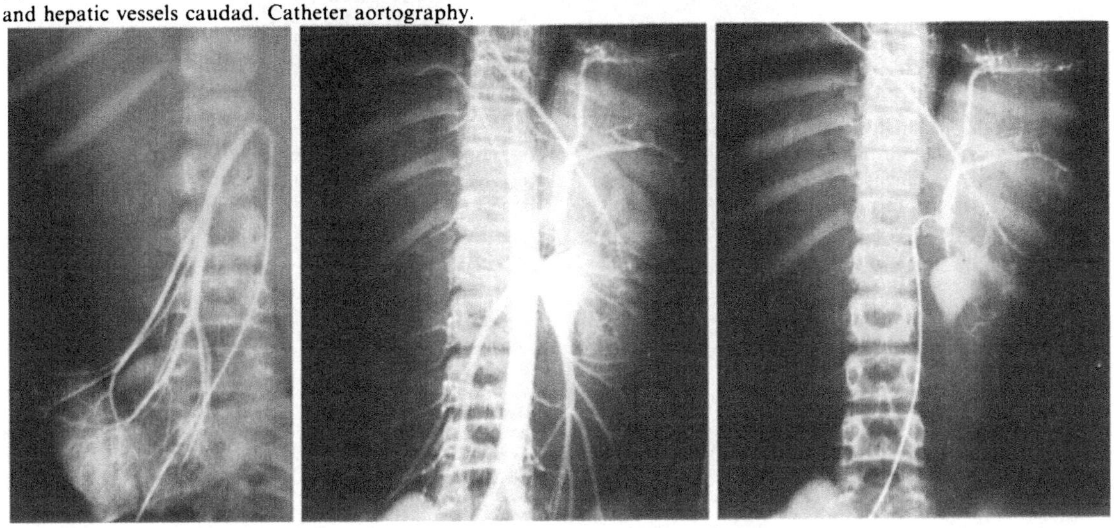

a b c

Fig. 105a–c. Giant cyst in right kidney. (a) Selective renal angiography. Right renal artery stretched caudad. The kidney is tilted and impressed by the large cyst. (b) Flush aortogram. Leftward displacement of celiac trunk. Marked displacement of right hepatic artery under diaphragm. The right kidney is seen in projection on right crest of ilium. (c) Celiac arteriogram. The celiac artery is deflected to the left. The right hepatic artery is displaced under the diaphragm. Surgery revealed a cyst of 5 L volume in the right kidney

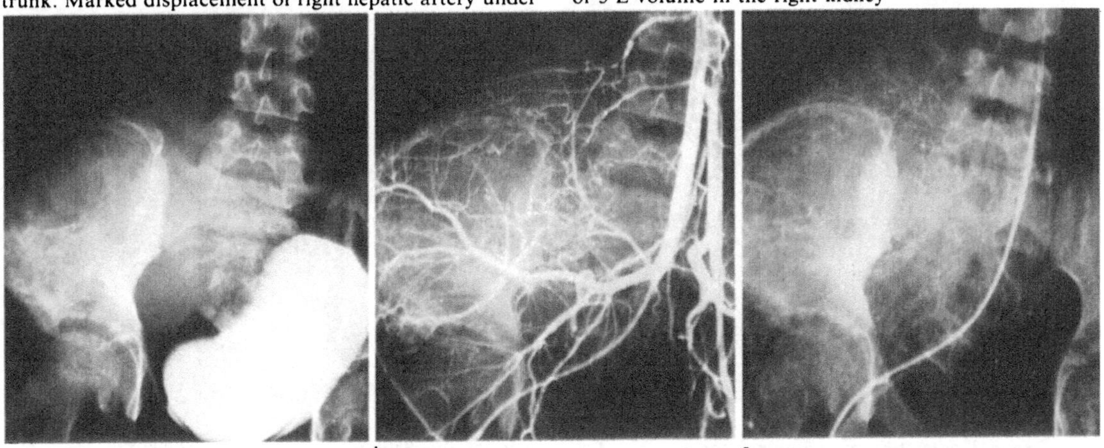

a b c

Fig. 106a–c. Hemangioblastoma of right pelvis. (a) Extensive osteolytic bone lesion of right upper part of ilium. Shadow of soft tumor tissue the size of a child's head with displacement of right bladder wall. (b) Marked vascularization of tumor via branches of internal iliac artery. Trunk of common iliac artery displaced leftward. Catheter aortogram. (c) Marked "tumor staining" in parenchymal phase

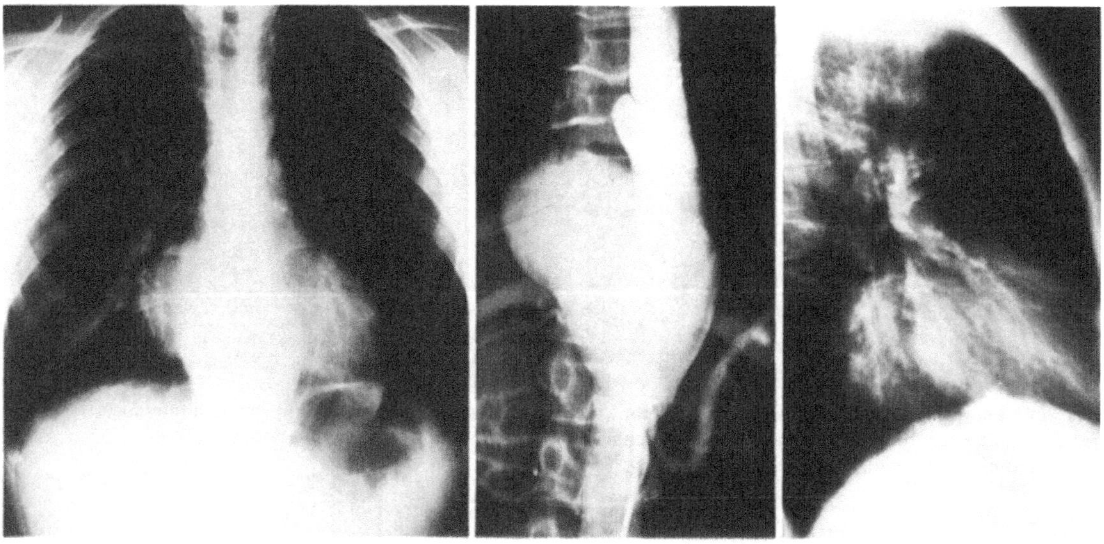

a b c

Fig. 107a–c. Congenital thoraco-abdominal aortic aneurysm (so-called aortic diverticulum). (a) Tumorous prominence at right margin of heart. Chest x-ray. (b) Fusiform aneurysm above origin of celiac artery extending mostly to the right. More proximally, circumscribed, bud-like prominence on descending aorta. Catheter aortogram. (c) The aneurysm shadow suggesting a tumor in lateral thoracic view

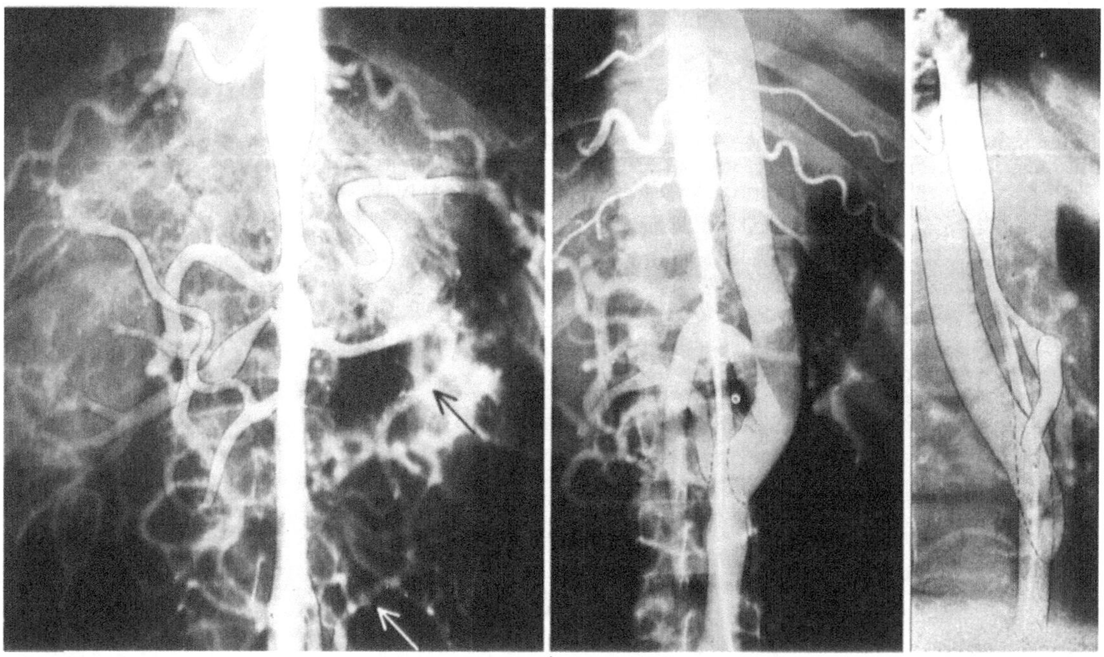

a b c

Fig. 108a–c. Coarctation of abdominal aorta. (a) Segmental, fusiform narrowing of aortic lumen involving origin of celiac artery. Stenosis of celiac and superior mesenteric arteries. Stenosis of right renal artery. Dilated collateral vessels (intercostal arteries and Riolan's anastomosis; see arrow). Catheter aortogram. (b) Bypass of stenosis with Dacron prosthesis (Dr. J. VOLLMAR). Catheter aortogram. (c) Lateral view

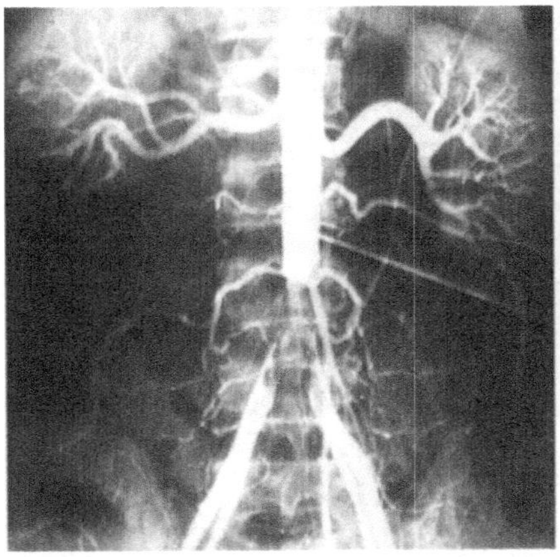

Fig. 109. Embolism at bifurcation ("straddling embolus"). Translumbar aortogram

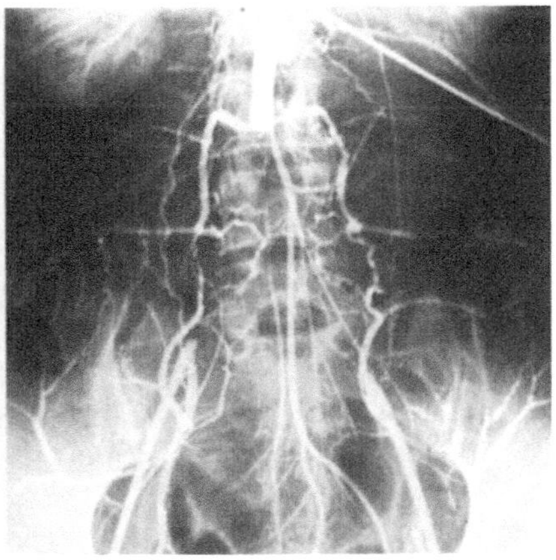

Fig. 110. Thrombosis of distal abdominal aorta and common iliac arteries. Collateralization mainly via lumbar branches. High translumbar aortogram

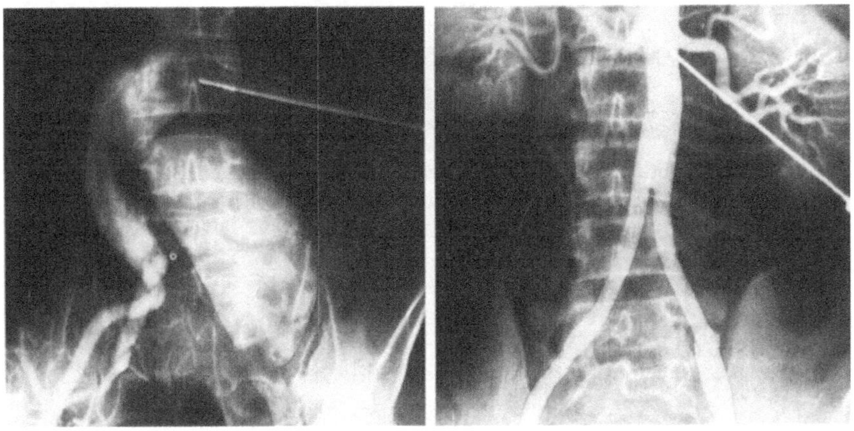

a b

Fig. 111a and b. (a) Aneurysm of aorta and common iliac artery. The aneurysm continues leftward to the inguinal region. Translumbar aortogram. (b) Postoperative angiogram after extirpation of aneurysm and aortofemoral bypass (Dr. VOLLMAR)

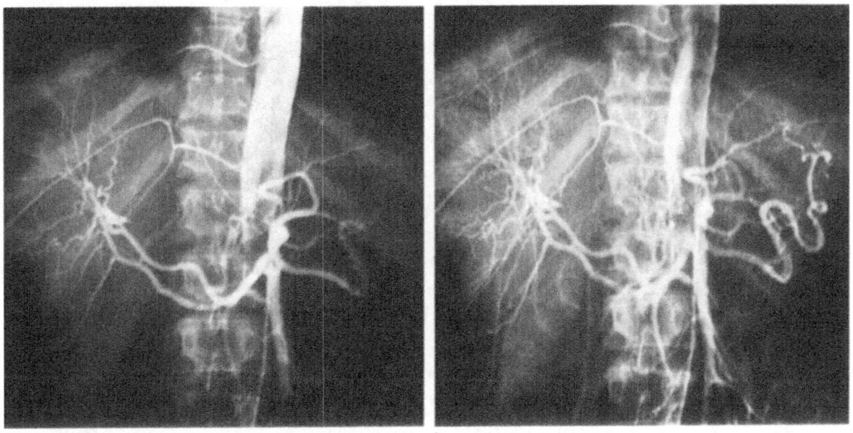

a b

Fig. 112a and b. (a) Dissecting aneurysm of aorta. Opacification of descending aorta, right intercostal arteries, celiac trunk, and superior mesenteric artery. Catheter aortogram. (b) Double lumen within thoracic aorta in late phase. No visualization of abdominal aorta and its branches below origin of superior mesenteric artery

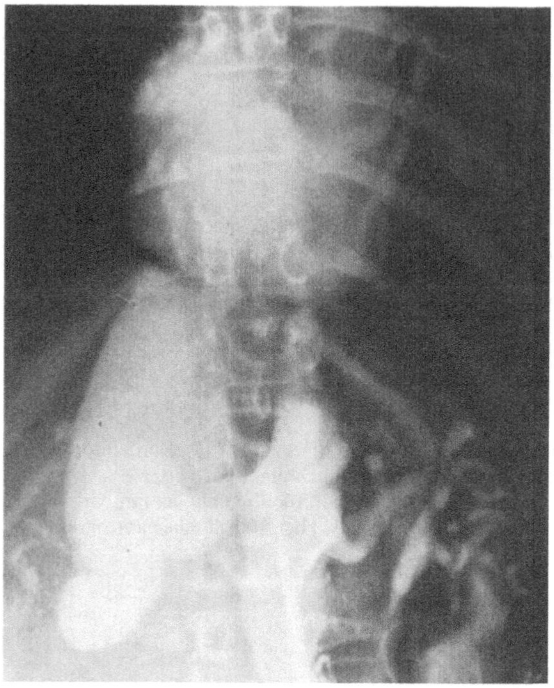

a

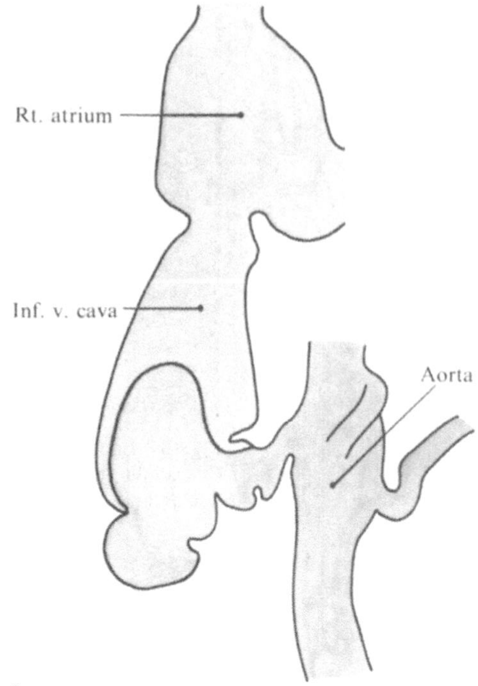

b

Fig. 113a and b. Aortocaval fistula. (a) 19 years after removal of right kidney. Bruit in middle abdomen. Angiographic demonstration of shunt between abdominal aorta and aneurysmally dilated inferior vena cava above stump of renal artery. Catheter aortogram. (b) Diagram

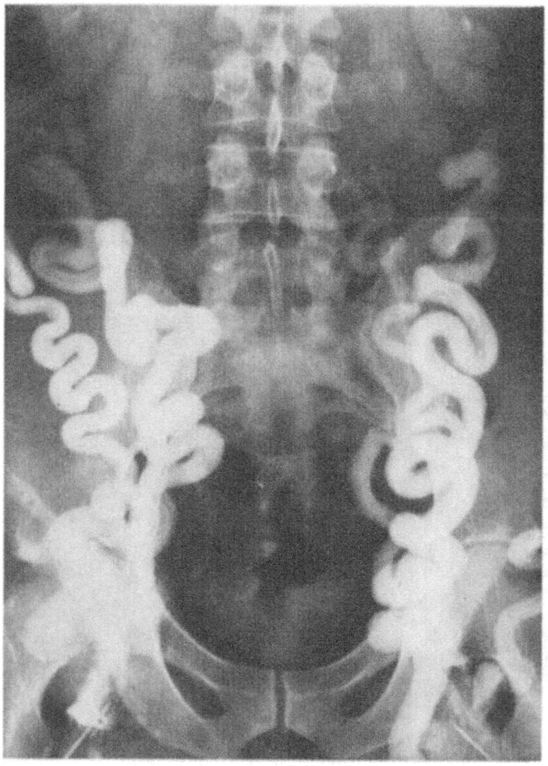

a

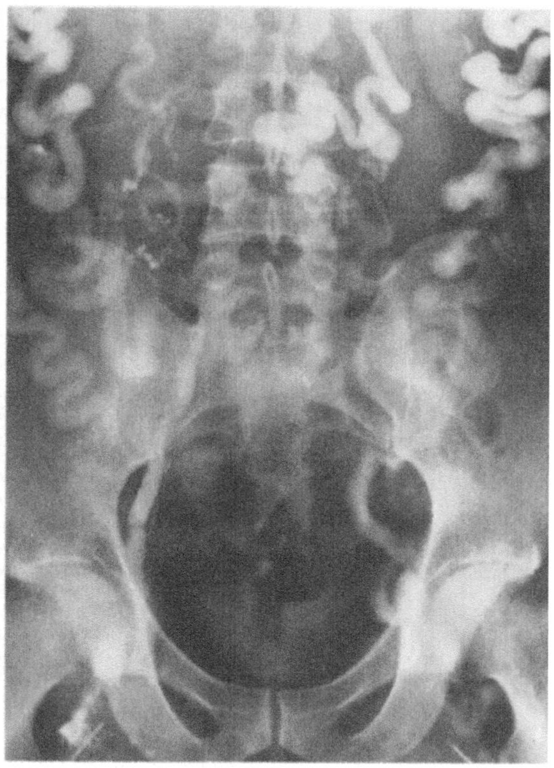

b

Fig. 114a and b. Total occlusion of inferior vena cava and pelvic arteries. (a) Picture of enormously dilated collaterals in abdominal wall, with garland-like filling in cranial direction. Angiogram of pelvic veins on both sides. (b) Still no visualization of ascending lumbar vein and vertebral veins in late phase

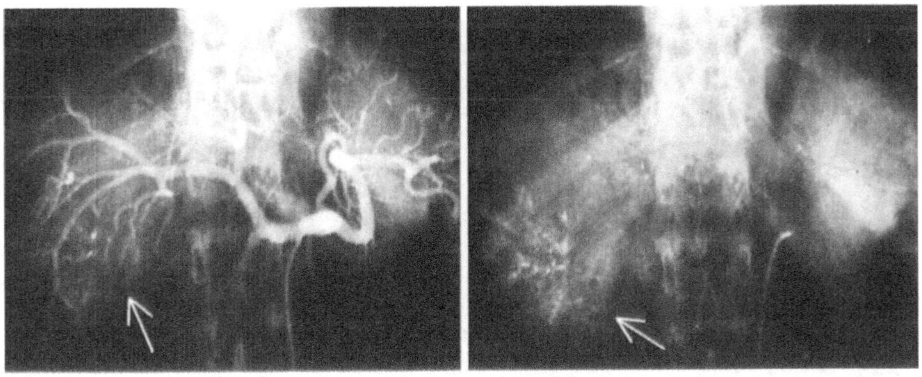

a b

Fig. 115a and b. Richly vascularized hepatic tumor (no histological examination).
(a) Arching of main branch of right hepatic artery. Abundant neovasculature with tiny pools of contrast medium. Poorly defined tumor profile (arrow). Celiac angiogram.
(b) Parenchymal phase with persistent pools of contrast medium

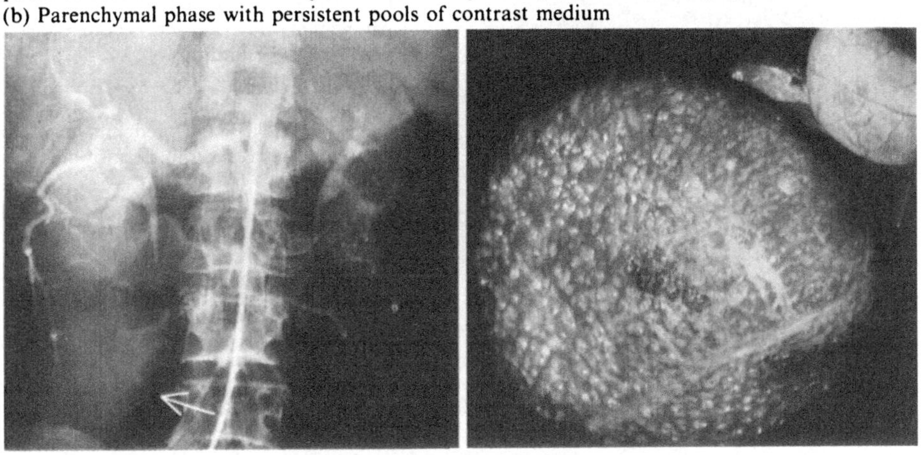

a b

Fig. 116a and b. Lymphosarcoma of liver. (a) The right hepatic artery arises from the superior mesenteric artery and extends a stretched branch into the extremely elongated right lobe of the liver as far as the crest of the ilium. As there is no parenchymal opacification, the right lobe appears more transparent than the rest of the liver. Selective angiography of superior mesenteric artery. (b) Operative specimen (Dr. E. GÖGLER): Tumor with small nodules spread over its surface, confined to the right liver lobe, and surprisingly found to be a lymphosarcoma histologically. Patient free of symptoms for three years

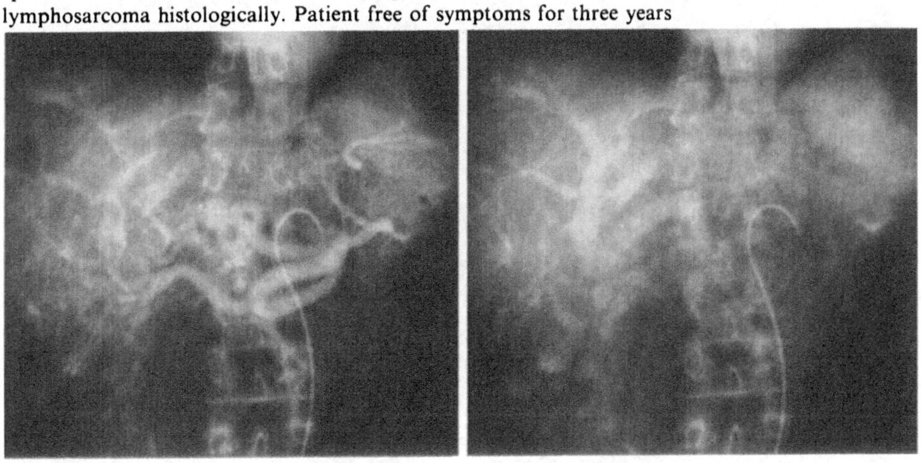

a b

Fig. 117a and b. Generalized hemangiomatosis of liver. (a) Liver enlarged to gigantic proportions. Dilated afferent arteries to left and right lobes of liver.
Relatively large, irregulary distributed spaces throughout the liver are visualized. Celiac angiogram. (b) Contrast medium persisted in vascular cavities in late phase. Diagnosis confirmed laparoscopically. Patient still living two years after diagnosis

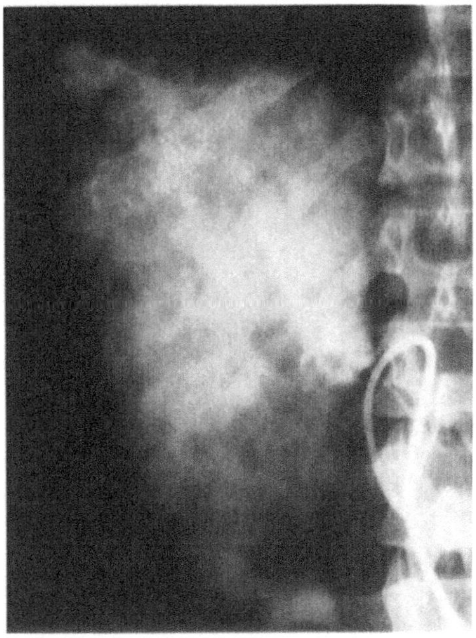

Fig. 118. Liver metastasis of bronchial carcinoma. Radiolucencies of hepatogram resembling Swiss cheese in late phase of omphaloportography. Infusions of cytostatic agents through catheter inserted into disobliterated umbilical vein followed

Fig. 119a and b. Liver abscess. (a) Egg-sized cavity (arrow) in right liver lobe during celiac angiography. (b) Parenchymal phase. Operation: Lancing of large abscess that had caused recurring bouts of fever with leukocytosis over a period of several weeks

Fig. 120a and b. Subcapsular liver hematoma after non-lacerating abdominal injury. (a) Displacement of liver parenchyma (arrow). Superselective angiography of hepatic artery. (b) The findings became even more distinct in the parenchymal phase. Parts of the compressed and displaced capsule can be differentiated. Laparotomy disclosed an extensive, predominantly subcapsular hematoma with subphrenic accumulation of blood

Fig. 119a

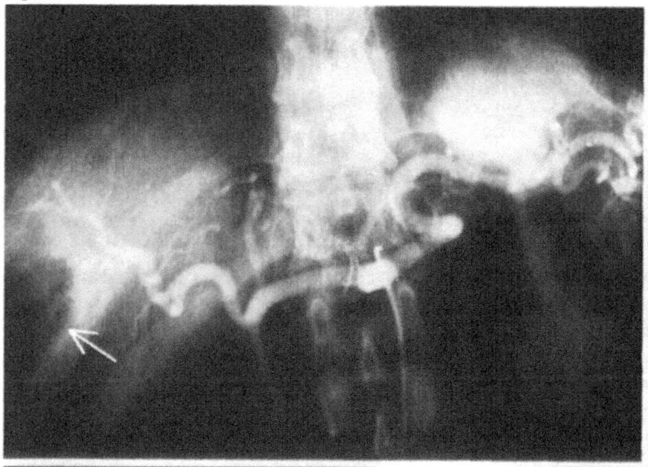

Fig. 119b

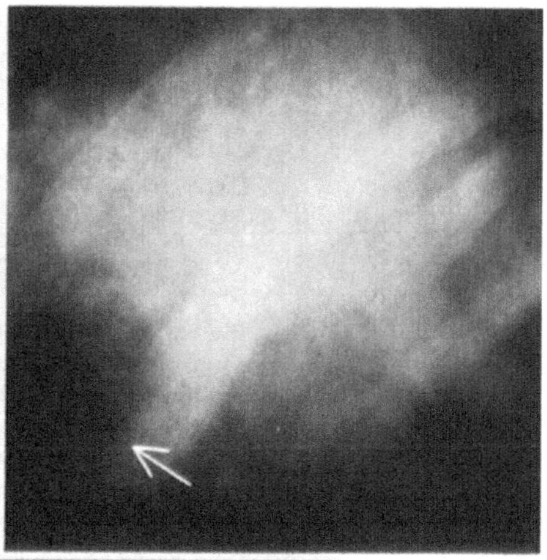

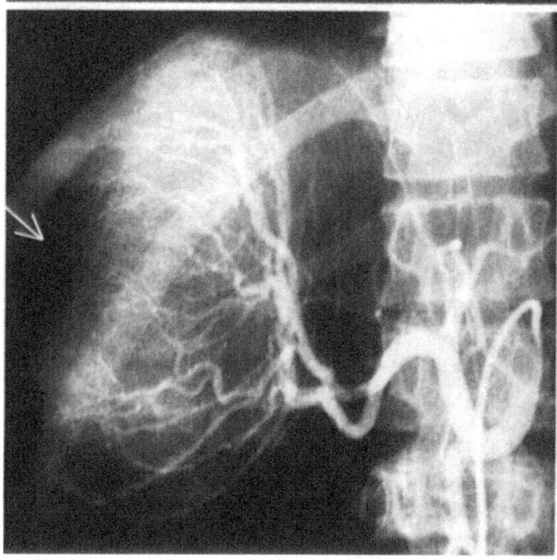

Fig. 120a

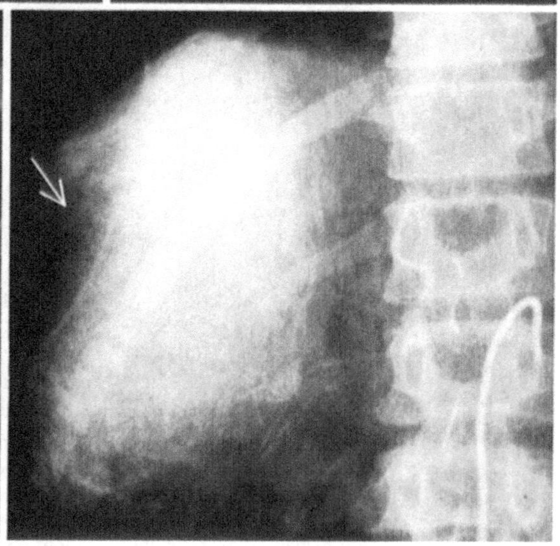

Fig. 120b

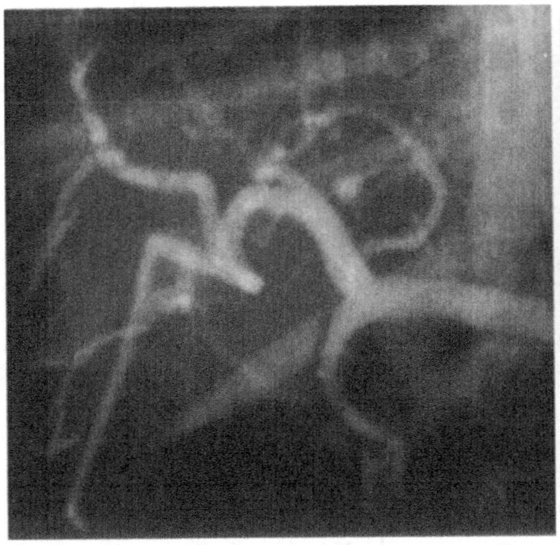

Fig. 121

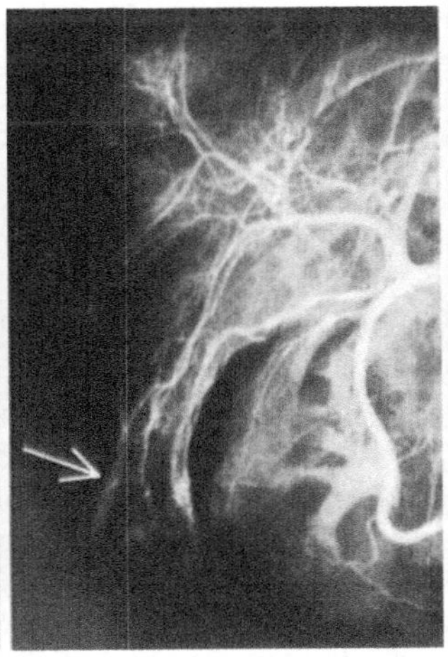

Fig. 122a

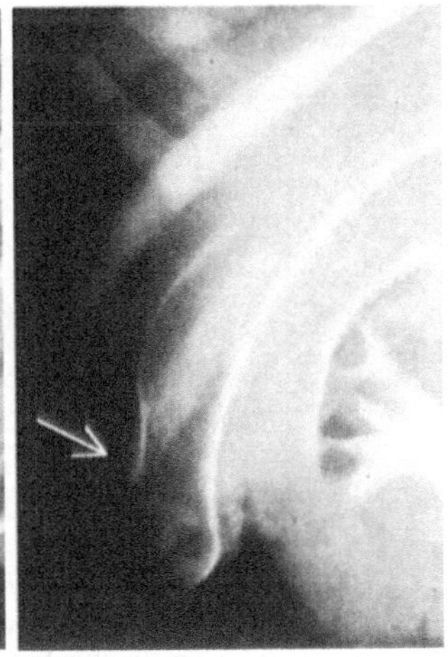

Fig. 122b

Fig. 121. Aneurysms of hepatic artery. Celiac angiography revealed several intrahepatic aneurysms in the hepatic artery, some cherry pit-sized

Fig. 122a and b. Angiogram of gallbladder. (a) Superselective angiogram of common hepatic artery. Origin of cystic artery from right hepatic artery with normal branching. (b) Parenchymal phase with good opacification of gallbladder wall (arrow)

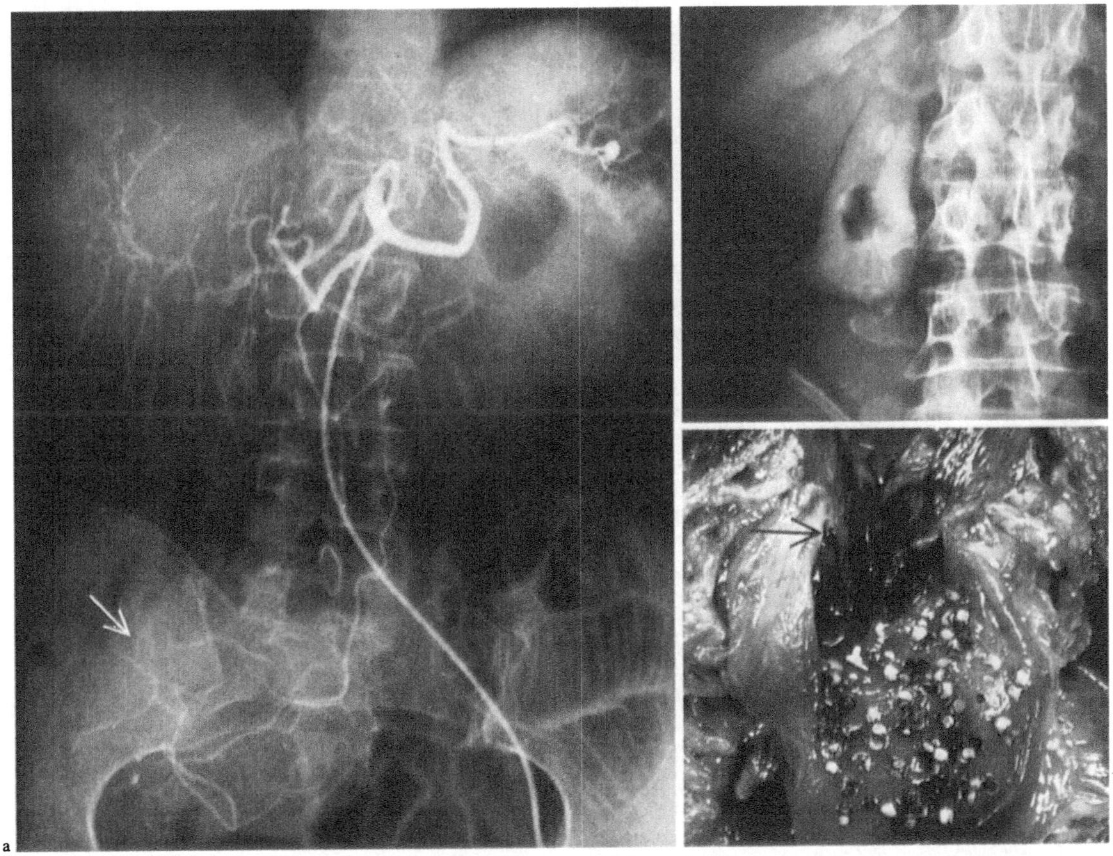

a c

Fig. 123a–c. Gallbladder carcinoma. (a) Unremarkable ramification of hepatic and splenic arteries; a branch arising from gastroduodenal artery extends caudad and is distributed in a palpable tumor projecting over the right sacroiliac joint (arrow). Celiac angiogram (b) Cholecystogram. Partial visualization of gallbladder with irregular contrast outline due to numerous concretions. Fundus of gallbladder not filled, fluoroscopically corresponds to a palpable tumor. (c) Surgical specimen. Extensive gallbladder carcinoma (arrow) in case of cholelithiasis

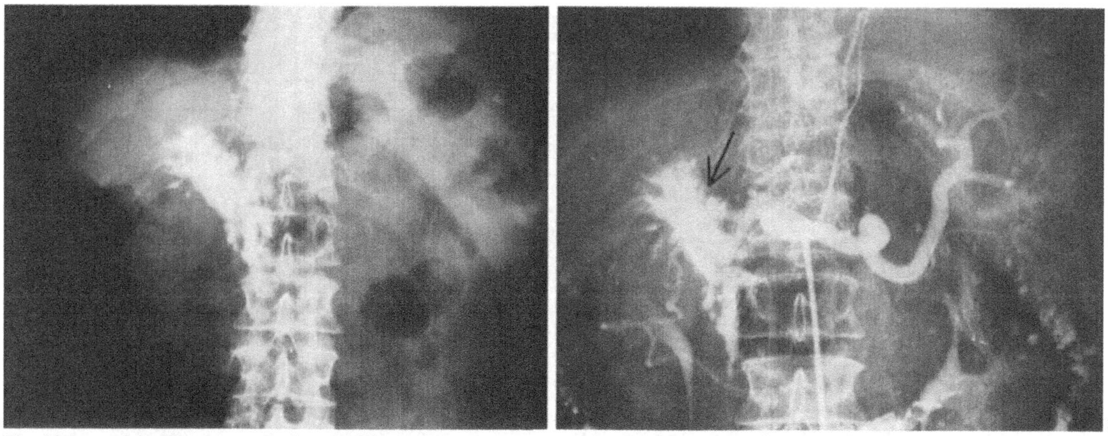

a b

Fig. 124a and b. Thorotrast-induced biliary duct carcinoma. (a) Thorotrast extravasate after unsuccessful intraoperative cholangiography 25 years previously. Plain abdominal x-ray. (b) Abrupt termination of hepatic artery at level of extravasation (arrow). Celiac angiography. Laparotomy disclosed an inoperable carcinoma emanating from the outer biliary ducts

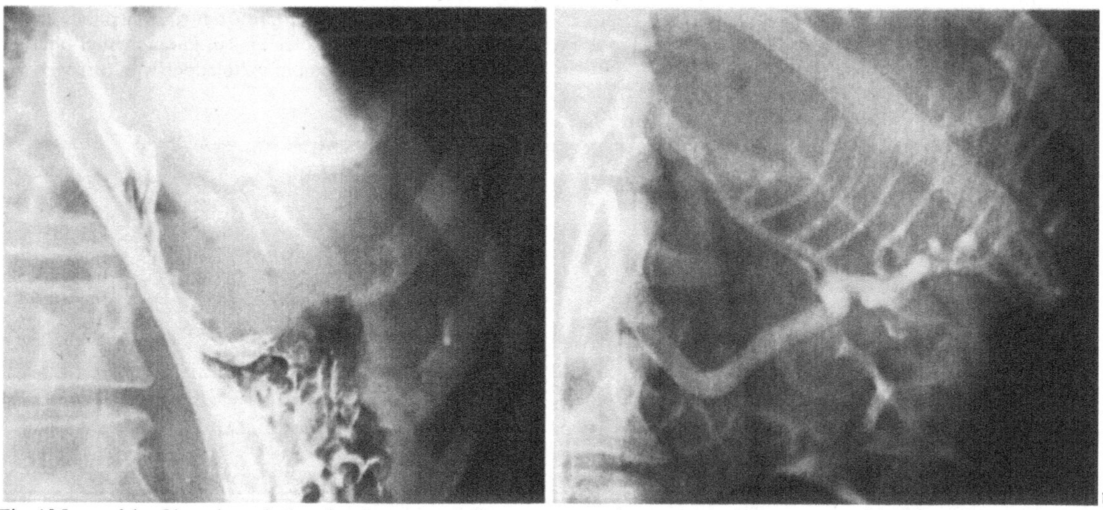

a b

Fig. 125a and b. Chronic, subphrenic abscess on left. (a) Spaceoccupying process of left hypochondrium with fist-sized filling defect at fundus of stomach. Moderate elevation of diaphragm. G. I. series. (b) Elongated splenic artery. The intrasplenic branches run a peculiar parallel course and seem to surround a cystic structure. They are notably blurred near the diaphragm. The spleen outline is indistinct. Celiac angiogram. Angiographic diagnosis of a cystic mass of the spleen. Laparotomy: detection of a chronic, putrescent subphrenic abscess in intact spleen

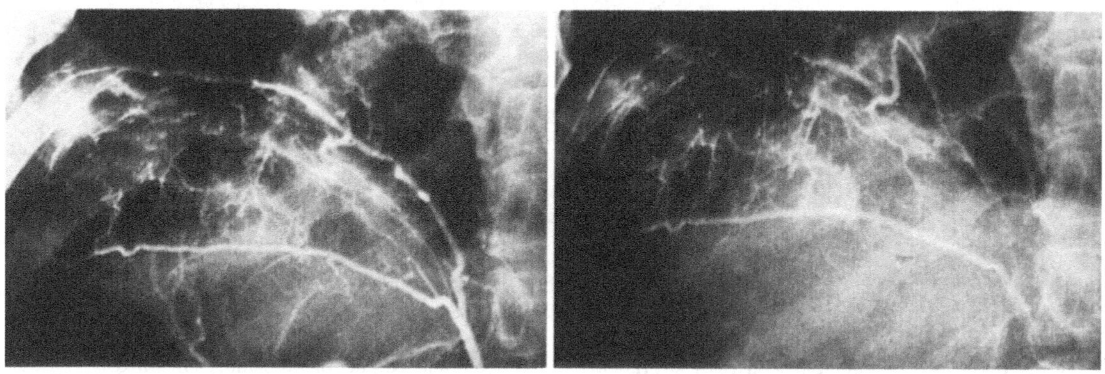

a b

Fig. 126a and b. Condition after subphrenic abscess. Selective angiography of right ascending phrenic artery which fans out over the entire diaphragmatic region. Anomalies in the course of the vessel and, in places, richly vascularized regions represent extensive residua after subphrenic abscess. A sizable cavernous system is not visualized

Fig. 127a and b. Metastasis of thyroid carcinoma in the spleen. Initial clinical finding of enlarged spleen. The patient lost weight rapidly and complained of pressure in left upper abdomen. (a) Picture of richly vascularized tumor supplied predominantly by splenic artery but also from left gastric artery. Celiac angiogram. (b) In late phase, pools of contrast medium in area of tumor, which had completely destroyed most of the spleen. Primary malignant tumor of spleen suspected on basis of angiographic evidence. Autopsy: Metastasis of small thyroid carcinoma

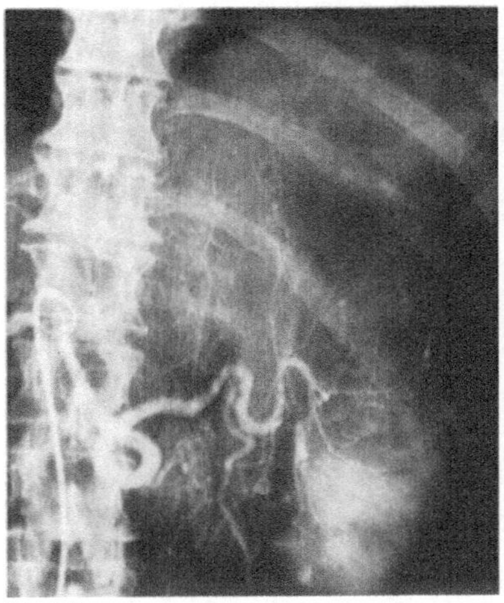

Fig. 127a

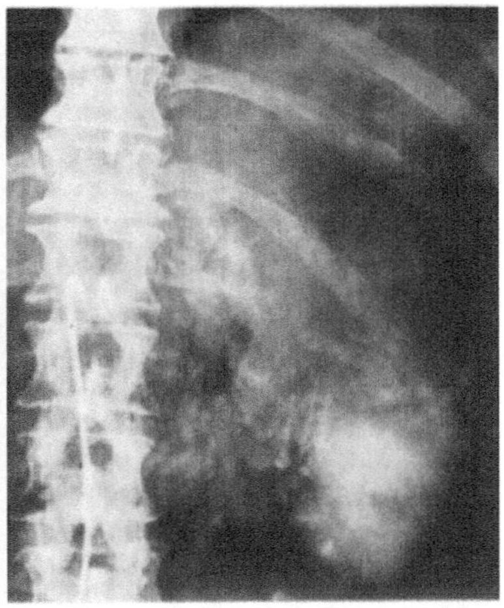

Fig. 127b

Fig. 128a and b. Hemangiomatosis of spleen. (a) Well-developed splenic artery with branches to organ considerably splayed. Spleen much enlarged. Superselective angiography of splenic artery. (b) Numerous cotton-like pools of contrast medium in parenchymal phase, with interspersed filling defects of varying size give the organ a checkerboard appearance. At this time the liver was not enlarged. One year later the patient died with extreme hepatosplenomegaly. Autopsy: Hemangiomatosis of spleen and liver

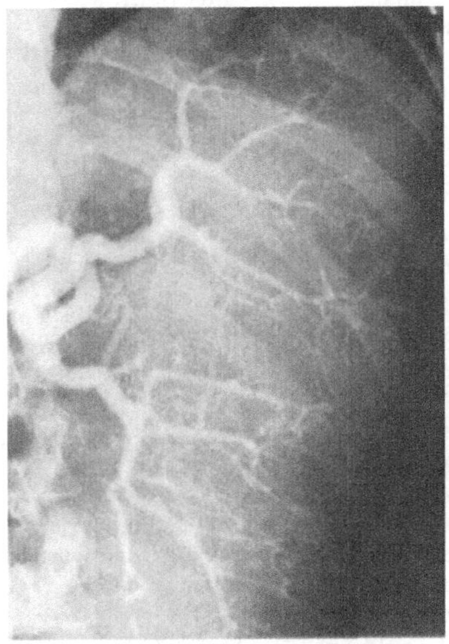

Fig. 128a

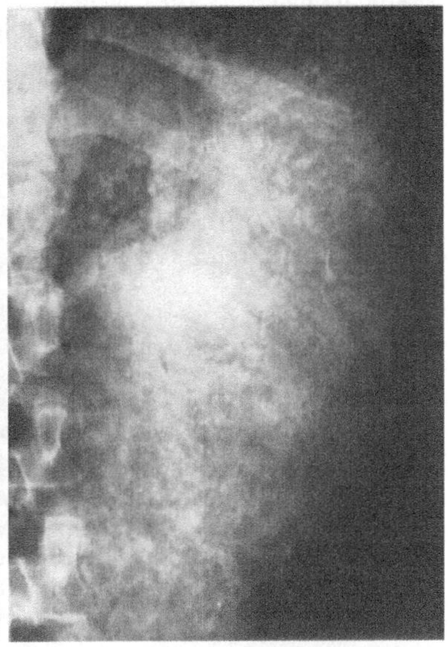

Fig. 128b

Fig. 129a and b. Splenic cyst. (a) Marked caudad displacement of splenic artery. The arterial branches are splayed and extend in a basketweave pattern into the capsule of an unvisualized tumor. Celiac angiogram. (b) Tumor the size of a child's head with well-formed capsule taking in upper part of spleen and entire hypochondrium on the left. Lower pole of spleen intact. Operation: Large splenic cyst

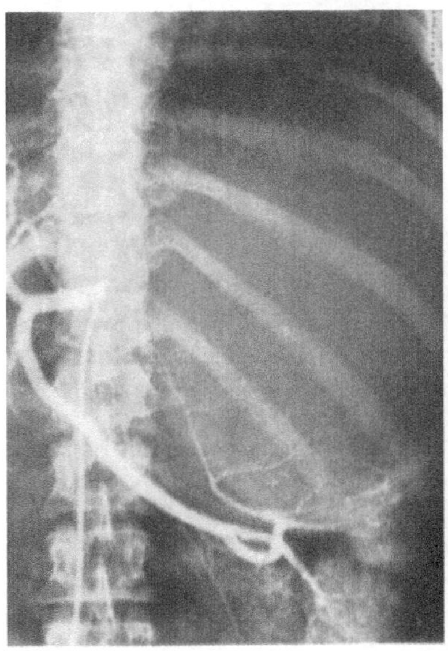

Fig. 129a

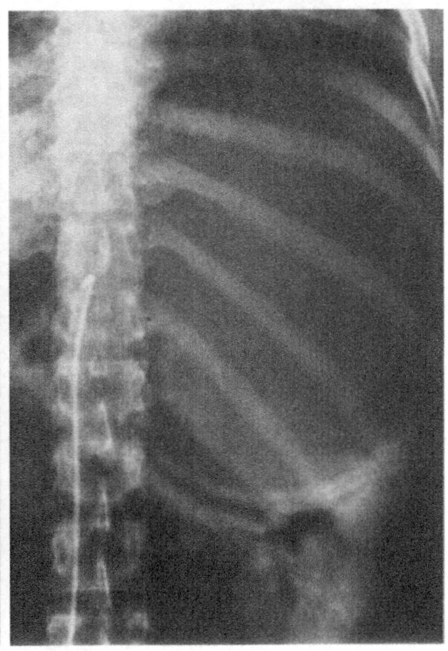

Fig. 129b

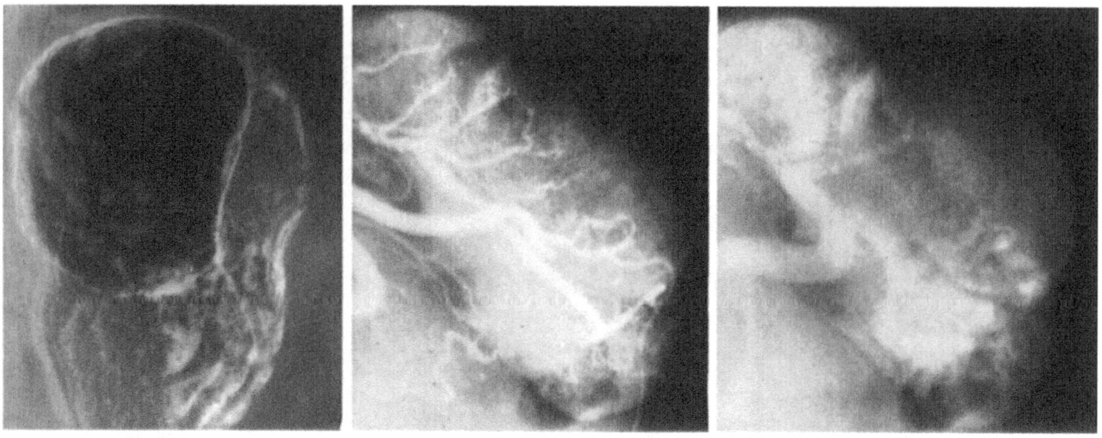

Fig. 130a–c. Traumatic cyst of spleen. (a) Constant impression of fundus of stomach from lateral view of gastrointestinal series. (b) Visualization of small spleen in typical location by selective splenoangiography. (c) An orange-sized cyst visible in lateral middle third of spleen in parenchymal phase. Condition after traffic accident with fall on lower left thorax

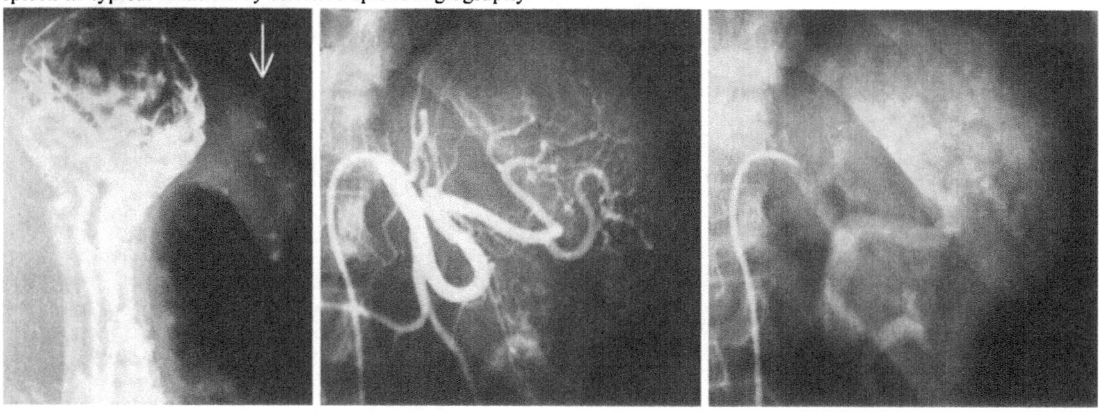

Fig. 131a–c. Tuberculosis of spleen. (a) Multiple calcareous densities, some pea-sized, to left of gastric fundus (arrow) revealed by G. I. series. (b) Normal arteriogram of spleen with increased tortuosity of artery. (c) Calcareous deposits visible within the spleen parenchyma. Otherwise, no pathological changes in parenchyma

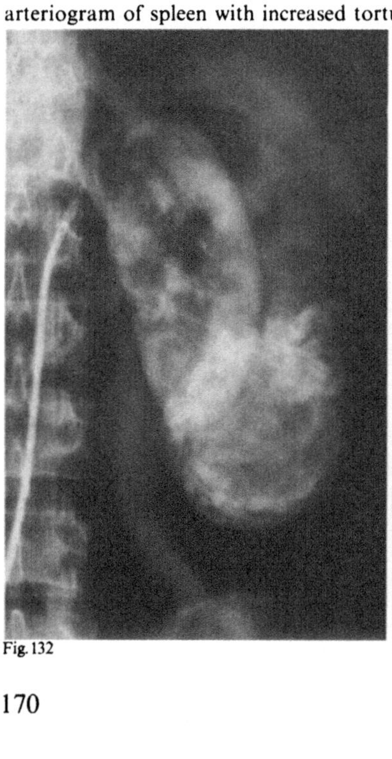

Fig. 132

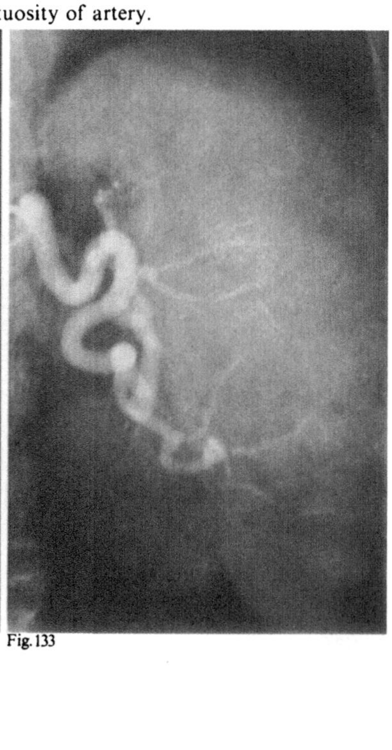

Fig. 133

Fig. 132. Tuberculoma at lower pole of spleen. Orange-sized calcified mass clearly delimited from the kidney and located at lower pole of spleen in late phase of catheter aortography. Splenectomy: Caseating tuberculosis of lower pole of spleen with pronounced calcification

Fig. 133. Malarial spleen with accessory spleen. Greek immigrant worker with liver cirrhosis and portal hypertension. History of malaria. Considerably enlarged spleen with kidney-shaped accessory spleen supplied by splenic artery; surgery showed it to be in apposition with lower third of spleen. Histological findings typical of malarial spleen with signs of congestion. Accessory spleen

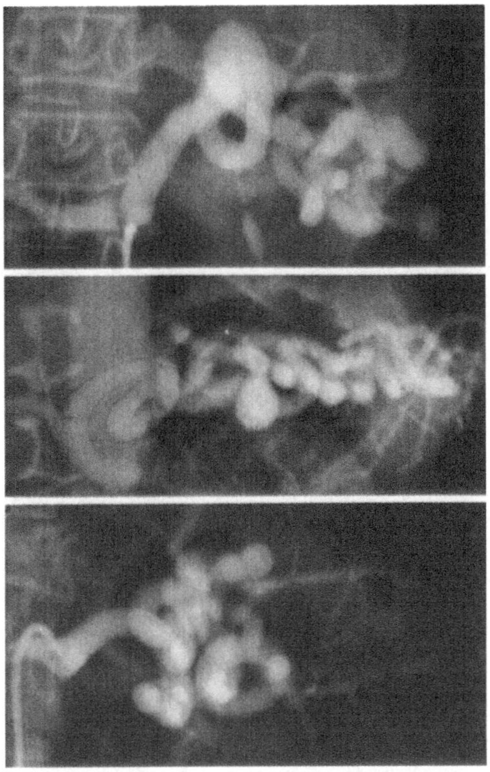

a
b
c

Fig. 134a–c. Variations in course of splenic artery. (a) Extrasplenic aneurysm of splenic artery with subtle calcareous infiltration in case of liver cirrhosis. Celiac angiogram. (b) Extremely tortuous splenic artery with incipient aneurysmal dilatation. Catheter aortogram. (c) Tortuosity and convoluted course of extrasplenic artery in splenomegally of obscure origin. Superselective angiography of splenic artery

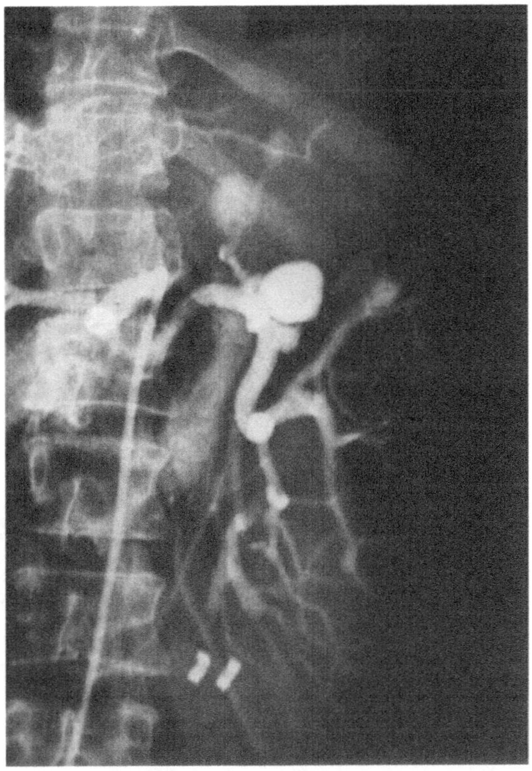

Fig. 135. Multiple extrasplenic and intrasplenic aneurysms with splenomegaly. Celiac angiogram

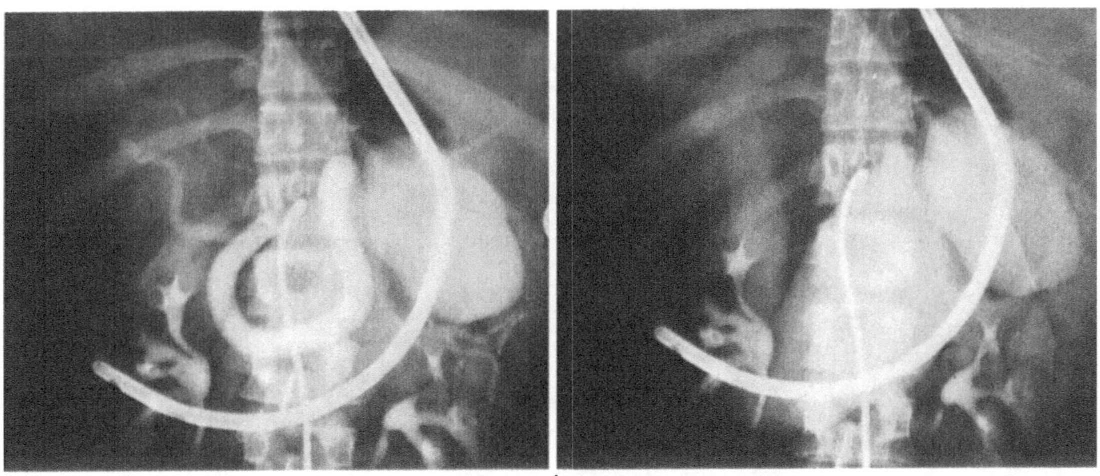

a b

Fig. 136a and b. Arterioportal fistula. (a) 27-year-old female patient with acute gastrointestinal bleeding. Bruit in left upper abdomen. Inflated Sengstaken tube in esophagus and stomach on account of bleeding varices. Dilated, tortuous splenic artery terminating in apple-sized aneurysmal sac. Superselective angiogram of splenic artery. (b) In venous phase, the contrast medium passed from the aneurysm into extremely dilated splenic vein and portal vein. Splenectomy with removal of aneurysm: Congenital fistula between splenic vein and artery (Dr. LINDER)

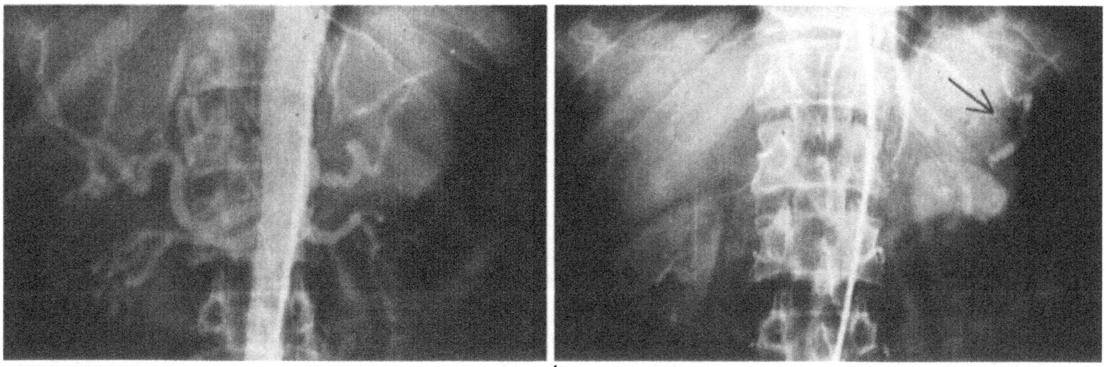

a b

Fig. 137a and b. Partial occlusion of splenic artery by stomach carcinoma. (a) Only proximal third of splenic artery is filled. Round tumor shadow extending from lesser curvature of stomach near splenic artery. Catheter aortogram. (b) In late phase, filling of intrasplenic splenic artery through collateral vessels with distinct delay (arrow)

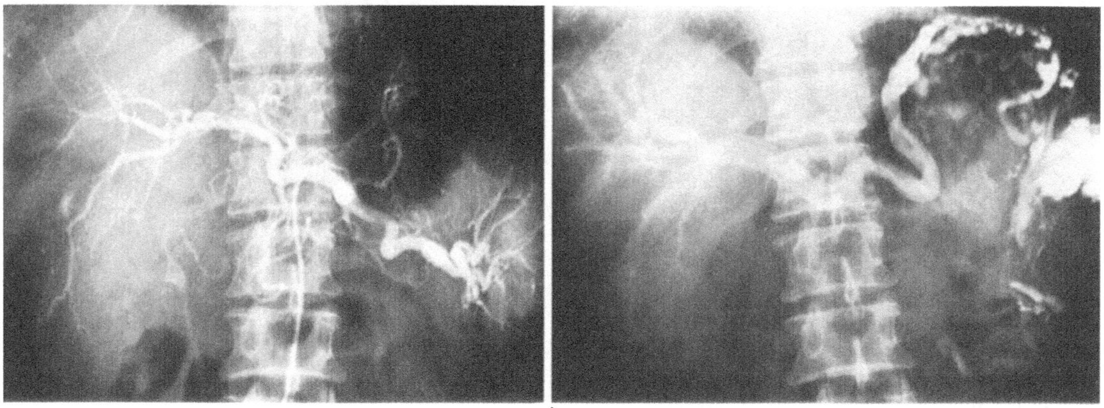

a b

Fig. 138a and b. Partial occlusion of splenic vein by carcinoma of tail of pancreas. (a) Distinct caudad displacement of spleen. Celiac angiogram.
(b) In splenoportogram, occlusion of principal vein near spleen. Collateralization via dilated gastric veins with complete filling of splenic vein in vicinity of portal vein. Orange-sized tumor in area of splenic vein interruption. Surgery: Carcinoma of tail of pancreas with encasement of splenic vein

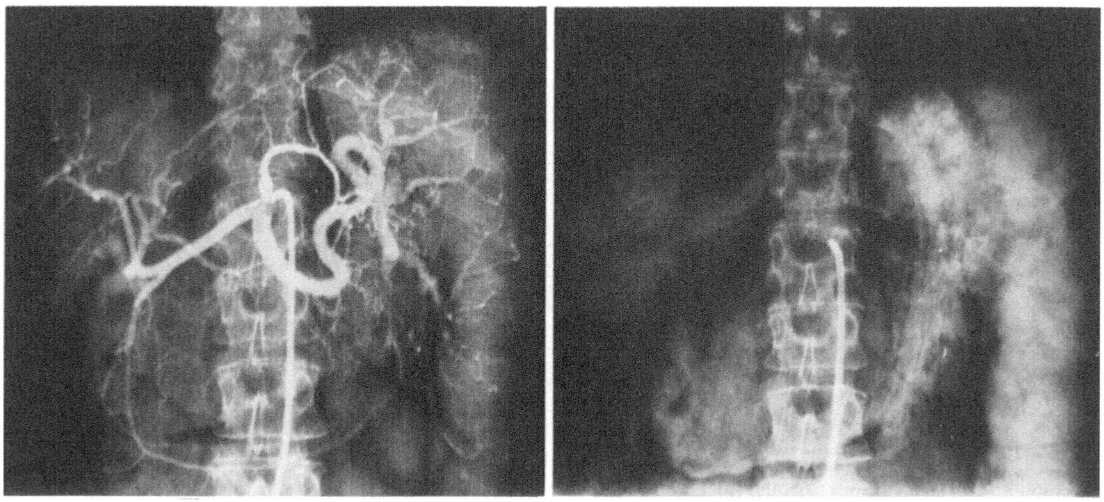

a. b

Fig. 138a and b. Cirrhosis of liver, portal hypertension, splenic vein thrombosis. (a) Arteriogram of considerably enlarged spleen; typical corkscrew course of pruned intrahepatic branches. Stenosis of left gastric artery at origin. Celiac angiogram.
(b) In late phase, persistence of contrast medium in enlarged spleen and in numerous veins along stomach. Surgery: Thrombosis of splenic vein

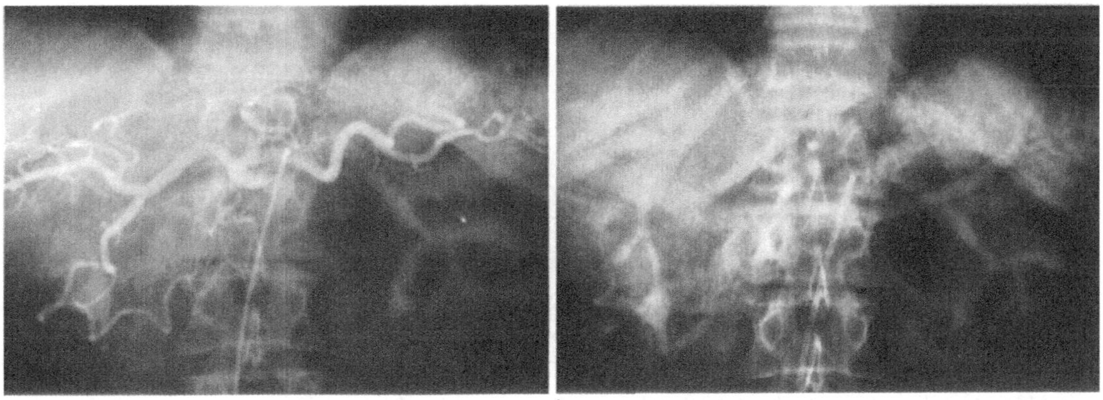

a b

Fig. 140a and b. Normal angiogram of pancreas. (a) Region around head of pancreas visualized in late arterial phase by filling of numerous small vessels from pancreatic arcades. Celiac angiogram. (b) Venous phase: Splenic and portal veins visualized. In addition to spleen and liver shadows, the soft tissue of the pancreas is opacified

a c

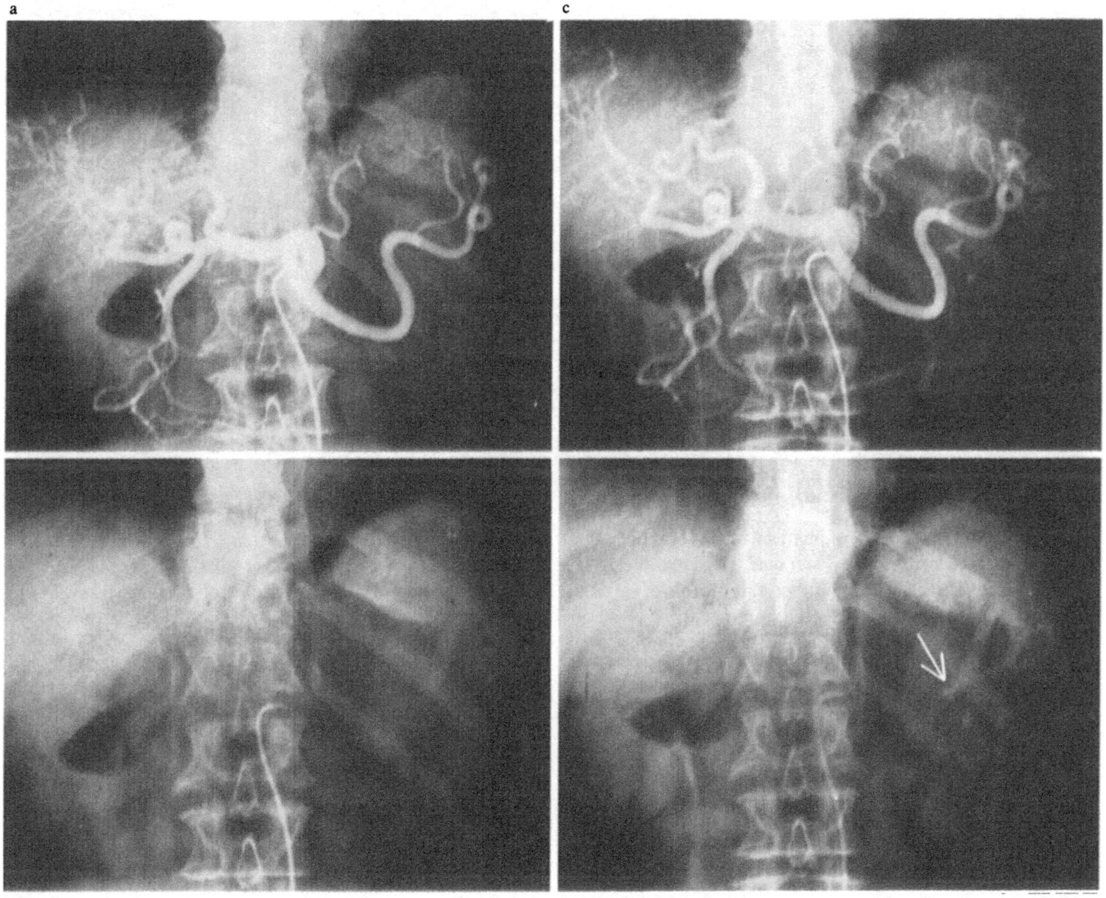

b d

Fig. 141a–d. Tumor in tail of pancreas, pharmacoangiogram. (a) Early arterial phase of celiac angiogram. (b) Venous phase. (c) Repeat of celiac angiography under the same technical conditions after glucose infusion which increased blood sugar level to 350 mg/100 ml. Sharper visualization of peripheral vessels with generally slightly dilated, larger tributaries. (d) Thrombosis of splenic vein, which is not clearly distinguishable in *b* is now (arrow) visualized. No improvement in visualization of pancreatic parenchyma

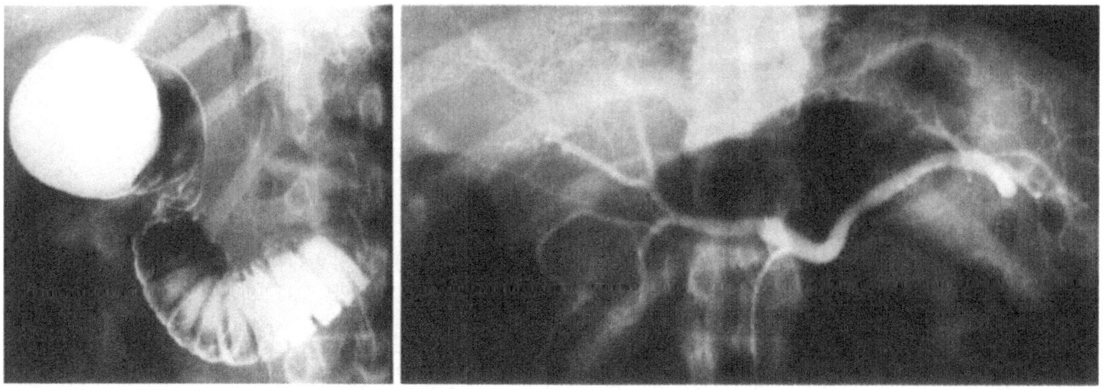

a b

Fig. 142a and b. Pancreatic annulus. (a) Typical postbulbar eccentric compression of descending duodenum. Hypotonic duodenography. (b) Annular course of pancreatic arcade. The pancreatico-duodenal arteries pass atypically from the gastroduodenal artery in an arch cranialward to the right. Celiac angiogram

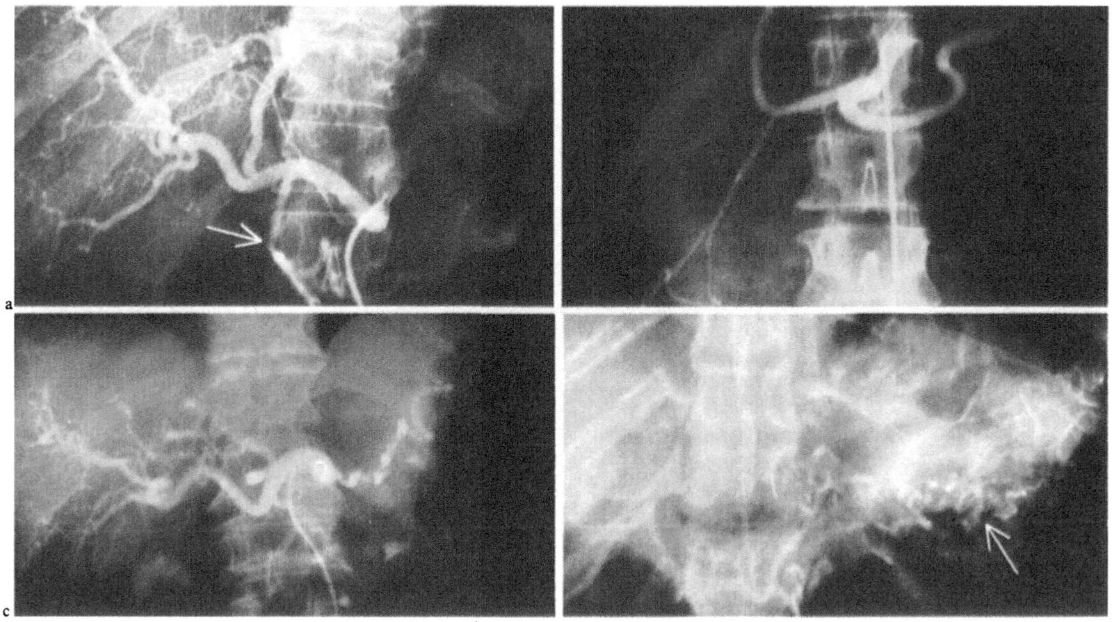

a b c d

Fig. 143a–d. Angiographic indication of pancreatic carcinoma. (a) Circumscribed stenosis of gastroduodenal artery as only objective evidence of carcinoma of head of pancreas (arrow). Superselective angiography of hepatic artery. (b) Stretching of gastroduodenal artery with impressions in the midsection in a case of carcinoma of head of pancreas. Celiac angiogram. (c) Stenosis in proximal portion of splenic artery in carcinoma of body of pancreas. Celiac angiogram. (d) Pathological vessels and contrast filling of tumor of tail of pancreas (arrow)

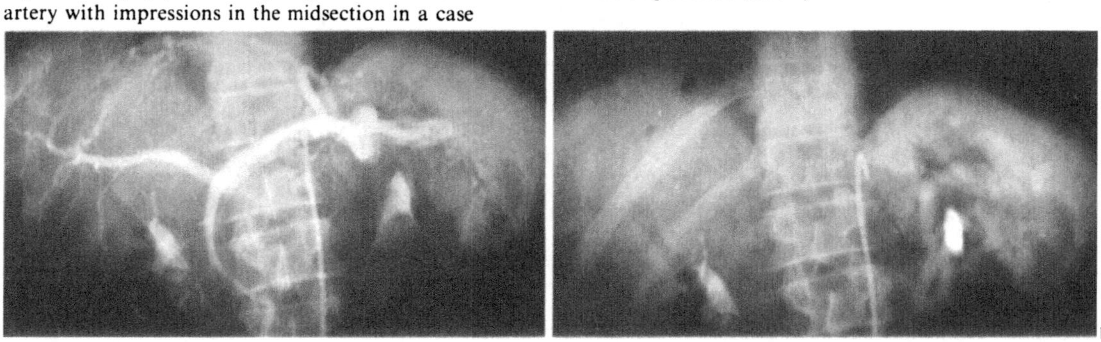

a b

Fig. 144a and b. Extensive pancreatic carcinoma. (a) Arcuate displacement of common hepatic artery and gastroduodenal artery. Celiac angiogram. (b) In venous phase, a convoluted cluster of tortuous veins adjacent to the splenic hilus in occlusion of splenic vein

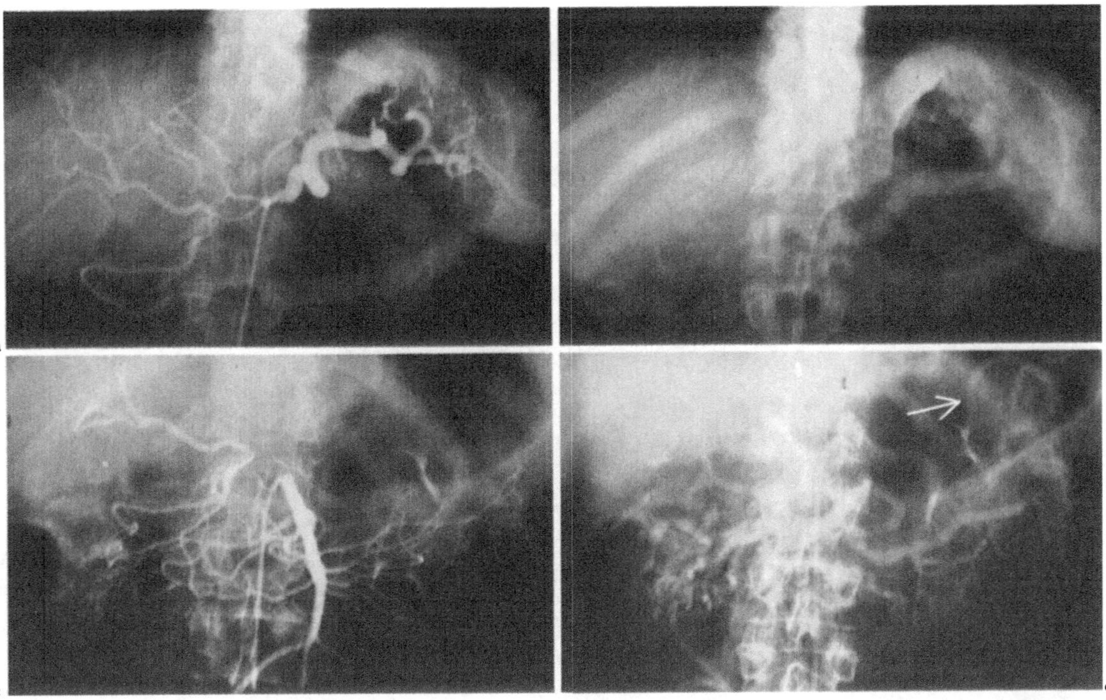
a b c d

Fig. 145a–d. Carcinoma of head of pancreas. (a) Marked stenosis of common hepatic and gastroduodenal arteries as well as of initial portion of left gastric and splenic arteries. Celiac angiogram. (b) In the venous phase no visualization of portal vein trunk. Drainage of contrast medium via pancreatic vein to vena coronaria ventriculi. (c) Collateral circulation from superior mesenteric artery through pancreatic arcades into stenotic part of hepatic artery. Selective angiography of superior mesenteric artery. (d) Venous phase: Obstruction of outflow from superior mesenteric artery. Dilated convolutions of mesenteric veins seeking an outlet in the direction of spleen and stomach (arrow)

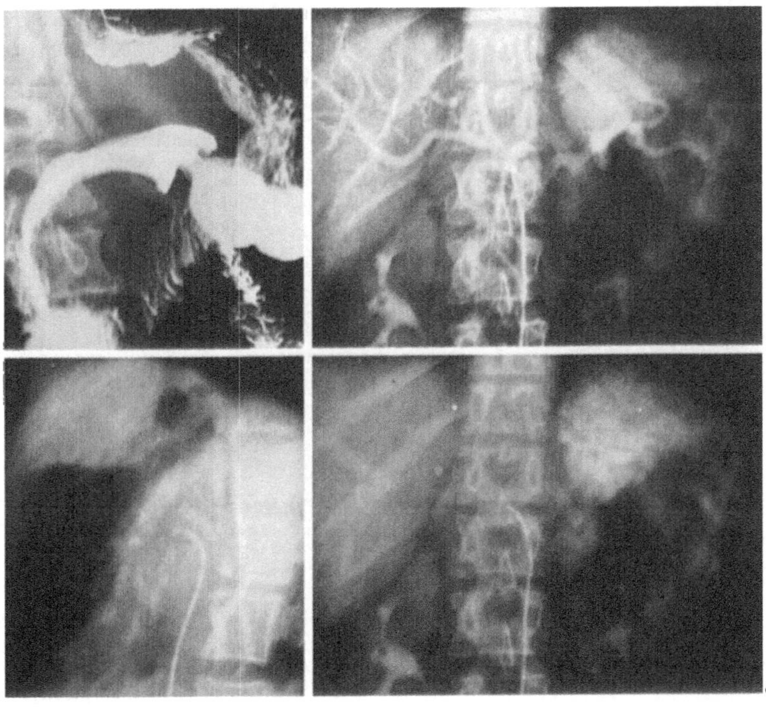
a c b d

Fig. 146a–d. Liposarcoma of pancreas. (a) Expansion of duodenal C-loop with impression effects. Gastrointestinal series. (b) Lateral view of space-occupying process in late phase of celiac angiogram. The stomach, inflated with air, is displaced ventrally. (c) Moderate elevation of common hepatic artery, with gastroduodenal artery remaining unfilled. Celiac angiogram. (d) Late phase: Numerous venous convolutions in left upper abdomen with splenic vein remaining unfilled. Surgery: Extensive liposarcoma beginning at head of pancreas; inoperable

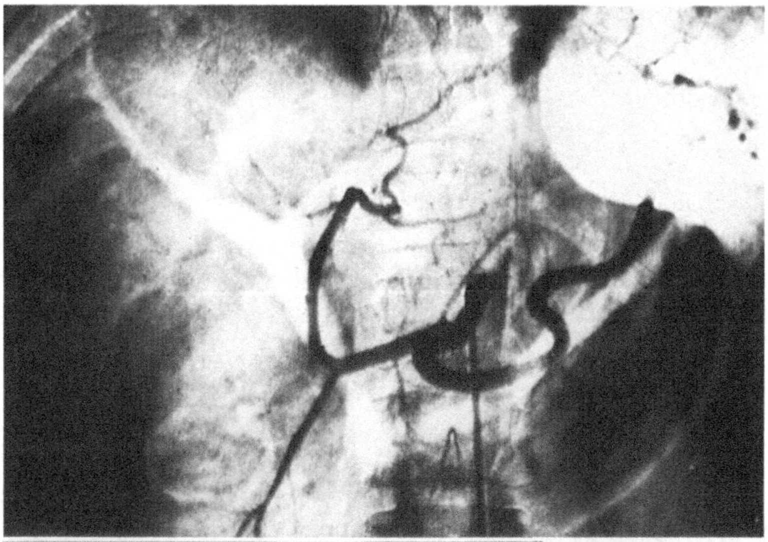

Fig. 147. Carcinoma originating in head of pancreas. Subtraction picture. Arterial and venous phases of celiac angiography pictured side by side. Note the considerably dilated gastroduodenal artery with multiple stenoses and the juxtaposition of the arterial vascular system and splenic and portal veins (tumor impression)

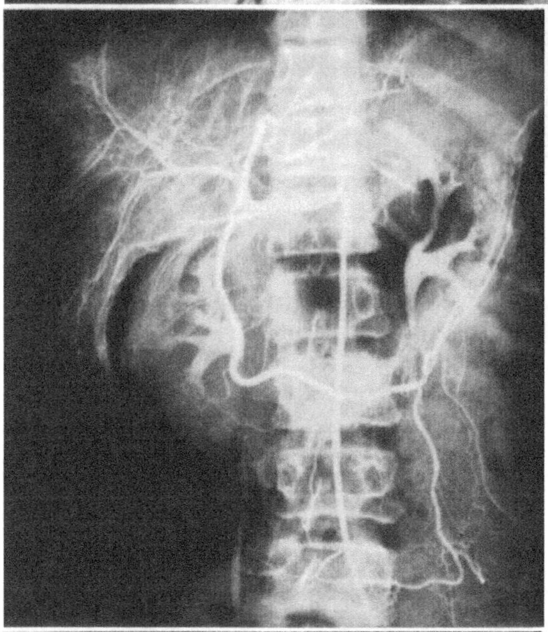

a

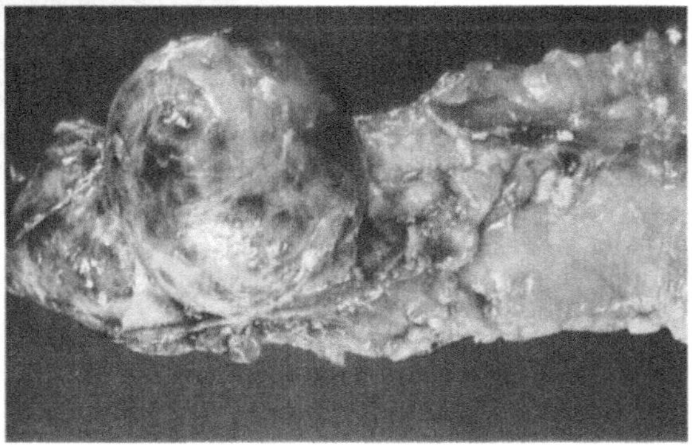

b

Fig. 148a and b. Pancreatic cystadenoma. (a) Widening of loop formed by gastroduodenal artery, which gives off numerous large-caliber arteries surrounding a round tumor. Superselective angiography of hepatic artery. (b) Surgical specimen

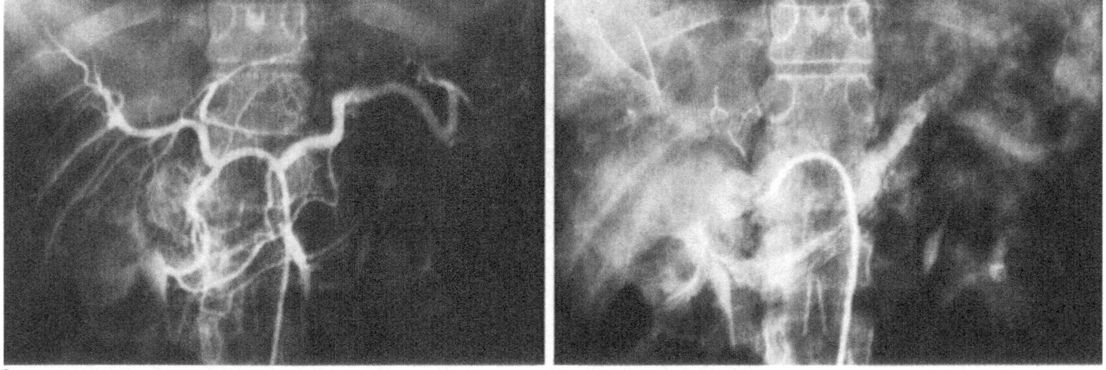

a b

Fig. 149a and b. Insulinoma. (a) Early tumor opacification in celiac angiogram. Considerable collateralization via pancreatic arcades to superior mesenteric artery, which is partially visualized. The catheter tip is situated proximal to origin of gastroduodenal artery. (b) Late phase: Good outline of circular, opacified tumor in head of pancreas (verified surgically)

Fig. 150. Chronic pancreatits with acute episode. Picture of whole pancreas at beginning of parenchymal phase

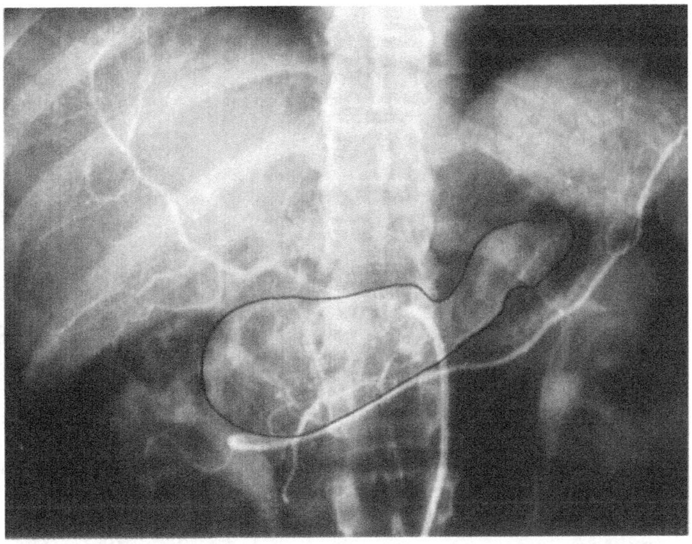

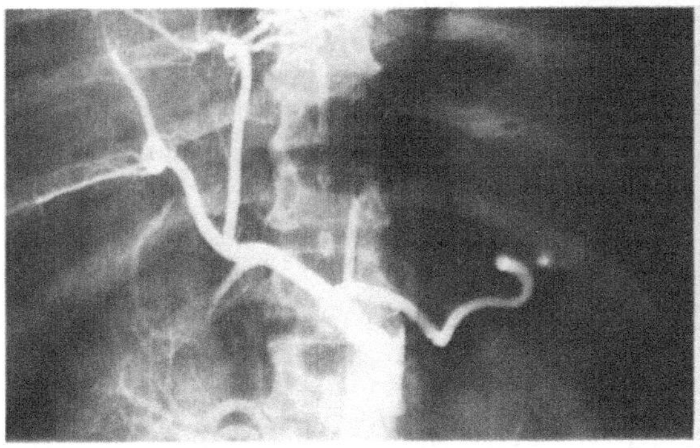

a

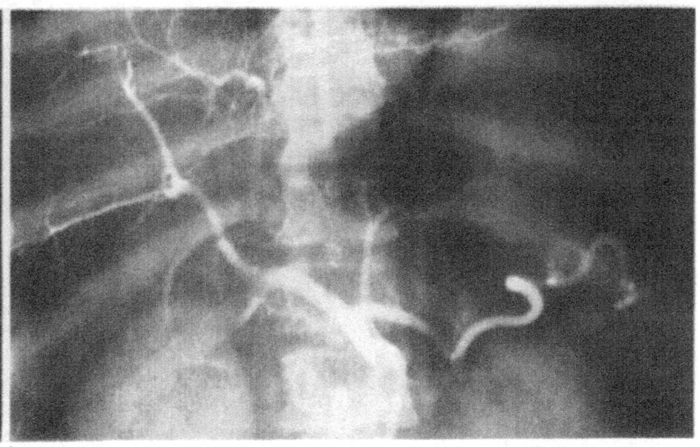

b

Fig. 151a and b. Acute necrotizing pancreatitis. (a) Marked pruning of vessel branches originating at celiac trunk. Celiac angiogram with massive contrast medium reflux into aorta. (b) 20 seconds after injection, the contrast medium is still present in the arterial trunk. Autopsy: Acute necrotizing pancreatitis with thrombosis of portal vein

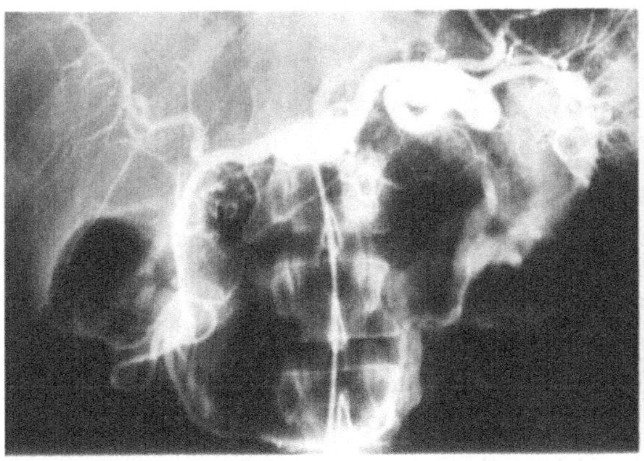

a

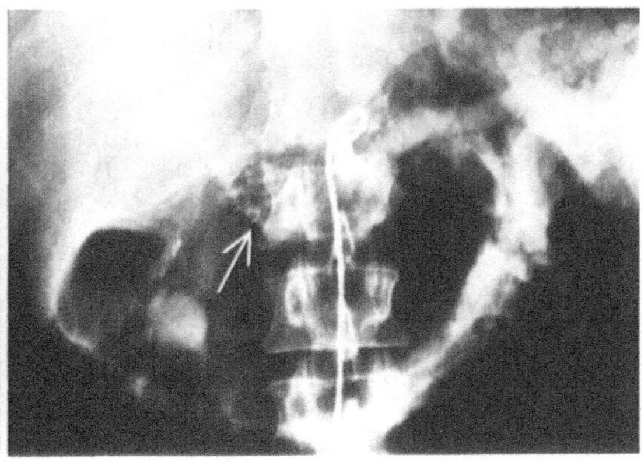

b

Fig. 152a and b. Acute pancreatitis. (a) Atonic distention of stomach and duodenum with corresponding dilation of associated arterial branches. Celiac angiogram. (b) Late phase; no visualization of pancreatic parenchyma. Portal vein system patent. Secondary finding: Plaque-like calcareous infiltrations in head of pancreas (arrow). Clinically, acute episode in chronic pancreatitis

a b c

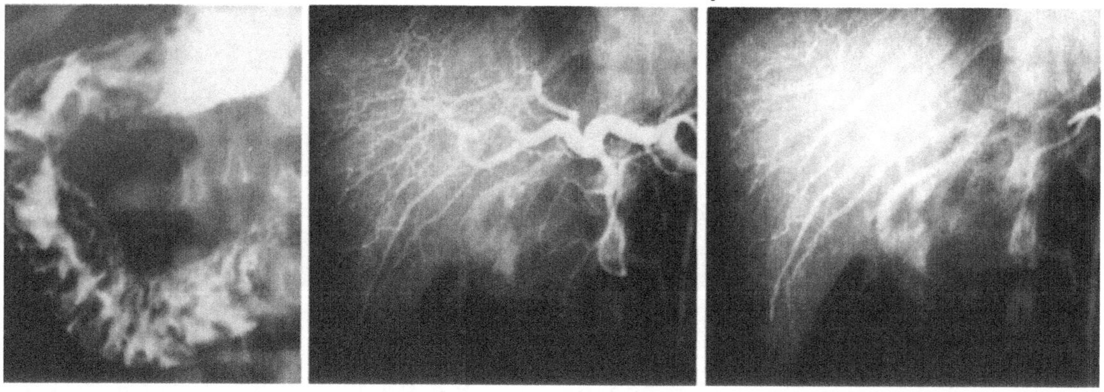

Fig. 153a–c. Chronic pancreatits with small cysts in head of the pancreas. (a) Hypotonic duodenogram with impression effect in upper duodenal bend and irregular outline of descending duodenum. (b) Leftward displacement of gastroduodenal artery. The vessels of the pancreatic arcade surround the enlarged head of pancreas in a basketweave pattern; cystic lucency in cranial right quadrant. Celiac angiogram. (c) Late arterial phase; the head of the pancreas, enlarged by inflammation, is well opacified

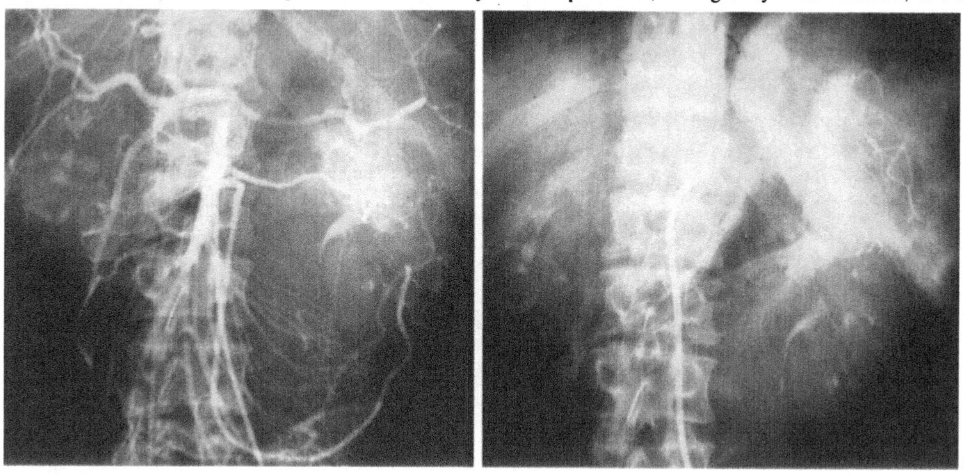

a b

Fig. 154a and b. Large postpancreatitic cyst. Child's head-sized tumor with smooth outlines in middle of left abdomen. (a) Marked dilatation and caudad displacement of superior jejunal branches. Simultaneous visualization of celiac artery via pancreatic arcades. Selective angiogram of superior mesenteric artery. (b) In venous phase, no visualization of splenic vein, which is greatly compressed by space-occupying process. Surgery: Splenomegaly owing to obstruction of splenic vein drainage by large cyst of pancreatic tail in chronic pancreatitis

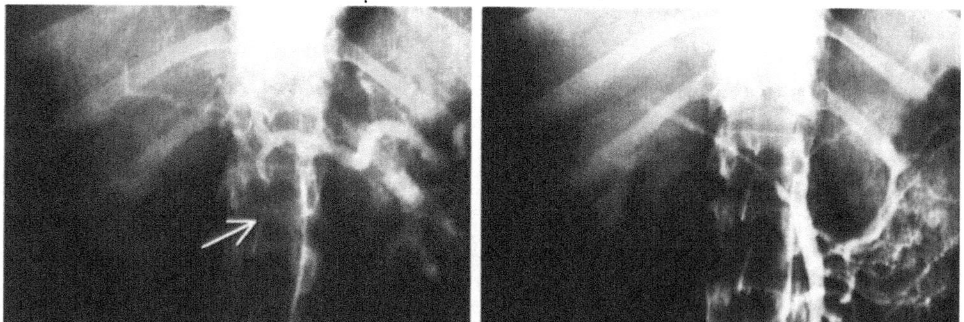

a b

Fig. 155a and b. Ruptured pancreas. Blunt abdominal injury. (a) Displacement and incomplete filling of gastroduodenal artery in celiac angiogram (arrow). (b) The right hepatic artery, originating at superior mesenteric artery, shows a filiform constriction near its origin and is not filled up to periphery. These alterations were interpreted as sequelae of injury at level of pancreatic head. Surgery: Partial avulsion of head of pancreas and its arteries, and the common bile duct (Dr. E. Gögler)

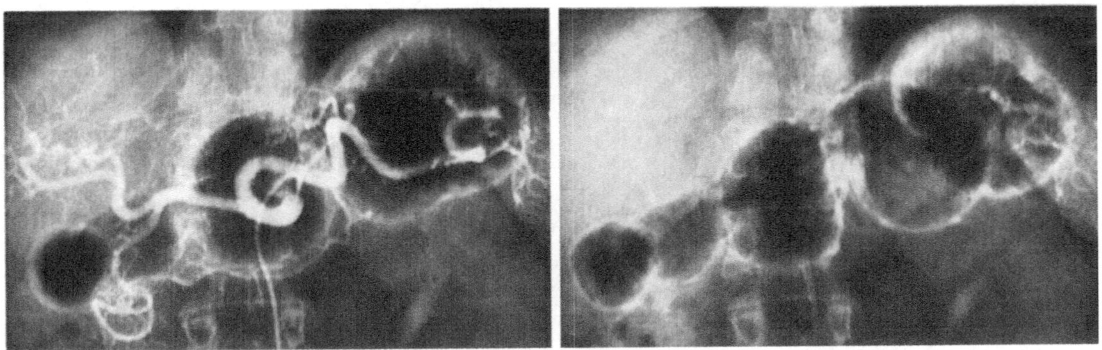

a b

Fig. 156a and b. Stomach and duodenum in angiogram. (a) Celiac angiogram. (b) Late phase with sharp visualization of wall of viscous

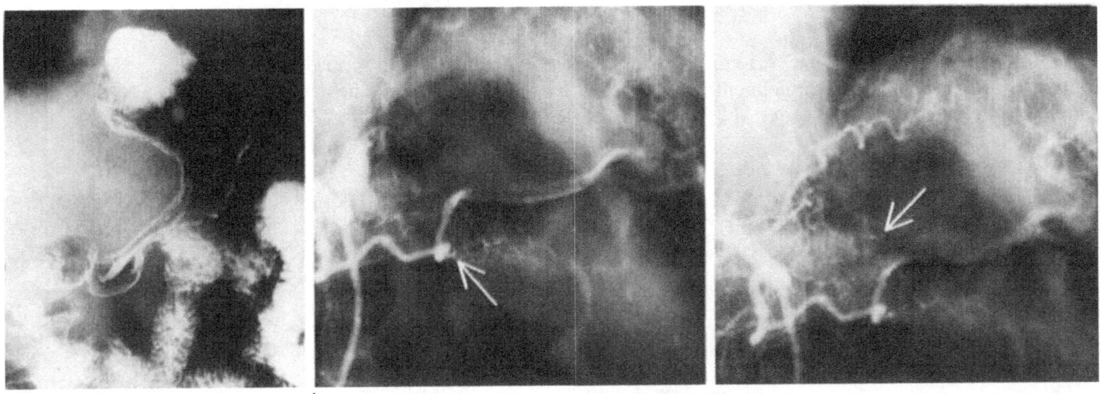

a b c

Fig. 157. Scirrhus of stomach. (a) Typical constriction in region of corpus and antrum with rigidity of stomach wall. Gastrointestinal series with double contrast. (b) Break at beginning of splenic artery (arrow) which is refilled peripherally via dorsal pancreatic artery. Celiac angiogram. (c) Pathological vessels in region of stomach tumor (arrow) in capillary phase

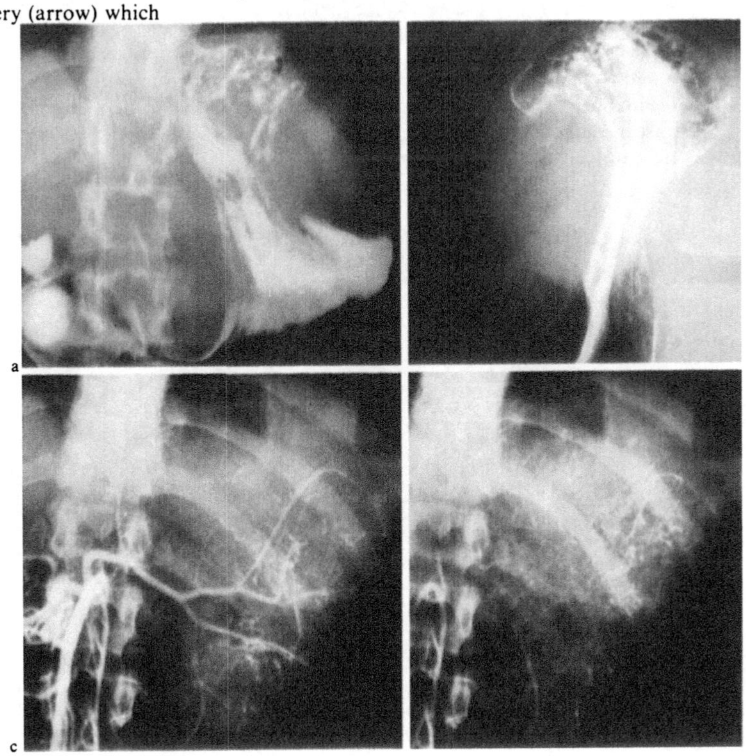

a b c d

Fig. 158a–d. Metastatic tumor in left lobe of liver. (a) Filling defect in lateral wall of body of stomach. Gastrointestinal series, anteroposterior view. (b) Tumor located on anterior side of stomach. Gastrointestinal series. Lateral view. (c) Atypical origin of left hepatic artery from superior mesenteric artery and visualization of giant tumor in left hypochondrium. Selective angiography of superior mesenteric artery.
(d) Pathological tumor vessels, irregular contrast medium extravasations, and unsharp tumor outlines indicating a richly vascularized sarcomatous tumor of left lobe of liver which, on G. I. series, was more suggestive of a stomach tumor

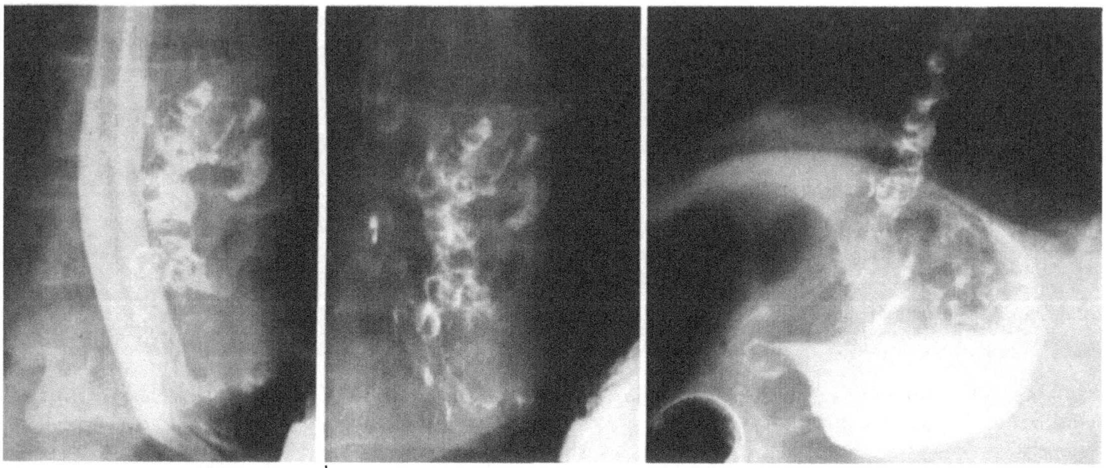

a b c

Fig. 159a–c. Boerhaave syndrome. (a) Paracardial rupture of stomach with mediastinal contrast medium extravasation. Gastrointestinal series. (b) Persistence of contrast medium in mediastinal abscess. (c) Lateral view. The acute incident was associated with gastric bleeding. Chronic abuse of alcohol

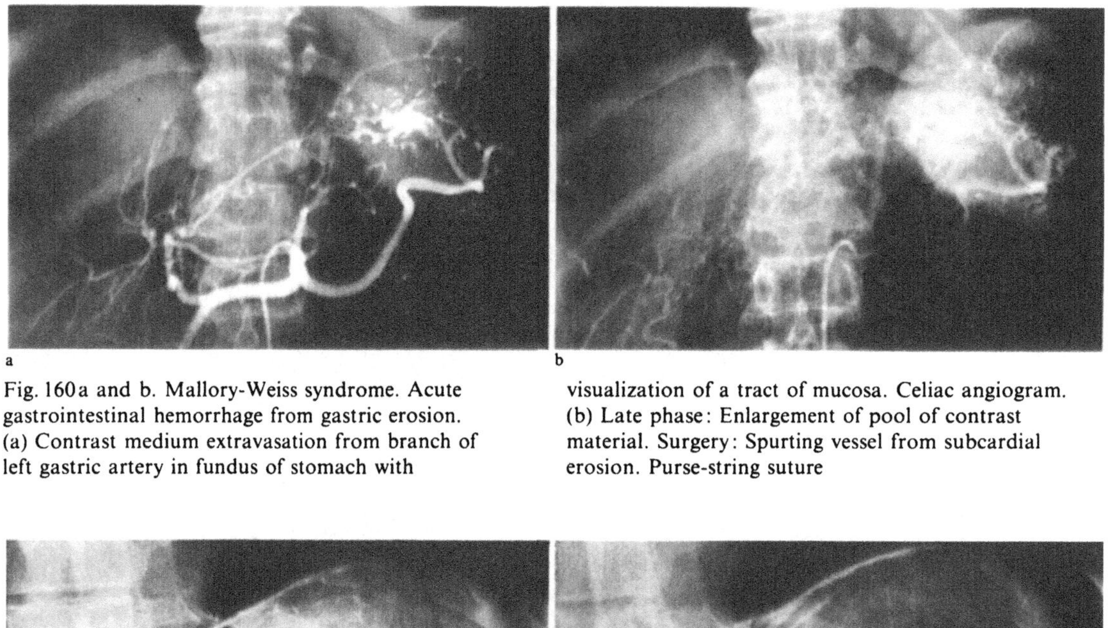

a b

Fig. 160a and b. Mallory-Weiss syndrome. Acute gastrointestinal hemorrhage from gastric erosion. (a) Contrast medium extravasation from branch of left gastric artery in fundus of stomach with visualization of a tract of mucosa. Celiac angiogram. (b) Late phase: Enlargement of pool of contrast material. Surgery: Spurting vessel from subcardial erosion. Purse-string suture

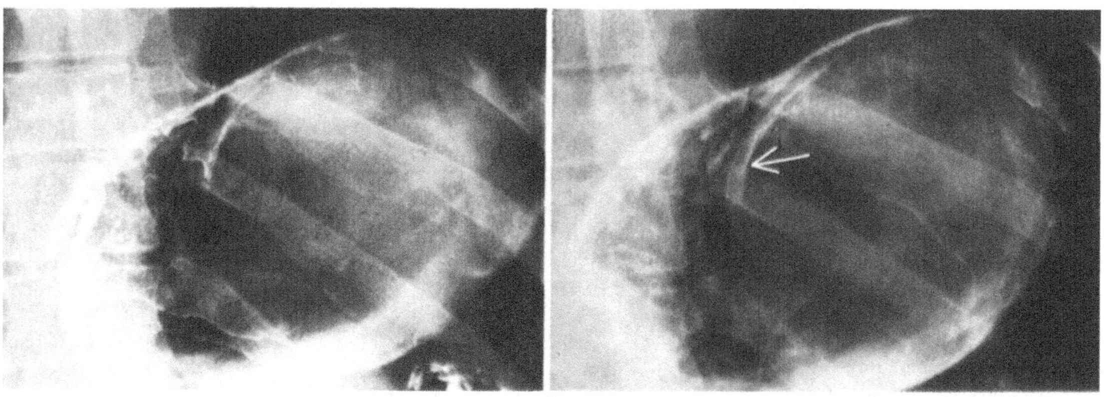

a b

Fig. 161a and b. Stomach bleeding in Dieulafoy ulcer. Hematemesis. Source of bledding not detected on laparotomy. (a) Visualization of vessels in fundus after air-inflation of stomach. Superselective angiography of left gastric artery. (b) Late phase: Contrast medium (arrow) is distributed aborally in a stomach fold. Relaparotomy and purse-string suture of vessel bleeding from acute erosin

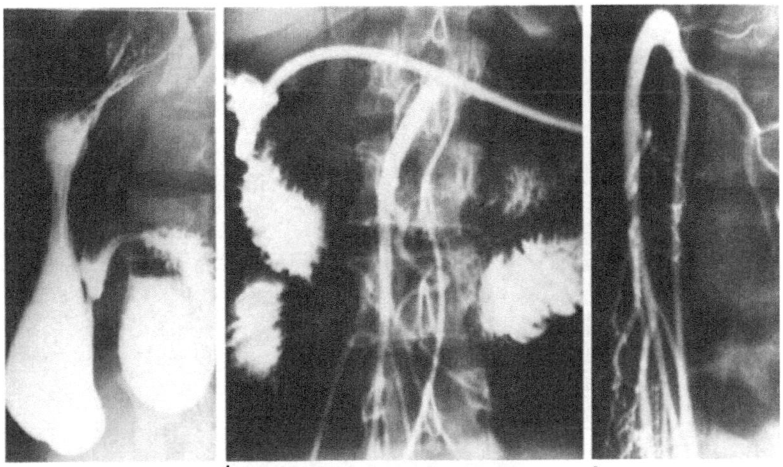

a b c

Fig. 162a–c. Compression of duodenum by mesenteric artery. (a) Distention and elongation of stomach and duodenum and retention of contrast medium in ascending duodenum. Gastrointestinal series, lateral view. (b) Compressive effect of superior mesenteric artery. Prone position. Simultaneous duodenography and angiography of superior mesenteric artery. (c) Acute angle between aorta and superior mesenteric. Lateral view

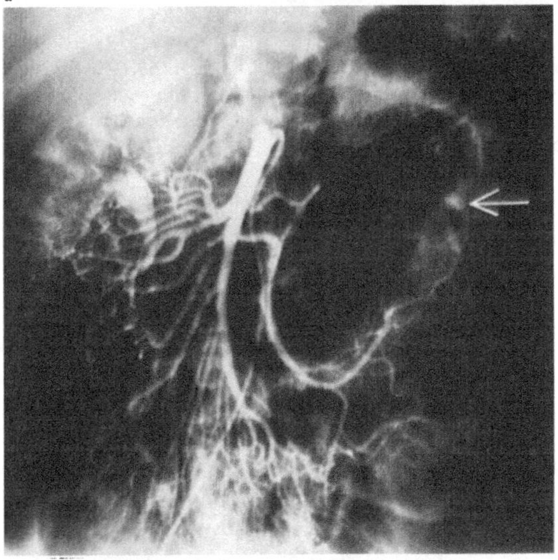

Fig. 163

Fig. 163. Appendiceal abscess in malrotation. Mirror-image reversal of locations of mesenteric branches. Circumscribed accumulation of contrast medium in territory of ileocolic artery in the left mid-abdomen (arrow); surgery revealed that it represented an appendiceal abscess in malrotation

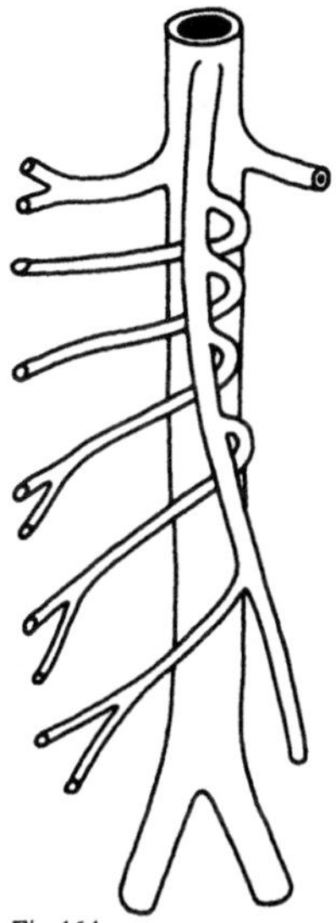

Fig. 164

Fig. 164. Diagram of course of superior mesenteric branches in paraduodenal hernia (Meyers, 1970)

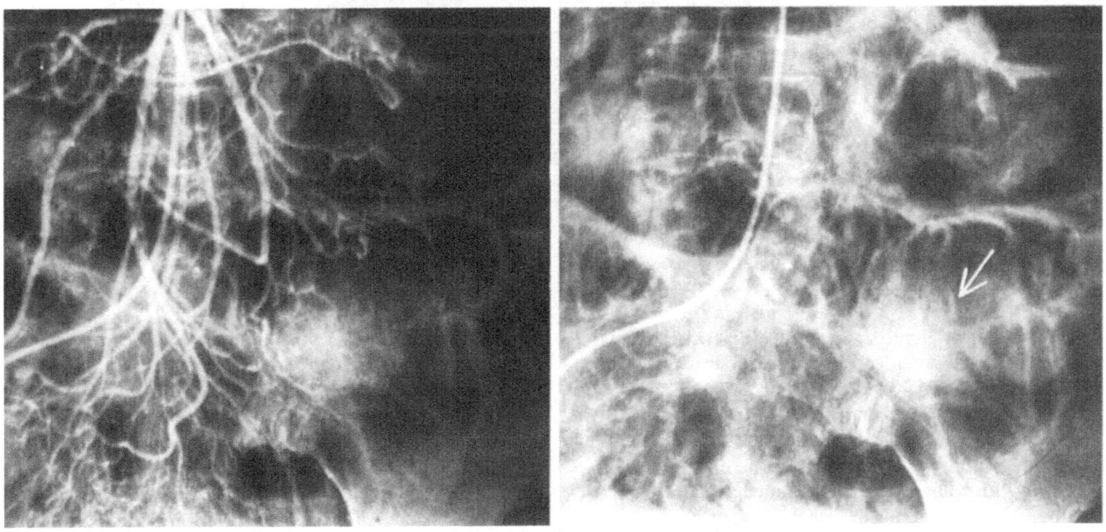

a b

Fig. 165a and b. Jejunal carcinoma. (a) Splaying and separation at junction between jejunal and ileal branches. Neoformation of minute vessels. Selective angiography of superior mesenteric artery. (b) Tumor visible in sharp outline in venous phase (arrow)

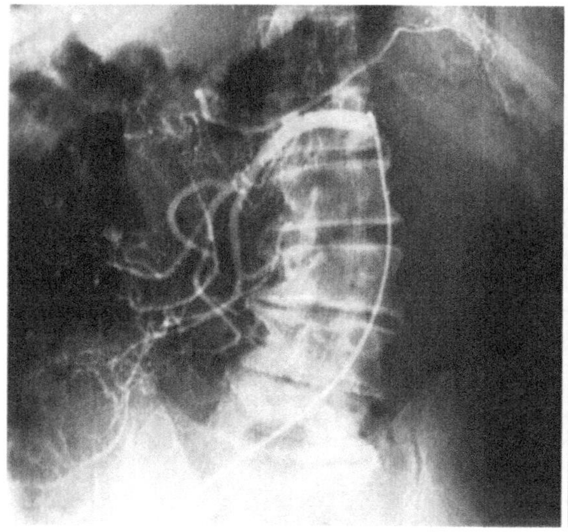

Fig. 166. Jejunal sarcoma. Giant tumor in left mid-abdomen with displacement of mesenteric branches toward the right beyond midline. Origin of vessels: jejunal branches. No tumor staining. Selective angiography of superior mesenteric artery

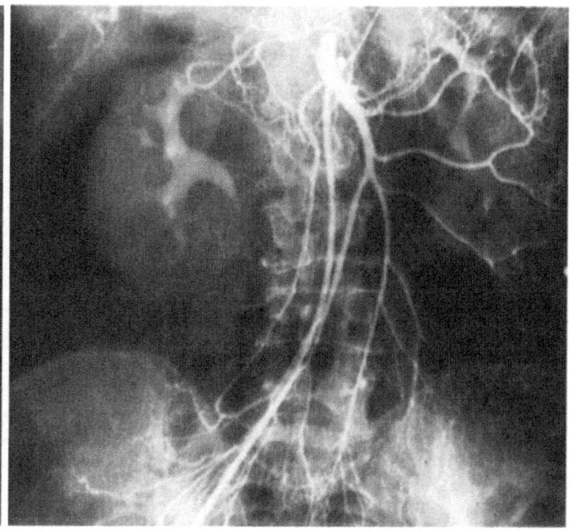

Fig. 167. Mesenteric sarcoma. Tumor of child's head-size in the right mid-abdomen; the tumor receives its vessels from the arcade network in right colon. No tumor staining in late phase. Selective angiography of superior mesenteric artery

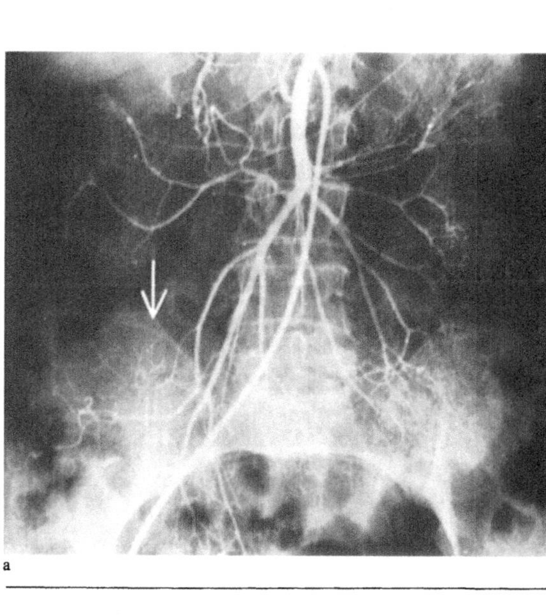

a

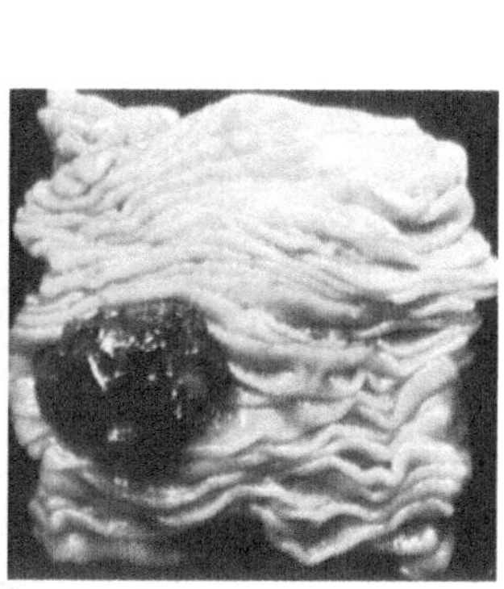

b

Fig. 168a and b. Metastasis of gemmangioma of terminal ileum. A 57-year-old woman with profuse gastrointestinal bleeding of uncertain origin. Twenty-six transfusions, 12 x-ray examinations of gastrointestinal tract, 10 endoscopies! (a) Circumscribed, lattice-shaped vasculature in territory of ileocolic artery (arrow). Selective angiography of superior mesenteric artery. (b) Surgical specimen with metastasis of a gemmangioma of the gluteal region operated on four years previously

Fig. 169a and b. Fistulizing enterocolitis. (a) Extensive fistula system between the rectosigmoid and the terminal ileum, which is considerably scarred. Severe inflammatory changes in mucosa. Barium enema. (b) No anomalies in angiogram other than moderate pruning of the arteries in the affected segment with splaying of a few branches. Selective angiography of superior mesenteric artery

Fig. 170a–d. Crohn's enteritis. (a) The ileocolic vessels are quite tortuous compared to the straight, faintly opacified arteries of the proximal segment of the small intestine; in some instances the former have a corkscrew appearance. Selective angiography of superior mesenteric artery. (b) Considerably augmented venous return from the ileocecal angle in an uneven parenchymal phase in this region. (c) Total rigidity of wall of terminal ileum with fistula formation. Stenosis of ileocecal valve and severe inflammatory changes in right colon. Barium enema. (d) Surgical specimen with air inflation and visualization of ileocolic artery. Right, normal conditions; left, vascular changes at the level of opaque pachymucosa

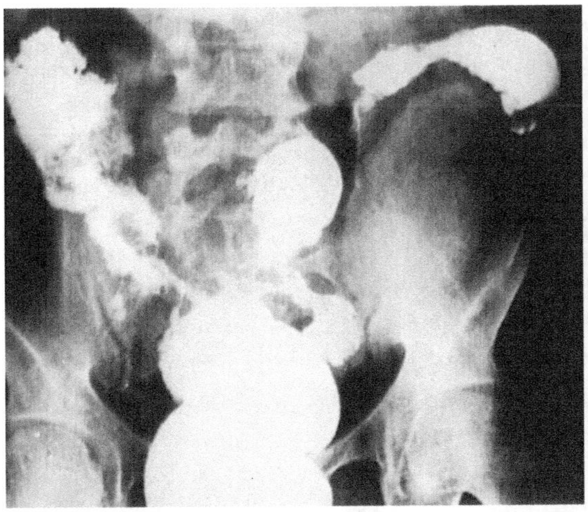

Fig. 169a (Legend see p. 182)

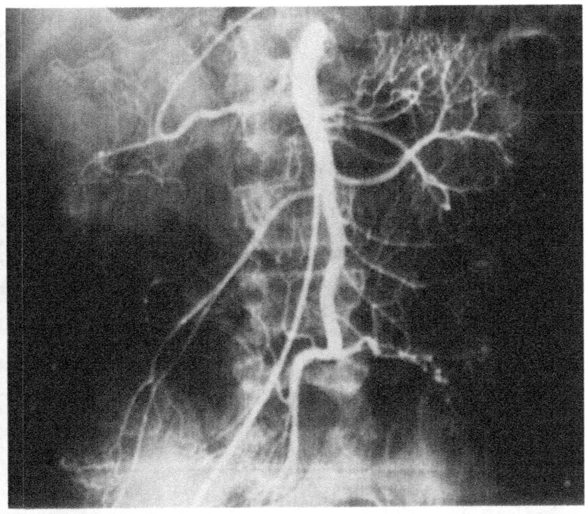

Fig. 169b

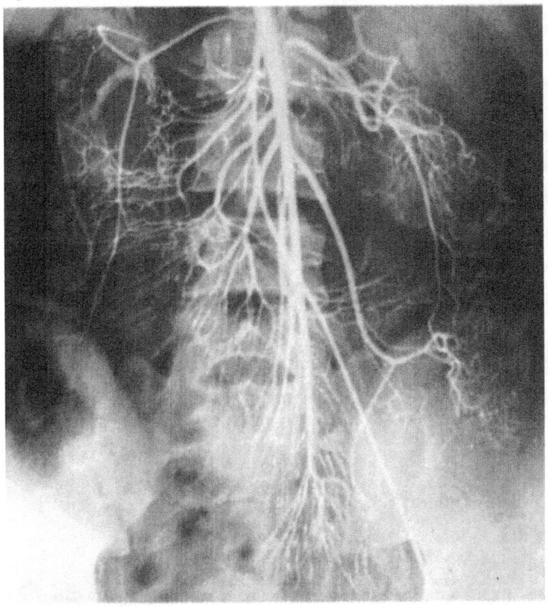

Fig. 170a (Legend see p. 182)

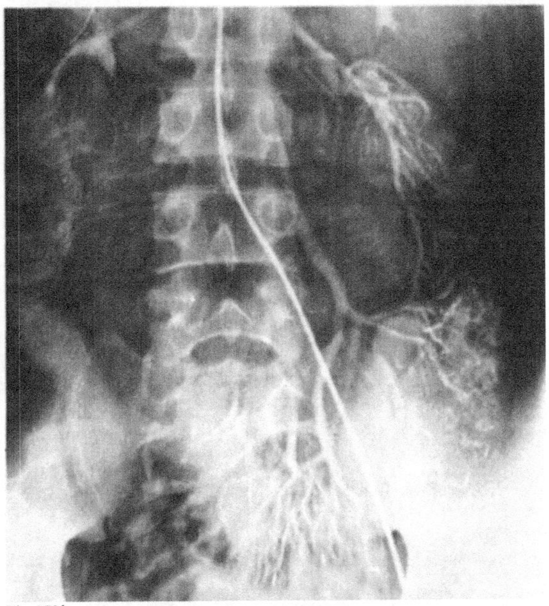

Fig. 170b

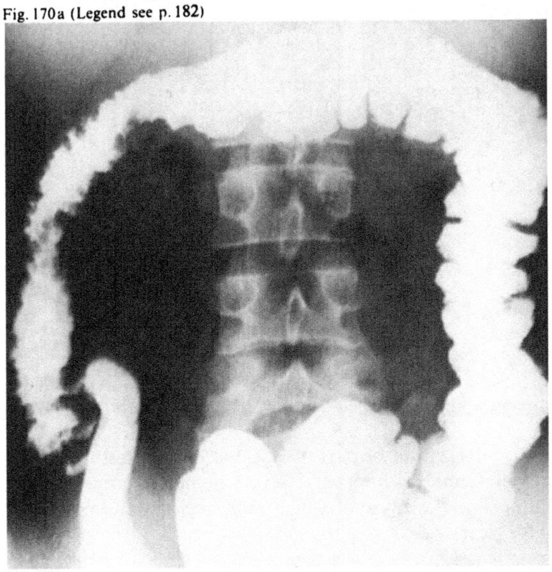

Fig. 170c

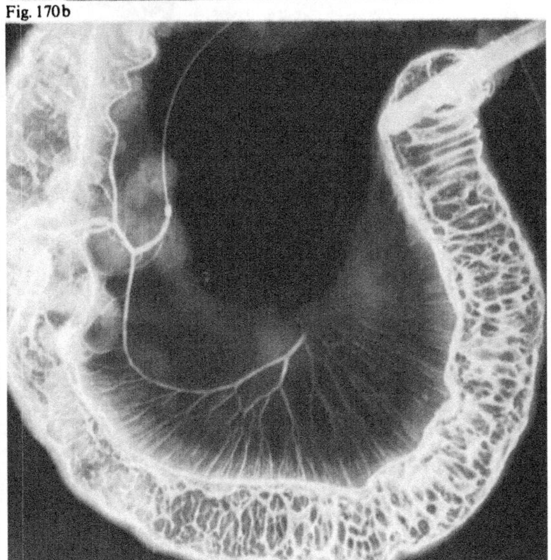

Fig. 170d

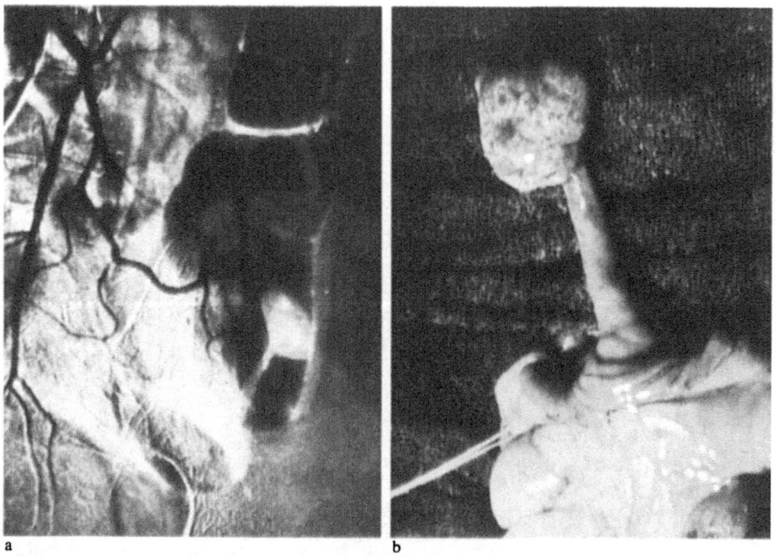

Fig. 171a and b. Sigmoid polyp. (a) Subtraction study; polyps in the air-filled left colon sharply defined. Selective angiography of inferior mesenteric artery. (b) Intraoperative appearance

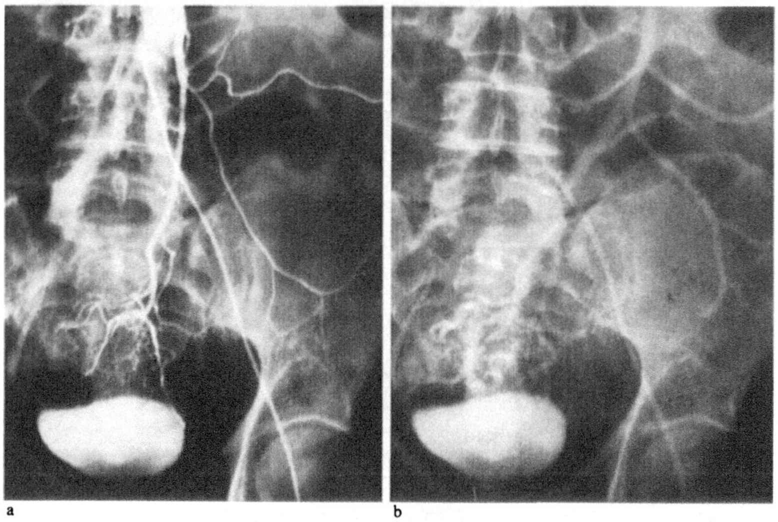

Fig. 172a and b. Richly vascularized rectal carcinoma. (a) Selective angiography of inferior mesenteric artery with visualization of richly vascularized tumor filling from the superior hemorrhoidal artery. The process is discernible above the opacified bladder. (b) Venous phase, with augmented contrast medium return through dilated tumor veins

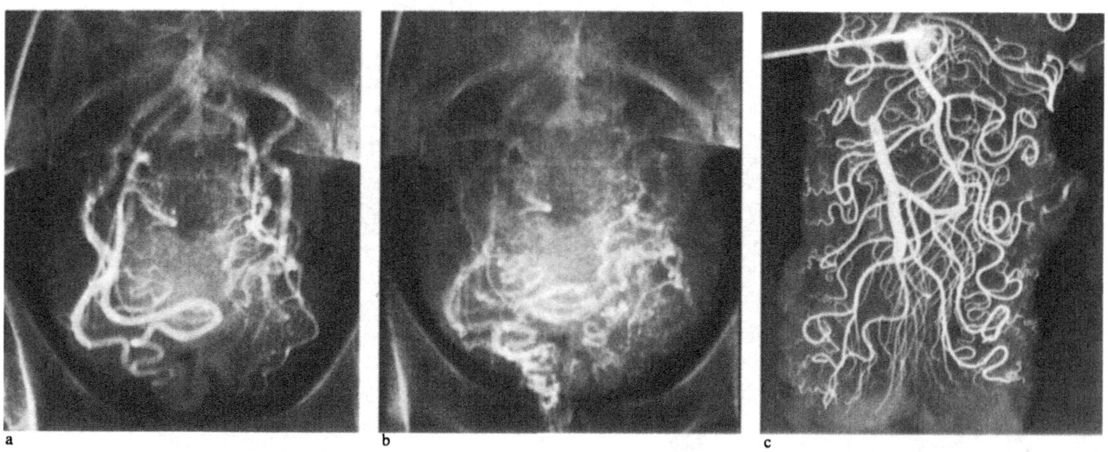

Fig. 173a–c. Arteriovenous deformity of rectum. (a) Dilated afferent arteries encircling the rectal ampulla. Selective angiography of inferior mesenteric artery. (b) Late phase: Array of arteries and veins in an extremely profuse pattern. (c) Rich arterial vascularization of part of resected large intestine wall. Clinical symptoms: Severe hemorrhaging of large intestine the cause of which remained undetermined for years

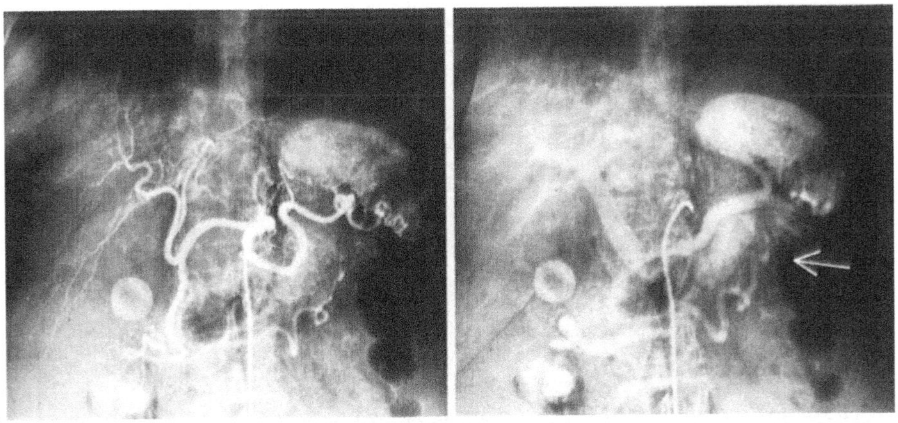

a b

Fig. 174a and b. Carcinomatous peritonitis. Ovarian carcinoma. Ascites. Single gallstone. (a) Unremarkable course of celiac branches. Celiac angiogram. (b) Late phase: Constant filling defect in left lateral splenic margin. Impression effect on the splenic vein. Circumscribed opacification of an oblong soft tissue growth extending along the splenic vein. Markedly dilated gastroepiploic vein with atypical course (arrow). Autopsy: Largenoduled carcinomatous peritonitis in ovarian carcinoma

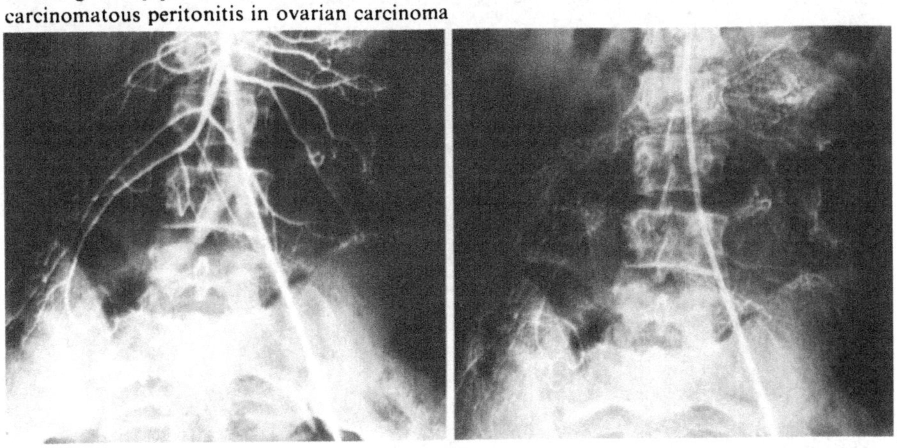

a b

Fig. 175a and b. Endometriosis. (a) Angiography of superior mesenteric artery performed on account of suspected mesenteric tumor. (b) In late phase, displacement of mesenteric branches by a process taking up almost the entire pelvis. Cause: Enlargement of uterus due to endometriosis

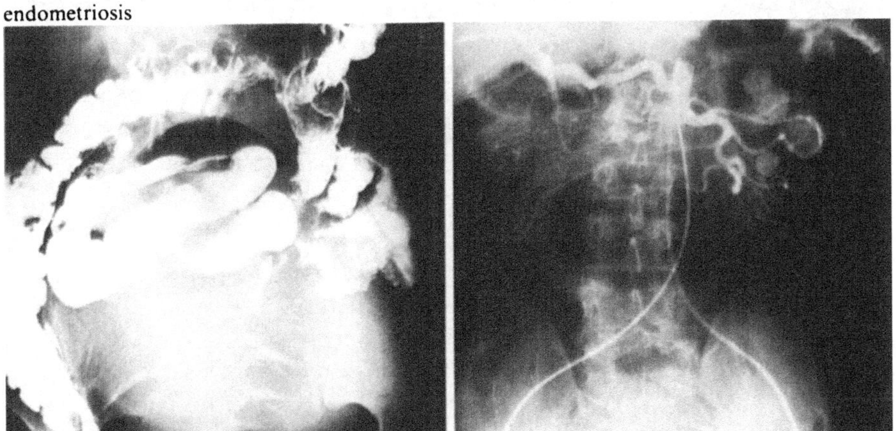

a b

Fig. 176a and b. Mesenteric cyst. (a) Displacement of colon and loops of small intestine by a process originating in middle lower abdomen. Gastrointestinal series. (b) Craniad displacement of branches supplied by superior mesenteric artery. No tumor opacification. Atypical origin of right hepatic artery from superior mesenteric artery. A second catheter has been inserted in the aorta to measure pressure. Surgery: Mesenteric cyst the size of a child's head

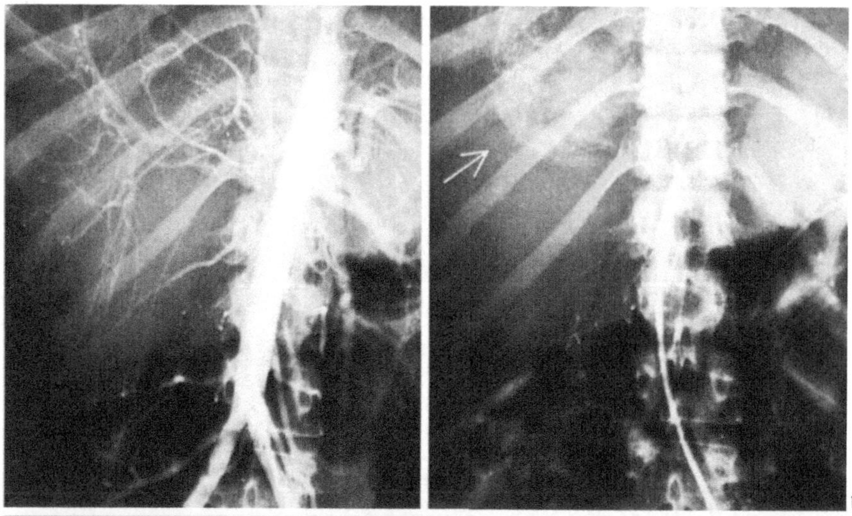

a b

Fig. 177a and b. Dystopic pheochromocytoma. (a) Atypical cluster of vessels projected over the liver shadow. Catheter aortogram. Lumbar dystopia of right kidney. (b) Circumscribed staining of richly vascularized apple-sized tumor in the same area (arrow). The surgeon (Dr. LINDER) removed a pheochromocytoma from the surrounding liver tissue

Legend to Fig. 178a–d see p. 187

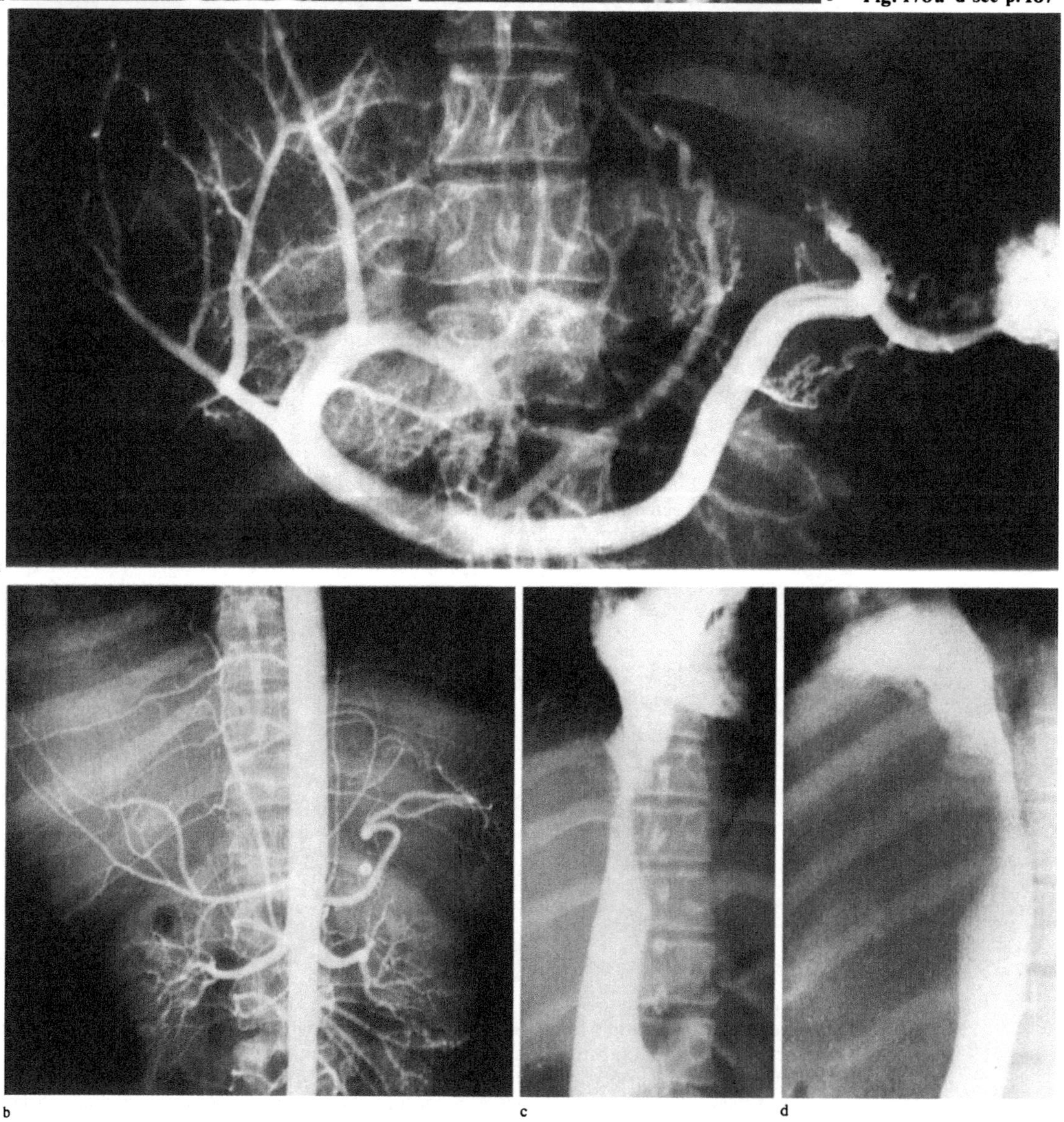

a b c d

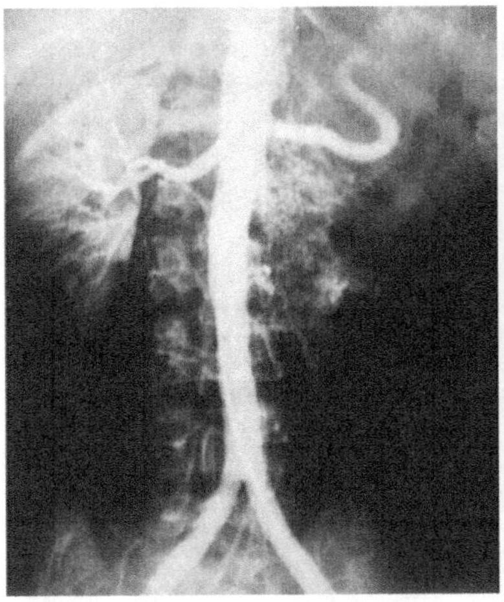

Fig. 179

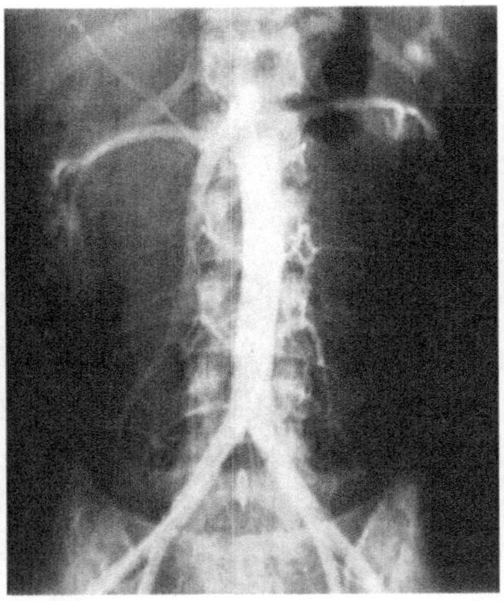

Fig. 180a

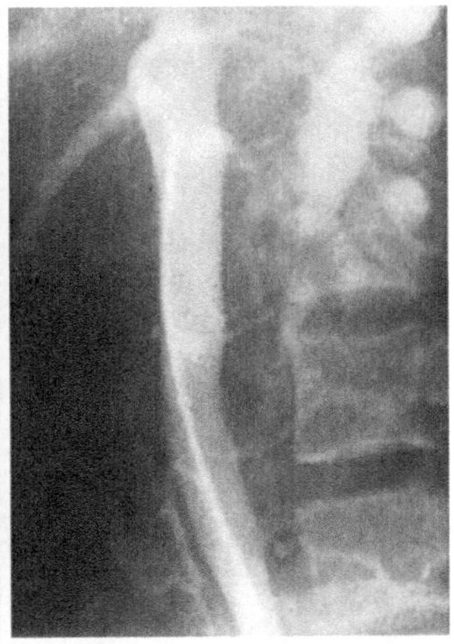

Fig. 180b

Fig. 179. Left-sided retroperitoneal carcinoma with complete obstruction in left renal artery and para-aortic pooling of contrast medium between splenic artery and third lumbar artery

Fig. 180a and b. Retroperitoneal sarcoma. (a) Symmetric elevation of both renal arteries by an active, bilateral spaceoccupying growth, with lateral displacement of kidneys. The tumor is supplied by lumbar arteries. Catheter aortogram. (b) Lateral view: Ventralward displacement of superior mesenteric artery. Histology: Fibrosarcoma

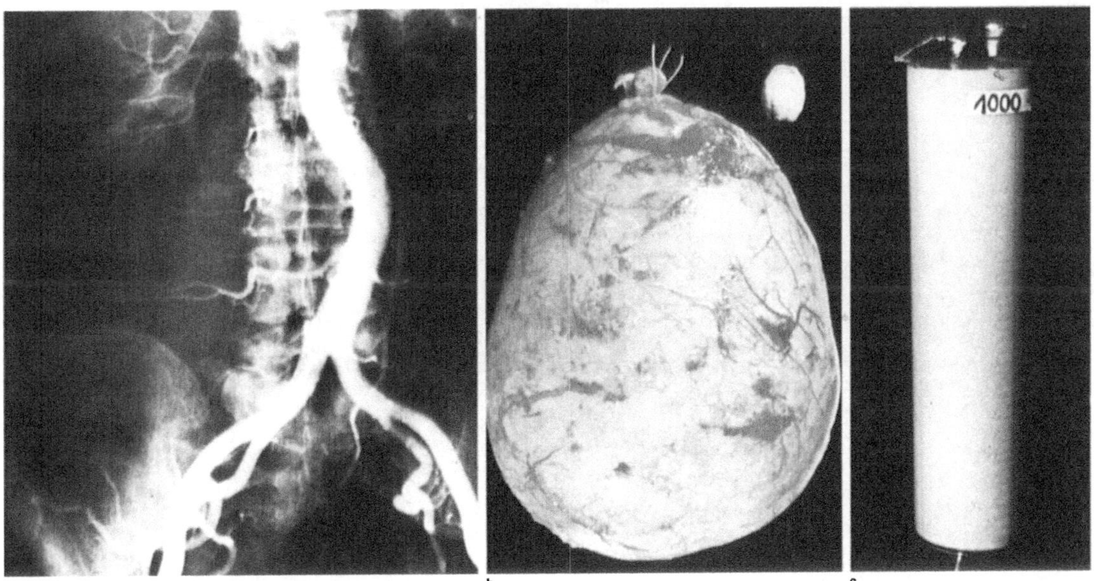

a b c

Fig. 181a–c. Gallbladder empyema misdiagnosed as retroperitoneal tumor. (a) Catheter aortogram with displacement away from the right. Large-caliber lumbar arteries. (b) The large gallbladder empyema with calculus from cystic duct. (Dr. LINDER). (c) The purulent contents

---

Fig. 178a–d. Budd-Chiari syndrome in presence of retroperitoneal tumor. (a) Bypass circulation via vena coronaria ventriculi owing to obstruction of venous outflow; portal hypertension. Splenoportogram. (b) Splaying of branches of hepatic artery in distinctly enlarged liver. Catheter aortogram. (c) Marked narrowing of inferior vena cava at origin of hepatic vein. Cavogram. (d) Ventral filling defect. Cavogram in lateral view. Surgery: Extensive retroperitoneal tumor encasing the vena cava at origin of hepatic vein

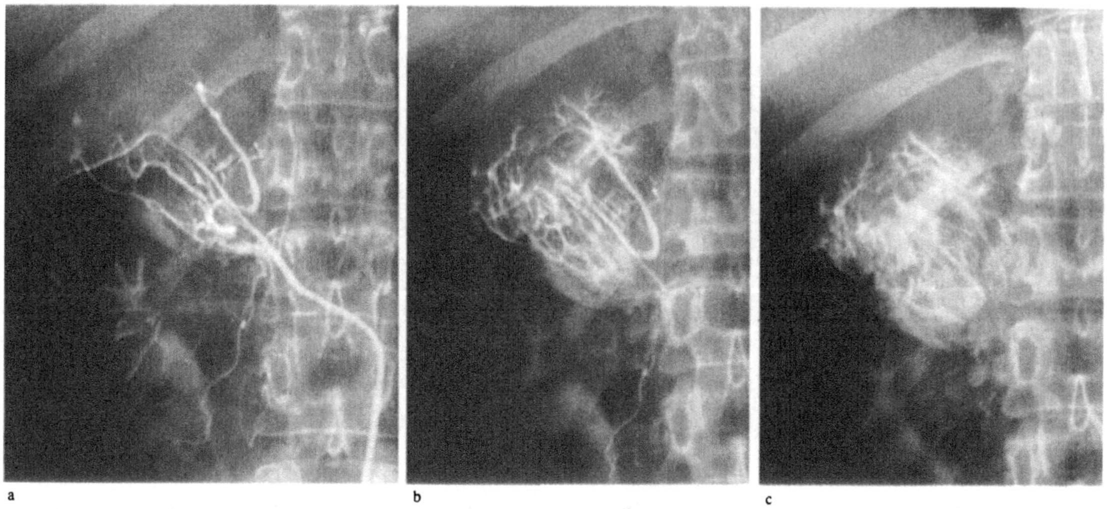

Fig. 182a–c. Adrenal carcinoma. (a) Superselective catheterization of right medial suprarenal artery. (b) Cluster of pathological vessels. Breaks in vessels, irregular outline of tumor. (c) Late phase: Strong opacification of tumor, which is poorly demarcated at its laterocranial margin. Avascular areas indicate necrosis. Histology: Adrenal carcinoma

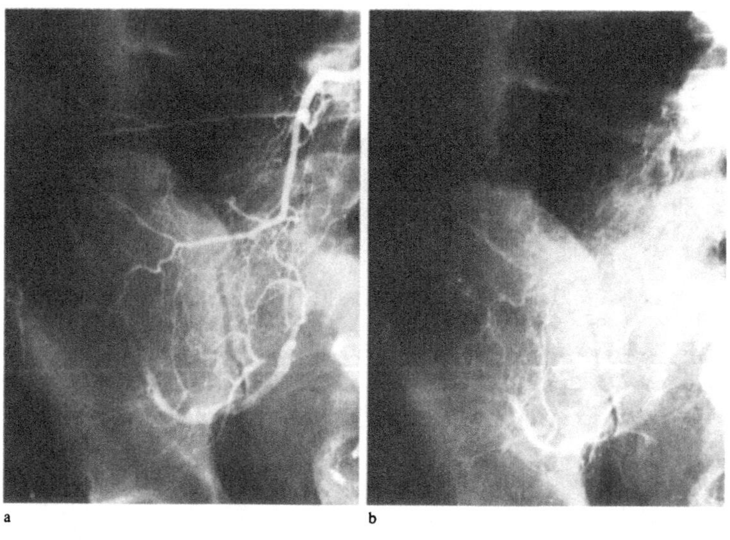

Fig. 183a and b. Transplant rejection. Condition after kidney transplant because of chronic nephritis. Disturbance of arterial blood flow. (a) Picture of richly vascularized capsule area supplied by a lumbar artery. Selective angiography of right lumbar artery (IV). (b) Late phase: No opacification of parenchyma of transplanted kidney

VIII Bibliography

AAKHUS, T.: The value of angiography in superior mesenteric artery embolism. Brit. J. Radiol. **39**, 928—932 (1966).

AAKHUS, T.: Angiography in experimental strangulating obstruction of the small intestine in dogs. Acta radiol. (Diagn.) **6**, 337—347 (1967).

AAKHUS, T., BRABRAND, G.: Angiography in acute superior mesenteric arterial insufficiency. Acta radiol. (Diagn.) **6**, 1—12 (1967).

AAKHUS, T., ENGE, J.: Angiography in traumatic rupture of the spleen. Brit. J. Radiol. **40**, 855—861 (1967).

AAKHUS, T., HOFSLI, M., VESTAD, E.: Angiography in acute pancreatitis. Acta radiol. (Diagn.) **8**, 119—128 (1969).

ABEATICI, S., CAMPI, L.: Visualizzazione radiologica della porta per via splenica. Minerva med. **92**, 593—598 (1951).

ABEATICI, S., CAMPI, L.: Les caractéristiques splénoportographiques des tumeurs du foie de l'abdomen supérior. Acta chir. belg. **59**, 803—834 (1960).

ABEATICI, S., CAMPI, L.: La morphologie de la porte dans les hépatides chroniques. Čs. Radiol. **19**, 318—323 (1965).

ABRAMS, H. L. (edit.): Angiography, vol. 1. 2. Boston, Mass.: Little, Brown & Comp. 1961.

ABRAMS, H. L.: Altered drug response of tumour in man. Nature (Lond.) **201**, 167 (1964).

ABRAMS, R. M., BERANBAUM, E. R., BERANBAUM, S. L., NGO, N. L.: Angiographic studies of benign and malignant cystadenoma of the pancreas. Radiology **89**, 1028—1032 (1967).

ABRAMS, R. M., BERANBAUM, E. R., SANTOS, J. S., LIPSON, J.: Angiographic features of cavernous hemiangioma of liver. Radiology **92**, 308—312 (1969).

ABRAMS, R. M., MENG, CH. H., FIROOZUIA, H., BERANBAUM, E. R., EPSTEIN, H. Y.: Angiographic demonstration of carcinoma of the gallbladder. Radiology **94**, 277—282 (1970).

ADOLPH, K.: Gallengangs- und Pankreasdiagnostik. Leitfaden der hypotonen Duodenographie und perkutanen, transhepatischen Cholangiographie. Stuttgart: Enke 1968.

AHLBERG, N. E., BARTLEY, O., CHIDEKEL, N.: Venous arteriography. A modified technique and indications for its use. Acta radiol. (Diagn.) **7**, 321—330 (1968).

ALFIDI, R. J., RASTOGI, H., BUONOCORE, E., BROWN, C. H.: Hepatic arteriography. Radiology **90**, 1136—1142 (1968).

ANACKER, H.: Röntgenanatomie des Pankreas. Fortschr. Röntgenstr. **94**, 1—13 (1961).

ANACKER, H.: Die pathologischen Veränderungen des Pankreasgangsystems im Röntgenbild. Fortschr. Röntgenstr. **96**, 455—470 (1962).

ANACKER, H.: Kritische Bewertung der röntgenologischen Untersuchungsmethoden zur Pankreasdiagnostik. Radiologe **5**, 312—318 (1965).

ANACKER, H.: Anomalien und Variationen des Pankreas. Radiologe **7**, 41—52 (1967).

ANACKER, H.: Schwerpunkte der röntgenologischen Pankreasdiagnostik. Dtsch. med. Wschr. **21**, 1127—1132 (1969).

ANACKER, H.: In: TESCHENDORF, W., Lehrbuch der röntgenologischen Differentialdiagnostik, Bd. 2. Erkrankungen der Bauchorgane. Stuttgart: Thieme 1964.

ANACKER, H., LINDEN, G., HUMPERT, R.: Die chronischen Pankreaskrankheiten im Splenoportogramm. Fortschr. Röntgenstr. **99**, 129—142 (1963).

ANACKER, H., MORINO, F., RÖSCH, J., SCHUMACHER, W., ZUPPINGER, A.: Röntgendiagnostik der Leber. Berlin-Göttingen-Heidelberg: Springer 1959.

ANDREN, L., FRIEDBERG, S., WELIN, S.: Roentgen diagnosis of small polyps in the colon and rectum. Acta radiol. (Stockh.) **43**, 201—208 (1955).

ANGERSTEIN, W., KRUG, W., RAKOW, A.: Eine Methode zur Erzeugung farbiger Röntgenbilder. Fortschr. Röntgenstr. **100**, 257—263 (1964).

ANNES, G., CAPLAN, L. H., HEIMLICH, H.: Upper gastrointestinal hemorrhage. Undetced site localized by selective arteriography. Arch. Surg. **94**, 44—45 (1967).

ARONSEN, K. F., LUNDERQUIST, A., NYLANDER, G.: The comparison of celiacography and direct portography in the diagnostic evaluation of liver diseases. Radiology **92**, 313—322 (1969).

ASANG, E., MITTELMEIER, H.: Die stenosierenden und obliterierenden Gefäßerkrankungen der inneren Organe. Münch. med. Wschr. **98**, 1604 (1956).

BACHMANN, D.: Arterieller Spasmus als Fehldeutungsmöglichkeit bei der Angiographie. Röntgen-Bl. **19**, 478—481 (1966).

BACHMANN, D.: Angiographie der Milz. Methoden und Ergebnisse. Internist **8**, 371—376 (1967).

BACHMANN, D., FRANKE, H.: Die Splenoportographie als diagnostische Sofortmaßnahme bei akuter Massenblutung aus Oesophagusvarizen. In: Angiographie und ihre Leistungen. Hrsg. von K. E. LOOSE, S. 139—141. Stuttgart: Thieme 1968.

BACHMANN, D., HAASNER, E., EL-SALLAB, R. A.: Zur Angiographie von Aortenaneurysmen. Fortschr. Röntgenstr. **104**, 670—676 (1966).

BACKMUND, H., DECKER, K., LOY, W.: Photographische Subtraktion — eine radiologische Routinemethode. Fortschr. Röntgenstr. **104**, 408 (1966).

BALTAXE, H. A., FLEMING, R. J.: The angiographic appearance of hydatid disease. Radiology **97**, 599—604 (1970).

BÁNG, I.: Ein angiographisch diagnostizierter Fall von Cystadenoma Pancreatis. Radiologe **5**, 287—288 (1965).

BARDSLEY, J. L., KOEHLER, P. R.: Pseudoxanthoma elasticum: angiographic manifestations in abdominal vessels. Radiology **93**, 559 (1969).

BARTEL, J., WIERNY, L.: Zur Agenesie der Vena cava caudalis. Fortschr. Röntgenstr. **99**, 467—473 (1963).

BARTLEY, O., EDLUND, Y., HELANDER, C.G.: Angiography in primary hepatic carcinoma. Acta radiol. (Diagn.) **6**, 81—90 (1967).

BARTLEY, O., BENGTSSON, U., CEDERBOM, G.: Die Nierenfunktion vor und nach Urographie und Angiographie mit großen Dosen von Kontrastmitteln. Acta radiol. (Diagn.) **8**, 9 (1969).

BARTLEY, O., HELANDER, C.-G., ROSENGREN, B., STATTIN, S.: Scintigraphy and angiography in demonstration of hepatic tumours. Acta radiol. (Diagn.) **8**, 161—167 (1969).

BAUM, S.: Hepatic arteriography. Amer. J. Gastroent. **51**, 151—153 (1969).

BAUM, S., ABRAMS, H.L.: A J-shaped catheter for retrograde catheterization of tortuous vessels. Radiology **83**, 436—437 (1964).

BAUM, S., GREENSTEIN, R.H., NUSBAUM, M., BLAKEMORE, W.S.: Diagnosis of ruptured noncalcified splenic artery aneurysm by selective celiac arteriography. Arch. Surg. **91**, 1026—1028 (1965).

BAUM, M., HOWE, C.T.: Hypotonic duodenography in the diagnosis of carcinoma of the pancreas and its further use when combined with percutaneous cholangiography and pancreatic scintiscanning. Amer. J. Surg. **115**, 519—525 (1968).

BAUM, S., NUSBAUM, M.: The control of gastrointestinal hemorrhage by selective mesenteric arterial infusion of vasopressin. Radiology **98**, 497—505 (1971).

BAUM, S., NUSBAUM, M., BLAKEMORE, W.S., FINKELSTEIN, A.K.: Preoperative radiographic demonstration of intra-abdominal bleeding from undetermined sites by percutaneous selective celiac and superior mesenteric arteriography. Surgery **58**, 797—805 (1965).

BAUM, S., NUSBAUM, M., KURODA, K., BLAKEMORE, W.S.: Direct serial magnification arteriography as an adjuvant in the diagnosis of surgical lesions in the alimentary tract. Amer. J. Surg. **117**, 170—176 (1969).

BAUM, S., ROY, R., FINKELSTEIN, A.K., BLAKEMORE, W.S.: Clinical application of selective celiac and superior mesenteric arteriography. Radiology **84**, 279—295 (1965).

BAUM, ST., STEIN, G.N., NUSBAUM, M., CHAIT, A.: Selective arteriography in diagnosis of hemorrhage in gastrointestinal tract. Radiol. Clin. N. Amer. **7**, 131—145 (1969).

BAUM, ST., WARD, ST., NUSBAUM, M.: Stress bleeding from mid-duodenum: often unrecognized source of gastrointestinal hemorrhage. Radiology **95**, 595—602 (1970).

BAYINDIR, S.: Angiographie der Leber und des Pankreas. In: Angiographie und ihre Leistungen. Hrsg. von K.E. LOOSE, S. 115—116. Stuttgart: Thieme 1968.

BAYINDIR, S.: Der Wert der kombinierten perkutanen transhepatischen Cholangiographie und Zöliakographie bei der Diagnostik des tumorbedingten Verschlußikterus. Fortschr. Röntgenstr. **109**, 16—23 (1968).

BAYINDIR, S., GRAEBNER, H.: Arteriovenöse Fistel zwischen Arteria und Vena lienalis nach Splenektomie. Fortschr. Röntgenstr. **105**, 279—282 (1966).

BAYINDIR, S., HEGER, N., SCHIRMER, H. F., STECKENMESSER, R.: Die percutane transhepatische Cholangiographie bei ikterischen und anikterischen Patienten. Bericht über 179 Untersuchungen. Fortschr. Röntgenstr. **111**, 315—329 (1969).

BAYINDIR, S., SCHULTIS, K.: Der Wert der perkutanen transhepatischen Cholangiographie in der präoperativen Diagnostik. In: Der Ikterus. Hrsg. von K. BECK, S. 373. Stuttgart-New York: Schattauer 1968.

BEALL, A. C., COOLEY, D. A., MORRIS, G. C., DEBAKEY, M. E.: Perforation of arteriosclerotic aneurysms into the vena cava. Arch. Surg. **86**, 809—818 (1963).

BEALL, A. C., Jr., MORRIS, G. C., Jr., GARRETT, H. E., HENLY, W. S., HALLMAN, G. L., CRAWFORD, E. S., COOLEY, D. A., DEBAKEY, M. E.: Translumbar aortography. Present indications and techniques. Ann. intern. Med. **60**, 843—856 (1964).

BECKER, V.: Leberstruktur und Blutkreislauf. Ärztl. Wschr. **11**, 829—835 (1956).

BEDUHN, D.: Röntgendiagnostik des Verschlußikterus mit experimentellen Untersuchungen zur röntgenologischen Symptomatologie. Med. Habil.-Schr. Heidelberg 1970.

BEDUHN, D.: Angiographischer Nachweis einer traumatisch bedingten Intimaeinrollung an der Nierenarterie. Fortschr. Röntgenstr. **112**, 828—829 (1970).

BEDUHN, D.: Angiographie beim kindlichen Trauma. Z. Kinderchir. **11** (Suppl.) 562—574 (1972).

BEDUHN, D., HALLWACHS, O.: Selektive Nierenangiographie über die implantierte Milzarterie. Fortschr. Röntgenstr. **113**, 133—137 (1970).

BEDUHN, D., VOLLMAR, J.: Arterio-portale Fistel nach Magenresektion. Radiologe **10**, 304—309 (1970).

BEDUHN, D., WENZ, W.: Abdominale Gefäßuntersuchungen im Kindesalter. Fortschr. Röntgenstr. **113**, 753—759 (1970).

BELAN, A., KOČANDRLE, V., POSPICHAL, J., BERÁNEK, J.: Komplikationen bei verschiedenen arteriographischen Untersuchungsmethoden. Fortschr. Röntgenstr. **110**, 57—64 (1969).

BENGMARK, S., ENGEVIK, L., ROSENGREN, K.: Angiography of the regenerating human liver after extensive resection. Surgery **65**, 590—596 (1969).

BENNEK, J.: Die diagnostische Bedeutung des Kavogramms bei retroperitonealen Tumoren im Kindesalter. Z. Kinderchir. **3**, 511—519 (1966).

BENNET, J., BIGOT, R.: Arteriography in primitive tumours of the liver. Ann. Radiol. **11**, 837—845 (1968).

BENNET, J., BRIAND, L., CHÉRIGIÉ, ED., DOYON, D.: Artériographie sélective du tronc coeliaque et tumeur splénique. J. Radiol. Électrol. **47**, 823—825 (1966).

BENNET, J., CHÉRIGIÉ, E., CAROLI, J., DOYON, D., ECONOMOPOULOS, P., PLESSIER, J., STOOPEN, M.: La pancréatographie après stimulation par la sécrétine intraarterielle; à propos de 33 cas. Ann. Radiol. **10**, 617—625 (1967).

BENNET, J., MUSSY, F.: Le diagnostic artériographie préopératoire des anévrismes de l'artère hépatique. Ann. Radiol. **13**, 33—41 (1970).

BENNET, J., CHALUT, J., PARAF, A., PROT, D.: L'artériographie hépatique dans le diagnostic des tumeurs du foie. Presse méd. **72**, 877—882 (1964).

BENKÖ, G.: Tumorähnliche Schatten des normalen Magens und des Zwölffingerdarms im Angiogramm. Fortschr. Röntgenstr. **110**, 322—328 (1969).

BENKÖ, G.: Das angiographische Bild des entzündlichen Netztumors und anderer Prozesse des Netzes. Röntgen-Bl. **24**, 289—292 (1971).

BENKÖ, G., SALT, J.: Malignes Paragangliom mit Riesenmetastasen in der Leber. Fortschr. Röntgenstr. **113**, 678—681 (1970).

BERCHTOLD, R., FUCHS, W.A.: Zur Lokalisationsdiagnostik einer recidivierenden, massiven Intestinalblutung. Helv. chir. Acta **33**, 56—58 (1966).

BERDON, W.E., BAKER, D.H.: Giant hepatic hemangioma with cardiac failure in the newborn infant. Value of high-dosage intravenous urography and umbilical angiography. Radiology **92**, 1523—1528 (1969).

BERGERHOFF, W.: Farbige Röntgenbilder. In: Handbuch der medizinischen Radiologie, Bd. III, S. 508—517. Berlin-Heidelberg-New York: Springer 1967.

BERK, R.N., WHOLEY, M.H.: The application of splenic arteriography in the diagnosis of rupture of the spleen. Amer. J. Roentgenol. **104**, 662—667 (1968).

BERKOWITZ, D.: (1954) zit. nach WENZ, W. (1969).

BERT, J.M., LAMARQUE, J.L., BALMES, J.L., GINESTIA, J.F.: La place de l'artériographie sélective dans l'identification des tumeurs digestives abdominales. Ann. Radiol. **11**, 788—791 (1968).

BIEBER, W.P., ALBO, R.J.: Cystadenoma of the pancreas: Its arteriographic diagnosis. Radiology **80**, 776 (1963).

BIERMAN, H.R., BYRON, R.L., Jr., KELLY, K.H., GRADY, A.: Studies on the blood supply of tumors in man. Vascular patterns of the liver by hepatic arteriography in vivo. J. nat. Cancer Inst. **12**, 107—132 (1951).

BIERMAN, H.R., KELLY, K.H., BYRON, R.L., Jr.: Hepatic arteriography. In: Angiography, vol. 2, Edit.: H.L. Abrams. Boston: Little, Brown & Comp. 1961.

BIERMAN, H.R., MILLER, E.R., BYRON, R.L., Jr., DOD, K.S., KELLY, K.H., BLACK, D.H.: Intraarterial catheterization of viscera in man. Amer. J. Roentgenol. **66**, 555—568 (1951).

BIRKE, G., ENGSTEDT, L.: Melena and hematemesis; follow-up investigation, with special reference to bleeding of unknown origin. Gastroenterologia (Basel) **85**, 97—115 (1956).

BÖCK, G.: Farbige Röntgenbilder im Dienst der Dosisminderung bei Aufnahmen im Gonadenbereich. Fortschr. Röntgenstr. **107**, 799—802 (1967).

BÖRGER, G.: Portaler Hochdruck. In: HELLNER, H., NISSEN, R., VOSSSCHULTE, K., Lehrbuch der Chirurgie, S. 722. Stuttgart: Thieme 1962.

BOIJSEN, E.: Selective visceral angiography using a percutaneous axillary technique. Brit. J. Radiol. **39**, 414—421 (1966).

BOIJSEN, E.: Angiographische Untersuchungen über die Wirkung vasoaktiver Substanzen auf die viscerale Zirkulation. In: Angiographie und ihre Leistungen. Hrsg. von K.E. LOOSE, S. 129—134. Stuttgart: Thieme 1968.

BOIJSEN, E., ABRAMS, H.: Roentgenologic diagnosis of primary carcinoma of the liver. Acta radiol. (Diagn.) **3**, 257—277 (1965).

BOIJSEN, E., EFSING, H.O.: Intrasplenic arterial aneurysms following splenoportal phlebography. Acta radiol. (Diagn.) **6**, 487—496 (1967).

BOIJSEN, E., EFSING, H.O.: Aneurysm of the splenic artery. Acta radiol. (Diagn.) **8**, 29—41 (1969).

BOIJSEN, E., EKMAN, C.A.: Angiography in portal hypertension. J. cardiovasc. Surg. (Torino), Suppl. 5—18 (1965).

BOIJSEN, E., EKMAN, C.A., LUNDH, G.: Selective splanchnic angiography. Adv. Surg. (Chic.) **3**, 13—73 (1968).

BOIJSEN, E., EKMAN, C.A., OLIN, T.: Coeliac and superior mesenteric angiography in portal hypertension. Acta chir. scand. **126**, 315—325 (1963).

BOIJSEN, E., GÖTHLIN, J., HALLBÖCK, T., SANDBLOM, P.: Preoperative angiographic diagnosis of bleeding aneurysms of abdominal visceral arteries. Radiology **93**, 781—791 (1969).

BOIJSEN, E., JUDKINDS, M., SIMAY, A.: Angiographic diagnosis of hepatic rupture. Radiology **86**, 66—72 (1966).

BOIJSEN, E., OLIN, T.: Zöliakographie und Angiographie der A. mesenterica superior. In: Ergebnisse der medizinischen Strahlenforschung, S. 112. Stuttgart: Thieme 1964.

BOIJSEN, E., REDMAN, H.C.: Effect of bradykinin of celiac and superior mesenteric angiography. Invest. Radiol. **1**, 422—430 (1966).

BOIJSEN, E., REDMAN, H.: Effect of epinephrine on celiac and superior mesenteric angiography. Invest. Radiol. **2**, 184—199 (1967).

BOIJSEN, E., REUTER, S.R.: Mesenteric angiography in the evaluation of inflammatory and neoplastic disease of the intestine. Radiology **87**, 1028—1036 (1966).

BOIJSEN, E., REUTER, S.R.: Angiography in the diagnosis of chronic unexplained melena. Radiology **89**, 413—419 (1967).

BOIJSEN, E., REUTER, M.S.: Combined percutaneous transhepatic cholangiography and angiography in the evaluation of obstructure jaundice. Amer. J. Roentgenol. **99**, 153—161 (1967).

BOIJSEN, E., WEILAND, P.O.: Dissecting aneurysm of the aorta in Marfan's syndrome. Acta radiol. (Diagn.) **3**, 89—96 (1965).

BOIJSEN, E., WILLIAMS, C.M., JUDKINS, M.P.: Angiography of pheochromocytoma. Amer. J. Roentgenol. **98**, 225—232 (1966).

BOISSON, J., HERNANDEZ, C., PARTURIER-ALBOT, M.: L'artériographié mésentérique dans la rectocolite ulcéro-hémorragique. (Incidences pratiques, diagnostiques, pronostiques et thérapeutiques, à propos de 10 cas.) Arch. Mal. Appar. dig. **55**, 63—76 (1966).

BOLEY, S.J., COHEN, M.I., WINSLOW, P.R., BECKER, N.H., TREIBER, W., MCNAMARA, H., VEITH, F.J., GLIEDMAN, M.L.: Mesenteric ischemia: a cause of increased gastric blood flow, hyperacidity, and acute gastric ulceration. Surgery **68**, 222—230 (1970).

BOLEY, S.J., SCHWARTZ, S., LASCH, J., STERNHILL, V.: Reversible vascular occlusion of the colon. Surg. Gynec. Obstet. **116**, 53—60 (1963).

BONAKDARPOUR, A.: Angiography of mesenteric arterial occlusion. Invest. Radiol. **5**, 316—328 (1970).

BONANN, L.J., DOWDY, A.H.: Log etronic simplification in simulated color radiography. Radiology **70**, 585—587 (1958).

BOOKSTEIN, J.J.: Vergrößerungstechnik, experimentelle Untersuchungen. In: Röntgendiagnostik. Hrsg. von W.A. FUCHS, E. VOEGELI. (Aktuelle Probleme der Röntgendiagnostik. Bd. 1, S. 12—23.) Bern-Stuttgart-Wien: Huber 1971.

BOOKSTEIN, J.J., OBERMAN, H.A.: Appraisal of selective angiography in localizing islet-cell tumors of the pancreas. Radiology **86**, 682—685 (1966).

BOOKSTEIN, J.J., REUTER, S.R., MARTEL, W.: Angiographic evaluation of pancreatic carcinoma. Radiology **93**, 757—764 (1969).

BOSNIAK, M. A., BYCK, W.: Wandering spleen diagnosed preoperativly by intravenous aortography. Amer. J. Roentgenol. **84**, 898—901 (1960).

BOSNIAK, M. A., WILLIAMS, L. F., Jr., HASIOTIS, CH. A., BYRNE, J. J., SCHAPIRO, J. H.: In vivo magnification arteriography of the bowel wall. Amer. J. Surg. **114**, 359—362 (1967).

BRAHME, F.: Mesenteric angiography in regional enterocolitis. Radiology **87**, 1037—1042 (1966).

BRAUNSTEIN, H.: Pathogenesis of dissecting aneurysm. Circulation **28**, 1071—1078 (1963).

BREEDIS, C., YOUNG, G.: The blood supply of neoplasms in the liver. Amer. J. Path. **30**, 969 (1954).

BREHM, H. v., HOEFFKEN, W., GEHL, H.: Präoperative angiographische Darstellung eines blutenden Dünndarmkarzinoms. Fortschr. Med. **85**, 233—235 (1967).

BREIT, A.: Angiographie der Uterustumoren und ihrer Rezidive. Stuttgart: Thieme 1967. (Fortschr. Röntgenstr. Erg.-Bd. **98**.)

BREIT, A.: Arteriographie vor und nach Tumorbestrahlung. Fortschr. Röntgenstr. **111**, 329—344 (1969).

BRICK, J. B., PALMER, E. D.: One thousand cases of portal cirrhosis of the liver. Implications of esophageal varices and their management. Arch. intern. Med. **113**, 501—511 (1964).

BRON, K. M., REDMAN, H. C.: Splanchnic artery stenosis and occlusion. Incidence; arteriography and clinical manifestations. Radiology **92**, 323—328 (1969).

BRON, K. M., RILEY, R. R., GIRDANY, B. R.: Pediatric arteriography in abdominal and extremity lesions. Radiology **92**, 1241—1255 (1969).

BRON, K. M., STROTT, C. A., SHAPIRO, A. P.: The diagnostic value of angiographic observations in polyarteritis nodosa. A case of multiple aneurysms in the visceral organs. Arch. intern. Med. **116**, 450—454 (1965).

BRON, K. M., WESTERMAN, M. P., JENKINS, J. L.: The diagnosis of a lienunculus. J. Amer. med. Ass. **203**, 1139—1140 (1968).

BROWN, R. B., RICE, B. H., SZAKAS, J. E.: Intestinal bleeding and perforation complicating treatment with vasoconstrictors. Ann. Surg. **150**, 790 (1959).

BROY, H.: Die Querschnittslähmung, eine fatale angiographische Komplikation, Kasuistik und Übersicht. Fortschr. Röntgenstr. **114**, 353—366 (1971).

BRÜNNER, S., LUNDERQUIST, A.: Arteriographische Probleme bei Crohn-Syndrom und Colitis ulcerosa. Ann. Radiol. **12**, R 224 (1969).

BÜCHELER, E.: Die direkte Angiographie der Vertebralplexus, der lumbalen Venen und des Azygosvenensystems. In: Ergebnisse der medizinischen Radiologie, Bd. III. Hrsg. GLAUNER, R., RÜTTIMANN, A., u. a. Stuttgart: Thieme 1971.

BÜCHELER, E., BELTZ, L., DÜX, A., THURN, P.: Zur Röntgenuntersuchung des Retroperitonealraumes. Radiologe **5**, 217—231 (1965).

BÜCHELER, E., DÜX, A.: Pathologische Veränderungen an den unpaaren Ästen der abdominellen Aorta und ihrer Verteilerarterien. Dtsch. Röntgenkongr. **48**, 53—55, 1967 (1968) (Fortschr. Röntgenstr. Beih.).

BÜCHELER, E., DÜX, A., ROHR, H.: Mesenteric-Steal-Syndrom. Fortschr. Röntgenstr. **106**, 313—320 (1967).

BÜCHELER, E., DÜX, A., SOBBE, A.: Die renolumbale Anastomose im direkten retroperitonealen Veno- und selektiven Azygogramm. Fortschr. Röntgenstr. **109**, 712—719 (1968).

BÜCHELER, E., DÜX, A., THURN, P.: Zur röntgenologischen Früherkennung lokaler Tumorrezidive im Retroperitonealraum. Fortschr. Röntgenstr. **105**, 448—457 (1965).

BÜCHELER, E., DÜX, A., THURN, P.: Die Stenose der abdominellen Aorta. Fortschr. Röntgenstr. **104**, 22—33 (1966).

BÜCHELER, E., DÜX, A., THURN, P.: Membranöser Verschluß und Agenesie der Vena cava inferior. Fortschr. Röntgenstr. **105**, 806—818 (1966).

BÜCHELER, E., DÜX, A., THURN, P.: Die Röntgendiagnostik der primären retroperitonalen Tumoren. Fortschr. Röntgenstr. **107**, 735—747 (1967).

BÜCHELER, E., SCHULZ, D., DÜX, A.: Angiographische Darstellung des Pfortadersystems nach Shunt-Operationen. Fortschr. Röntgenstr. **114**, 740—752 (1971).

BÜCHELER, E., THELEN, M.: Superselektive Angiographie der Äste des Truncus coeliacus. Röntgen-Bl. **24**, 11—25 (1971).

BÜCHELER, E., THELEN, M., THURN, P.: Indikationen und Ergebnisse der Coeliacographie. Dtsch. med. Wschr. **96**, 43—46 (1971).

BULGRIN, J. G., JACOBSEN, G.: Aortographic demonstration of an aortocaval fistula. A case report. Radiology **71**, 409—411 (1958).

BUNNAG, T. S., KAOPARISUTHI, V., ARTHACHINTA, S., CHIENPRADIT, K., BINBAKAYA, L.: Percutaneous splenic portography in amebic liver abcess. Amer. J. Roentgenol. **80**, 324—329 (1958).

BUONOCORE, E., MEANY, T. F., SKILLERN, P. G., GUIK, G.: Functioning pancreatic islet-cell adenoma diagnosed preoperatively by means of splanchnic arteriography. Arch. intern. Med. **116**, 824—827 (1965).

BURCKHARDT, D., VERA, C. A., LADUE, J. S., STEINBERG, I.: Enzyme activity following angiography. Amer. J. Roentgenol. **22**, 446—450 (1968).

BURCKHARDT, H., MÜLLER, W.: Versuche über die Punktion der Gallenblase und ihre Röntgendarstellung. Dtsch. Z. Chir. **162**, 168—197 (1920/21).

BURGENER, F., FUCHS, W. A., BETTEX, W.: Die angiographische Diagnostik der abdominellen Neuroblastome. Fortschr. Röntgenstr. **114**, 752—758 (1971).

BURY, P.: In: A. KAPPERT: Lehrbuch und Atlas der Angiologie, 4. Aufl. Bern-Stuttgart-Wien: Huber 1969.

CACCIARI, C., PISI, E., CAVALLI, G.: Splenoportographie. Sci. med. ital., (dtsch. Ausg.) **7**, 349—402 (1958).

CANDY, J., GRAINGER, K., GRUYER, P. B.: Aortoduodenal fistula complicating translumbar aortography. Brit. J. Surg. **52**, 312—313 (1965).

CAPLAN, L. H., SIMON, M.: Nonparasitic cysts of the liver. Amer. J. Roentgenol. **96**, 421—428 (1966).

CARTER, R. F., SAYPOL, G. M.: Transabdominal cholangiographie. J. Amer. med. Ass. **148**, 253—255 (1952).

CASTIGLIONI, G. C., PETRONIO, R.: Percutaneous intrahepatic cholangiography as a diagnostic aid in post hepatic jaundice. Surgery **56**, 635—643 (1964).

CELLINA, M.: Medionecrosis disseminata aortae. Virchows Arch. path. Anat. **280**, 65—86 (1931).

CEN, U., KÄMMERER, K., NEEF, H.: Verschluß der drei unpaaren Eingeweidearterien ohne klinische Symptomatik. Dtsch. med. Wschr. **97**, 197—199 (1972).

CEN, U., ROSENBUSCH, G.: Zöliakographie mit Adrenalin. (Möglichkeiten der Pharmakoangiographie in der Pankreasdiagnostik.) Fortschr. Röntgenstr. **111**, 82—92 (1969).

CEN, U., ROSENBUSCH, G., DIHLMANN, W., FRICK, W.: Cavographie, indirekte und direkte Nephrophlebographie nach intraarterieller Adrenalinapplikation und ihre Anwendung beim Nierenkarzinom. Dtsch. med. Wschr. **95**, 1251—1254 (1970).

CEN, U., ROSENBUSCH, G., FRICK, W., KALFF, G.: Pharmakoangiographie des Pankreas mit Sekretin und Adrenalin. Dtsch. med. Wschr. **94**, 1970—1972 (1969).

CHAIT, A., MARGULIES, M.: Splenic arteriovenous fistula following percutaneous splenoportography. Radiology **87**, 518—520 (1966).

CHAVÉZ, C. M.: Aorto-arteriography and splenoportography with a teflon catheter-needle. J. cardiovasc. Surg. (Torino) **9**, 319—322 (1968).

CHAVÉZ, C. M., MORA, L. O., CONN, J. H., FAIN, W. R.: Congenital atresia of the celiac axis. Arch. Surg. **93**, 667—670 (1966).

CHAVÉZ, C. M., MORA, L. O., FAIN, W. R., CONN, J. H.: Imagenes tumorales intra-abdominales falsas en la angiografia. Radiologia (Panamá) **17**, 145—150 (1967).

CHAVÉZ, C. M., MORA, L. O., FAIN, W. R., CONN, J. H.: False intra-abdominal tumoral images with angiography. Angiology **18**, 248—255 (1967).

CHÉRIGIÉ, E., DOYON, D., BIGOT, R., MOYON, S.: Intérêt de la soustraction éléctronique en radiologie vasculaire abdominale. Ann. Radiol. **10**, 537—542 (1967).

CHÉRIGIÉ, E., MELLIÈRE, D., BENNET, J., DOYON, D., CHENARD, J. C.: Anatomie radiologique de la vascularisation du pancréas. J. Radiol. Électrol. **48**, 346—352 (1967).

CHEVROT, L., ROUX, G., DOR, P., CHERRY, M., KANDELMAN, M., KREUZER, J.: La couleur en radiodiagnostic. (Techniques et essais en radiologie thoracique.) J. Radiol. Électrol. **50** (Suppl.) 11—13 (1969).

CHIENE, J.: Complete obliterations of the coeliac and the mesenteric arteries, the viscera receiving their blood supply through the extraperitoneal system of vessels. J. Anat. (Paris) **3**, 65 (1968).

CHILDERS, R. W., RANNIGER, K., RABINOWITZ, M.: Intrahepatic arteriovenous fistula with pulmonary vascular obstruction in Osler-Rendu-Weber disease. Amer. J. Med. **43**, 304—312 (1967).

CHOU, C. C., FROHLICH, E. D., TEXTER, E. C.: A comparative study of the effects of Bradykinin, Kallidin II, and Eledoisin on segmental superior mesenteric resistance. J. Physiol. (Lond.) **176**, 1—11 (1965).

CHUDÁČEK, Z.: Zum splenoportographischen Bild des Budd-Chiari-Syndroms. Fortschr. Röntgenstr. **100**, 644—666 (1964).

CHUDÁČEK, Z.: Zöliakographie und Angiographie der Arteria mesenterica superior bei ikterischen Kranken. Fortschr. Röntgenstr. **108**, 1—9 (1968).

CHUDÁČEK, Z.: Grenzen der transparietalen Cholangiographie und die Möglichkeit einer Kombination dieser Cholangiographie mit anderen Röntgenuntersuchungsmethoden. Fortschr. Röntgenstr. **110**, 601—615 (1969).

CHVOJKA, J.: Ein Beitrag der gezielten Angiographie zur Diagnostik der Pankreasverletzungen. Fortschr. Röntgenstr. **113**, 336—339 (1970).

CITRON, B. P., HALPERN, M., MCCARRON, M., LUNDBERG, G. D., PINCUS, I. J., TATTER, D., HAVERBACK, B. J.: Necrotizing angiitis associated with drug abuse. New Engl. J. Med. **283**, 1003 (1970).

CLARA, M.: Die arteriovenösen Anastomosen. Leipzig: Barth 1939.

CLARK, R. A., RÖSCH, J.: Arteriography in the diagnosis of large bowel bleeding. Radiology **94**, 83—88 (1970).

CLEMETT, A. R., PARK, W. M.: Arteriographic demonstration of pancreatic tumor in the Zollinger-Ellison syndrome. Radiology **88**, 32—34 (1967).

COLAPINTO, R. F.: Arteriography in the diagnosis of liver tumors. Canad. med. Ass. J. **99**, 1175—1185 (1968).

COOK, F. E., Jr., FLAHERTY, R. A., WILLMARTH, C. L., LANGELIER, P. R.: Chylothorax. A complication of translumbar aortography. Radiology **75**, 251—253 (1960).

COPE, D. J.: The radiographic management of closed injuries to the chest and abdomen. Radiography **35**, 55—61 (1969).

CORDAY, E., IRVING, D. W., GOLD, H., BERNSTEIN, H., SKELTON, R. B. T.: Mesenteric vascular insufficiency. Intestinal ischemia induced by remote circulatory disturbances. Amer. J. Med. **33**, 365—376 (1962).

CORMIER, J. M., HERNANDEZ, C., KIENY, R., NATALI, J.: Aortographie abdominale. Tronc et collatérales. Paris: Masson 1966.

COUTINHO, S. G., SAAD, E. A., DA SILVA, J. R.: Segmental hepatic angiography. A prelim. report. Amer. J. dig. Dis., N.S. **12**, 685—695 (1967).

CRUVEILHIER, J. C.: Anatomie pathologique du corps humain, T. 1—2. Paris: Baillière 1829/42.

CZEMBIREK, H., GRÖZINGER, K. H.: Nachweis einer „Malrotation" im Angiogramm. Wien. klin. Wschr. **82**, 917—918 (1970).

CZEMBIREK, H., KÜHN, P. M., ROTH, F.-J., WENZ, W.: Das Mesenterikogramm im experimentellen haemorrhagischen Schock. Fortschr. Röntgenstr. **114**, 43—49 (1971).

DALICHAU, H., UNGEHEUER, E., SCHADE, G.: Die massive Ulkusblutung. Fortschr. Med. **86**, 686—689 (1968).

DANFORD, R. O., DAVIDSON, A. J.: The use of glucagon as a vasodilator in visceral angiography. Radiology **93**, 173—175 (1969).

DAUM, R.: Straßenunfälle: offene und stumpfe Verletzungen von Thorax und Bauch. Therapiewoche **21**, 3599—3607 (1971).

DE BAKEY, M. E., HENLY, W. S., COOLEY, D. A., CRAWFORD, E. S., MORRIS, G. C., Jr.: Surgical treatment of dissecting aneurysm of the aorta. Analysis of 72 cases. Circulation **24**, 290—303 (1961).

DEBRAY, A., LEYMARIOS, J.: L'artère mésentérique supérieure. Paris: Masson 1965.

DEBRAY, C., LEYMARIOS, J., HERNANDEZ, C.: L'artériographie sélective dans les tumeurs de l'estomac, du grêle et du colon. Ann. Radiol. **11**, 806—812 (1968).

DEBRAY, CH., LEYMARIOS, J., HERNANDEZ, CL., MARCHE, CL., HARDOUIN, J.-P., PIRONNEAU, A.: Tumeur bénigne de l'intestin grèle (Léiomyome) diagnostiquée par artériographie mésentérique supérieure. Presse méd. **72**, 3005—3008 (1964).

DEBRAY, CH., LEYMARIOS, J., MORIN, G., HERNANDEZ, CL.: La splénoportographie par artériographie sélective coelique. Sem. Hôp. Paris **41**, 1347—1349 (1965).

DEBRUN, G., GASQUET, C.: Explorations vasculaires des tumeurs abdominales de l'enfant. [Ann. Radiol. (Paris) Monogr. 4.]. Paris: Expansion Scient. Franç. 1970.

DECKER, K., BACKMUND, H.: Angiographie des Hirnkreislaufs. Stuttgart: Thieme 1968.

DECKER, K., LINCKE, H. O., OOSTERKAMP, W. J.: Die Beurteilung von Röntgenbildern und ihre Erleichterung durch Farbsubstraktion. Deutsch. Röntgenkongr. **48**, 78—79, 1967 (1968). (Fortschr. Röntgenstr., Beih.)

DEIMER, E.: Die perkutane Hepatographie. Fortschr. Röntgenstr. **114**, 84—102 (1971).

DELORME, G., STAFFEN, J., TAVERNIER, J., MAS, J. P., ROUSSEAU, J.: La phlébographie sushépatique par cathéterisme fémoral. Ann. Radiol. **6**, 581—587 (1963).

DENNIS, E. W., KINARD, S. A., Jr., MCCALL, B. W., DE BAKEY, M. E., HOWELL, J. F., GARRET, H. E.: Aneurysms of the aorta. A consideration of pre- and postoperative medical management. Progr. cardiovasc. Dis. **7**, 544—564 (1965).

DESGREZ, H., LEDOUX-LEBRARD, G., HEITZ, F.: Manuel d'anatomie radiologique. Paris: Masson 1962.

DEUTSCH, V.: Cholecysto-angiography. Visualization of the gallbladder by selective celiac and mesenteric angiography. Amer. J. Roentgenol. **101**, 608—616 (1967).

DIEMEL, H., RAU, G., SCHMITZ-DRÄGER, H.-G.: Die Riolansche Kollaterale. Ihre diagnostische Bedeutung für die Angiographie bei Verschlußkrankheiten der Mesenterialarterien. Fortschr. Röntgenstr. **101**, 253—264 (1964).

DIEMEL, H., SCHMITZ-DRÄGER, H.-G.: Intraabdominale Kollateralbahnen bei Verschlußkrankheiten der Eingeweidearterien. Zugleich ein Beitrag zur Auswertungsmethodik der abdominalen Aortographie. Fortschr. Röntgenstr. **103**, 652—664 (1965).

DIEMEL, H., SCHMITZ-DRÄGER, H.-G.: Komplikationen der abdominalen Aortographie. Vergleichende Gegenüberstellung der translumbalen und transfemoralen Technik. Radiologe **8**, 54—65 (1968).

DINGENDORF, W., SWART, B., HABERICH, H.: Inkomplette Mesenterialgefäßverschlüsse als mögliche Ursache der Enteritis regionalis Crohn. Radiologe **11**, 37—42 (1971).

DINSMORE, R. E., ROURKE, J. A., DE SANCTIS, R. D., HARTHORNE, J. W., AUSTEN, W. G.: Angiographic findings in dissecting aortic aneurysms. New Engl. J. Med. **275**, 1152—1157 (1966).

DI RIENZO, A. J.: Langzeittherapie. Radiologe **10**, 342—344 (1970).

DJINDJIAN, R., FAURE, C.: Accidents médullaires de l'aortographié. J. belge Radiol. **50**, 207—213 (1967).

DOERR, W.: Spezielle pathologische Anatomie II. (Heidelberger Taschenbücher. 70a.) Berlin-Heidelberg-New York: Springer 1970.

DOERR, W., QUADBECK, G.: Allgemeine Pathologie. (Heidelberger Taschenbücher. 68.) Berlin-Heidelberg-New York: Springer 1970.

DOMBROWSKI, H.: Zur Kathetertechnik bei der direkten Splenoportographie. Radiologe **8**, 95—97 (1968).

DOMBROWSKI, H., HUPE, K., KORB, G.: Zur differentialdiagnostischen Bedeutung angiographischer Untersuchungen bei entzündlichen Dünn- und Dickdarmerkrankungen. Langenbecks Arch. klin. Chir. **327**, 103—109 (1970).

DOPPMAN, J. L., FRIED, L. C., DICHIRO, G.: Absent constrictive response of wound vessels to intra-arterial vasopressors: angiographic observations. Radiology **93**, 57—62 (1969).

DOPPMAN, J., SHAPIRO, R., CONTE, M.: Aneurysm of the hepatic artery. The importance of angiographic visualization. Amer. J. Roentgenol. **90**, 578—582 (1963).

DOROSHOW, L. W., YOON, H. Y., ROBBINGS, M. A.: Intrathecal injection, an unusual complication of translumbar aortography: case report. J. Urol. (Baltimore) **88**, 438—439 (1962).

DOS SANTOS, R.: Arteriography in bone tumors. J. Bone Jt Surg. **32**b, 17—29 (1950).

DOS SANTOS, R., LAMAS, A., PEREIRA-CALDAS, J.: Arteriographia da Aorta dos abdominais. Med. contemp. **47**, 93 (1929).

DOS SANTOS, R., LAMAS, A. C., CALDOS, J. P.: Artériographie des membres et de l'aorte abdominale. Paris: Masson 1931.

DOS SANTOS, R., DOS SANTOS, J. C.: Aspects normeaux de l'artériographie des membres de l'aorte abdominale sur le vivant. C.R. Ass. Anat. 599—611 (1933).

DOTTER, C. T., FRISCHE, L. H., JUDKINS, M. P., MUELLER, R.: The "non-surgical" treatment of iliofemoral arteriosclerotic obstruction. Radiology **86**, 871—875 (1966).

DOUTRE, L.-P., DELORME, G., TAVERNIER, J., PÉRISSAT, J., PACCALIN, J.: Complications thromboemboliques de l'artériographie rétrograde transcutanée par la méthode de Seldinger. Arch. Mal. Appar. dig. **59**, 703—708 (1970).

DOW, J., ROEBUCK, E. J., COLE, F.: Dissecting aneurysms of the aorta. Brit. J. Radiol. **39**, 915—927 (1966).

DRAPANAS, TH., YATES, A. J., BRICKMAN, R., WHOLEY, M.: Syndrome of occult rupture of spleen. Arch. Surg. **99**, 298—306 (1969).

DUBARRY, J. J., BLANQUET, P., TAVERNIER, J., BÉRAUD, CL., BECK, CL., LE BRAS, M., PIGNEUX, A., QUINTON, A.: Intérêt de l'examen couplé dans l'exploration pancréatique: artériographie et scintigraphie pancréatique. J. Radiol. Électrol. **50**, 703—706 (1969).

DÜX, A.: Splenoportographie. In: Lehrbuch der Röntgendiagnostik. Hrsg. SCHINZ, H. R., BAENSCH, W., u. a. 6. Aufl., Bd. 1, S. 355—362. Stuttgart: Thieme 1965.

DÜX, A.: Die Röntgendiagnostik der Leber. Dtsch. med. Wschr. **91**, 1669—1673 (1966).

DÜX, A.: Fortschritte in der Diagnostik chirurgischer Krankheitsbilder durch selektive Angiographie. Langenbecks Arch. klin. Chir. **327**, 65—88 (1970).

DÜX, A., BÜCHELER, E., BARTSCH, W. M., SOBBE, A.: Die direkte lumbale Venographie bei Magentumoren. Fortschr. Röntgenstr. **109**, 1—15 (1968).

DÜX, A., BÜCHELER, E., DOHMEN, U., FELIX, R.: Die direkte retrograde Azygographie. Fortschr. Röntgenstr. **107**, 309—328 (1967).

DÜX, A., BÜCHELER, E., THURN, P.: Der arterielle Kollateralkreislauf der Leber. Fortschr. Röntgenstr. **105**, 1—17 (1966).

DÜX, A., BÜCHELER, E., THURN, P.: Die indirekte Splenoportographie: Methodik, Indikationen und Ergebnisse. Fortschr. Röntgenstr. **106**, 183—197 (1967).

DÜX, A., WINKLER, C., ESSER, G., BÜCHELER, E.: Vergleichende angiographische und szintigraphische Untersuchungen bei Lebertumoren. Fortschr. Röntgenstr. **106**, 502—524 (1967).

EATON, S. B., FLEISCHLI, D. J., POLLARD, J. J., NEBESAR, R. A., POTSAID, M. S.: Comparison of current radiologic approaches of the diagnosis of pancreatic disease. New Engl. J. Med. **279**, 389—396 (1968).

ECOFFIER, J.: La practique de l'angiographie. Méthode anatomo-clinique d'exploration de l'appareil circulatoire et techniques opératoires. Paris: Masson 1966.

EDSMAN, G.: Malignant tumour of the spleen diagnosed by lienal arteriography. Acta radiol. (Stockh.) **42**, 461–464 (1954).

EFSEN, F.: Spinal cord lesion as a complication of abdominal aortography. Report of 4 cases. Acta radiol. (Diagn.) 47—61 (1966).
EFSEN, F., MUNKNER, T.: Influence of abdominal aortography on arterial blood pressure, cardiac output and heart rate. Invest. Radiol. **1**, 6—14 (1968).
EGER, H., FIEHRING, H.: Die abdominale Aortenkoarktation in der Differentialdiagnose der Oberbaucherkrankungen. Radiol. diagn. (Berl.) **8**, 557—564 (1967).
EMMRICH, J., FRENCHS, H.: Klinische und angiographische Befunde bei Inselzelladenomen. Fortschr. Röntgenstr. **110**, 358—365 (1969).
ENCKE, H. J., ROTH, F.-J., LOHÖLTER, H., DRÜNER, H. U.: Röntgenologische Nachuntersuchungen der Rektumresthöhle nach sacro-abdominaler Rektumexstirpation 1972 (im Druck).
ENGE, I., KNUTRUD, O., NORMANN, R.: Central rupture of the liver with traumatic haemobilia. A pre- and postoperative angiographic study. Brit. J. Radiol. **41**, 789—791 (1968).
ENGEVIK, L., BENGMARK, S.: Einwirkung auf die Leber nach selektiver Leberangiographie. Langenbecks Arch. klin. Chir. **313**, 917—922 (1965).
EPSTEIN, H. Y., ABRAMS, R. M., BERANBAUM, E. R., LOCALIO, S. A.: Angiographic localization of insulinomas: high reported success rate and two additional cases. Ann. Surg. **169**, 349—354 (1969).
ERDHEIM, S.: (1929) zit. nach DOERR, W. (1970).
ERIKSON, U., FAGERBERG, S., KRAUSE, U., OLDING, L.: Angiographic studies in Crohn's disease and ulcerative colitis. Amer. J. Roentgenol. **110**, 385—392 (1970).
ERNST, D.: Elektronische Bildsubtraktion bei der Coeliaco- und Mesenteriacographie. Med. Diss. Heidelberg 1971.
EYLER, W. R., CLARK, M. D.: Dissection aneurysms of the aorta: roentgen manifestations including a comparison with other types of aneurysms. Radiology **85**, 1047—1057 (1965).
FADHLI, H. A.: Congenital diaphragmatic obstruction of the aorta and the celiac artery. A new surgical Entity. J. thorac. cardiovasc. Surg. **55**, 431—433 (1968).
FAHRLÄNDER, H., GLOOR, F.: Akute regionäre Enteritis. Dtsch. med. Wschr. **92**, 1891—1896 (1967).
FARMAN, J.: Vascular lesions of the colon. Brit. J. Radiol. **39**, 575—582 (1966).
FELIX, R., HAHN, N., DÜX, A., BECKER, H., DRAZININ, N.: Hämodynamik nach Kontrastmittelinjektion in den rechten Vorhof. Tierexperimentelle Untersuchungen mit Urovison und Urografin. Fortschr. Röntgenstr. **110**, 164—177 (1969).
FINE, J.: Vergleich verschiedener Formen des experimentellen Schocks. In: Schock, Pathogenese und Therapie. Hrsg. BOCK, K. D., S. 27. Berlin-Göttingen-Heidelberg: Springer 1962.
FISCHER, A. W.: Über die Röntgenuntersuchung des Dickdarms mit Hilfe einer Kombination von Lufteinblasung und Kontrasteinlauf (kombinierte Methode). Langenbecks Arch. klin. Chir. **134**, 209—269 (1925).
FISCHER, H., SPANN, W.: Pathologie des Trauma. München: Bergmann 1967.
FISCHER, H. W.: Viscosity, solubility and toxicity in the choice of an angiographic contrast medium. Angiology **16**, 759—766 (1965).
FISCHER, H. W.: Hemodynamic reactions to angiographic media; a survey and commentary. Radiology **91**, 66—73 (1968).
FISCHER, J. F., GERSHON-COHEN, J.: Color translation and contrast enhancement of roentgenograms by television techniques. J. A. Einstein med. Cent. **5**, 116—176 (1957).
FISCHER, J. F., GERSON-COHEN, J.: Television techniques for contrast enhancement and color translation of roentgenograms. Amer. J. Roentgenol. **79**, 342 (1958).
FODA, M. T., CASTILLO, C. A., CORLISS, R. J., MCKENNA, D. H., CRUMPTON, C. W., ROWE, G. G.: The intravascular pressure response in man to contrast substance used for angiocardiography. Amer. J. med. Sci. **50**, 390 (1965).
FOEX, P., LAMBERT, H., MENTHA, C.: Les complications médullaires de l'aortographie abdominale. Arch. Mal. Cœur **57**, 142—157 (1964).
FOLKOW, B.: Vom Nervensystem ausgehende Einflüsse auf die Strombahn unter besonderer Berücksichtigung der vasomotorisch wirkenden Nervenfasern. In: Schock, Pathogenese und Therapie. Hrsg. BOCK, K. D., S. 69. Berlin-Göttingen-Heidelberg: Springer 1962.
FONTAINE, R., KIENY, R., JAPY, CL., WARTER, P.: Etude angiographique des oblitérations de l'artère mésentérique supérieure. J. Radiol. Électrol. **47**, 6 (1966).
FONTAINE, R., PIETRI, J., JAPY, C., BABIN, S., LAMPERT, M.: L'angiographie sélective dans le diagnostic des traumatismes fermes de la rate. J. Chir. (Paris) **95**, 587—598 (1968).
FORSSMANN, W.: (1928) entnommen aus: SAVORY, P. B.: Arteriography: Principles and techniques. Illinois med. J. **138**, 215—221 (1970).
FREDENS, M.: Angiography in primary hepatic tumors in children. Acta radiol. (Diagn.) **8**, 193—200 (1969).
FREDENS, M., EGEBLAD, M., HOLST-NIELSEN, F.: The value of selective angiography in the diagnosis of tumors in pancreas and liver. Radiology **93**, 765—769 (1969).
FREEARK, R. J., LOVE, L., BAKER, R. J.: The role of aortography in the mangement of blunt abdominal trauma. J. Trauma **8**, 557—571 (1968).
FREY, C. F., ERNST, C., LINDENAUER, M., BARLETT, J., BOOKSTEIN, J.: Use of arteriography in the diagnosis of occult gastrointestinal and traumatic intraabdominal hemorrhage. Amer. J. Surg. **113**, 137—148 (1967).
FREY, CH. F., REUTER, ST. R., BOOKSTEIN, J. J.: Localization of gastrointestinal hemorrhage by selective angiography. Surgery **67**, 548—555 (1970).
FREY, H. S., NORMAN, A.: Radiographic substraction by color addition. Radiology **84**, 123 (1965).
FRICK, W.: Farbszintigraphie und farbige Röntgenbilder. Fortschr. Röntgenstr. **103**, 227—228 (1965).
FRIEDENBERG, H. J., POLK, H. C., Jr., MCALISTER, W. H., SHOCHAT, S. J.: Superior mesenteric arteriography in experimental mesenteric venous thrombosis. Radiology **85**, 38—45 (1965).
FRIEDMAN, P. J., GREENSPAN, R. H.: Observations on magnification radiography. Visualisation of small blood vessels and determination of focal spot size. Radiology **92**, 549—557 (1969).
FUCHS, W. A.: Der diagnostische Wert der Cavographie. Radiol. clin. (Basel) **30**, 129—149 (1961).

FUCHS, W. A.: Vena cava inferior. In: Handbuch der medizinischen Radiologie. Hrsg. von L. DIETHELM, O. OLSSON u.a. Bd. X, 3, S. 371—399. Berlin-Göttingen-Heidelberg: Springer 1964.

FUCHS, W. A., MESSERSCHMID, U.: Die elektronische Detailverdeutlichung beim Röntgenfernsehen. Fortschr. Röntgenstr. **105**, 260—273 (1965).

FUCHS, W. A.: Elektronische Detailverdeutlichung bei der Röntgenfernsehdurchleuchtung. In: Röntgentechnik. Hrsg. von W. A. FUCHS, E. VOEGELI. (Aktuelle Probleme der Röntgendiagnostik. Bd. 1, S. 7—11.) Bern-Stuttgart-Wien: Huber 1971.

FUCHS, W. A., VÖGELI, E., SCHWEGLER, N., HÜNIG, R., RÖSLER, H.: Angiographie, Szintigraphie und Ultraschalltomographie der Leber. Schweiz. med. Wschr. **101**, 1180—1186 (1971).

GAJEWSKI, H., GOERING, U., WENZ, W.: Eine technisch einfache Röntgen-Stereo-Einrichtung und ihr diagnostischer Wert für die viszerale Serienangiographie. In: Abstr. 2nd Congr. Europ. Assoc. Radiol. Amsterdam 1971. Amsterdam: Excerpta Medica 1971.

GAZES, P. C., HOLMES, C. R., MOSELEY, V., PRATT-THOMAS, H. R.: Acute hemorrhage and necrosis of the intestines associated with digitalization. Circulation **23**, 358—364 (1961).

GEINDRE, M., VALOIS, J., COULOMB, M.: Exploration artériographique et splénoportographique du «syndrome bantien». Presse méd. **75**, 2229—2234 (1967).

GEINDRE, M., VALOIS, J., RACHAIL, M., COULOMB, M.: Variations des aspects artériographiques dans les cirrhoses hépatiques. Ann. Radiol. **10**, 373—381 (1967).

GEORGI, M., SCHEIDEL, A., AKISADA, M.: Experimentelle und klinische Untersuchungen zur stereometrischen Auswertung von Angiographien. Fortschr. Röntgenstr. **113**, 157—163 (1970).

GEORGI, M., ZUM WINKEL, K., PRPIC, B.: Zöliakographie und Szintigraphie in der radiologischen Diagnostik von Lebermetastasen. Strahlentherapie **127**, 405—417 (1965).

GEORGI, U., BECKER, J., JAHUS, E.: Untersuchungen über die Kontrastmittelpassagezeit von intraarteriell applizierten ^{131}J-Urografin bei der Leberarteriographie. Fortschr. Röntgenstr. **108**, 482—486 (1968).

GIRARD, J. C., ECOIFFIER, J.: Stereo-angiographie des petits vaisseaux. Nouvelle approche technique. Abstr. Int. Congr. Radiol. **12**, 260 (1969).

GÖBBELER, T., LÖHR, E.: Abdominelle Aortenverschlüsse und deren Umgehungskreisläufe unter besonderer Berücksichtigung angiographischer Untersuchungstechnik. Fortschr. Röntgenstr. **109**, 471—478 (1968).

GÖGLER, E.: Unfallopfer im Straßenverkehr. Series chirurgica. Documenta Geigy No. 5, Basel 1962.

GOERTTLER, KL.: Das Gefäßsystem im Bauchraum aus der Sicht des Pathologen. In: Aktuelle Gastroenterologie. Hrsg. BARTHELHEIMER, H., HEISIG, N. Stuttgart: Thieme 1968.

GOERTTLER, KL., PFLIEGER, H., ZAHN, D. G. H.: Lokalisation arteriosklerotischer Schäden an den großen Eingeweideschlagadern und begünstigende Wandfaktoren. Verh. Dtsch. Ges. Path. **53**, 441—447 (1969).

GORE, I.: Pathogenesis of dissecting aneurysm of the aorta. Arch. Path. **53**, 142—159 (1952).

GORE, I., SEIWERT, V. J.: Dissecting aneurysm of the aorta. Arch. Path. **53**, 121—141 (1952).

GOULD, H. R., CLEMETT, A. R., ROSSI, P.: Radiologic diagnosis of splenic metastasis. Amer. J. Roentgenol. **109**, 755—760 (1970).

GRAHAM, J. C., WEIDNER, W. A., VINIK, U.: Angiographic features of organizing splenic hematoma. Amer. J. Roentgenol. **107**, 430—433 (1969).

GRAY, R. K., RÖSCH, J., GROLLMANN, J. H.: Arteriography in diagnosis of islet-cell tumors. Radiology **97**, 39—44 (1970).

GREEN, W. H., KERNISH, A. J., WOHL, G. T.: Percutaneous selective arteriography in abdominal emergencies. Amer. J. Roentgenol. **107**, 803—811 (1969).

GRENZMANN, M., THURN, P.: Der Wert der Röntgenuntersuchung bei inkretorisch wirksamen Nebennieren-Erkrankungen. Fortschr. Röntgenschr. **111**, 353—374 (1969).

GRÖZINGER, K.-H., JANSEN, H. H., WENZ, W.: Solitäre pseudocystische Spätmetastase der Milz. Ein Beitrag zur Differentialdiagnose der Milzzysten. Bruns' Beitr. klin. Chir. **216**, 88—95 (1968).

GRÖZINGER, K.-H., WENZ, W.: Arterielle Perfusion des Pankreas mit Trasylol bei akuter Pankreatitis. Z. Gastroent. **3**, 77—80 (1965).

GROH, F., HAENDLE, J.: Harmonisierung und Farbsubtraktion. Electromedica **3**, 71—74 (1968).

GROSSE-BROCKHOFF, F.: Pathologische Physiologie. Berlin-Heidelberg-New York: Springer 1969.

GRÜNERT, R. D.: Lebervenenkatheterung und Splenoportographie in der Diagnostik des portalen Hochdrucks. Chirurg **31**, 534—539 (1960).

GRUSS, J. D., WENZ, W., HEILMANN, K.: Zur Problematik der retrograden Aortendissektion. Dtsch. med. Wschr. **96**, 338—343 (1971).

GSELL, O.: Wandnekrosen der Aorta als selbständige Erkrankung und ihre Beziehung zur Spontanruptur. Virchows Arch. path. Anat. **270**, 1—36 (1928).

GUIEN, CL., HODGKINSON, J., PADOVANI, J., LEGRÉ, J.: Variations anatomiques découvertes par angiographie sélective du tronc cœliaque et de l'artère mésentérique supérieure. J. Radiol. Électrol. **48**, 203—206 (1967).

HABIGHORST, L. V., ALBERS, P., ZEITLER, E.: Die Gefäße der Gallenblase im postmortalen Angiogramm. Fortschr. Röntgenstr. **103**, 63—70 (1965).

HABIGHORST, L. V., WELKER, H., ZEITLER, E.: Vergleichende postmortale Untersuchungen zur Leberangiographie. Fortschr. Röntgenstr. **100**, 681—701 (1964).

HABIGHORST, L. V., WELKER, H., ZEITLER, E.: Zur Technik der vergleichenden post-mortal-angiographischen Darstellung der Lebergefäßsysteme. Acta hepato-splenol. (Stuttg.) **11**, 341—346 (1964).

HÄRTEL, M.: Die Röntgendiagnostik des Aneurysma dissecans der Aorta. Schweiz. med. Wschr. **101**, 965—968 (1971).

HAFFERL, A., THIEL, W.: Lehrbuch der topographischen Anatomie. Berlin-Heidelberg-New York: Springer 1969.

HAGER, C., MICHAELSEN, L.-M., SCHMID, F.: Zur Problematik der intravasalen Kontrastmittelanwendung. Fortschr. Med. **84**, 961—964 (1966).

HALES, M. R., ALLEN, J. S., HALL, E. M.: Injection-corrosion studies of normal and cirrhotic livers. Amer. J. Path. **35**, 909—927 (1959).

HALL, B.: Blutdruckänderungen während der Aorto-Arteriographie. Med. Diss. Heidelberg 1970.

HALL, K., HARTWEG, H., KAUTHEIM, J., MÜHRER, A., SCHMID, E., WINKLER, E.: Atraumatische komplette Ruptur des terminalen Oesophagus. (Boerhaave-Syndrom). Z. Gastroent. **9**, 23—35 (1971).

HALLORAN, J. F., KAHN, P. C.: Concomitant aortography and inferior vena cavography in patients with abdominal masses. Arch. Surg. **98**, 341—343 (1969).

HALPERN, M.: Percutaneous transfemoral arteriography. An analysis of the complications in 1000 consecutive cases. Amer. J. Roentgenol. **92**, 918—934 (1964).

HALPERN, M., TURNER, A., CITRON, P.: An angiographic study of abdominal visceral angiodysplasias associated with gastrointestinal hemorrhage: hereditary, hemorrhagic telangiectasia. Radiology **90**, 1143 (1968).

HAMMERSEN, F., GROSS, D.: (Hrsg.) Aktuelle Probleme in der Angiologie. 2. Bd. Die arterio-venösen Anastomosen. Anatomie, Physiologie, Pathologie, Klinik. Bern-Stuttgart: Huber 1968.

HANNAN, J. R., JACKSON, B. F., PIPIK, P.: Fibrosis and stenosis of the descending colon and sigmoid following occlusion of the inferior mesenteric artery. Amer. J. Roentgenol. **91**, 826—832 (1964).

HANSER, R.: Atrophie, Nekrose, Ablagerungen und Speicherungen. In: Handbuch der speziellen pathologischen Anatomie und Histologie, Hrsg. von F. HENKE, O. LUBARSCH. Bd. 5, 1, S. 132—243. Berlin: Springer 1930.

HASSE, H. M.: Diskussion. In: Die Gefäßthrombosen nach Katheterangiographie. Hrsg. von E. ZEITLER. (Aktuelle Probleme in der Angiographie. Bd. 10.) Bern-Stuttgart-Wien: Huber 1970.

HAUBRICH, R.: Zwerchfellpathologie im Röntgenbild. Berlin-Göttingen-Heidelberg: Springer 1956.

HAUBRICH, R.: Zwerchfell. In: Handbuch der medizinischen Radiologie, Hrsg.: DIETHELM, L., OLSSON, O., u. a. Bd. IX, 6, S. 1—192. Berlin-Heidelberg-New York: Springer 1970.

HEBERER, G., GIESSLER, R., MARQUARDT, H.: Zur Erkennung und Behandlung von Bauchaortenaneurysmen. Erfahrungsbericht über 100 Kranke in 11 Jahren. Dtsch. med. Wschr. **94**, 699—708 (1969).

HEBERER, G., RAU, G., LÖHR, H. H.: Aorta und große Arterien. Berlin-Heidelberg-New York: Springer 1966.

HEGER, N., BAYINDIR, S., RISTIG, W.: Zur angiographischen Lokalisation von Inselzellgeschwülsten des Pankreas. Med. Welt., N. F. **20**, 1999—2003 (1969).

HEGER, N., BAYINDIR, S., STECKENMESSER, R., HEBERLEIN, H.: Komplikationen bei Katheterarteriographien nach Seldinger-Technik. Fortschr. Röntgenstr. **111**, 124 (1969).

HEGER, N., MUSSMANN, J., SCHIRMER, H.: Angiographischer Nachweis eines hypoglykämisierenden sekundären Lebersarkomes. Fortschr. Röntgenstr. **111**, 809—814 (1969).

HEINRICH, P., OSCHATZ, R.: Chirurgisch behandelte Komplikationen bei der indirekten Angiographie nach dem Seldinger-Verfahren. Zbl. Chir. **94**, 12—22 (1969).

HEINZ, E. R.: Stereoangiography. A simple system. Amer. J. Roentgenol. **104**, 220—222 (1968).

HELENON, CH.: L'artériographie en pathologie digestive abdominale. Cah. Méd. **11**, 1165—1189 (1970).

HELLNER, H., NISSEN, R., VOSSSCHULTE, K. (Hrsg.): Lehrbuch der Chirurgie. 5. Aufl. Stuttgart: Thieme 1967.

HENTSCHEL, M.: Untersuchungen zur Blutversorgung des Pankreas. In: Angiographie und ihre Leistungen, hrsg. von K. F. LOOSE, S. 223. Stuttgart: Thieme 1968.

HEPP, J., HERNANDEZ, C., MOREAUX, J., BISMUTH, H.: L'artériographie dans les affections chirurgicales du foie, du pancréas et de la rate. Paris: Masson 1968.

HEPP, J., MOREAUX, J., BISMUTH, H., HERNANDEZ, C.: L'intérêt de l'artériographie sélective dans la chirurgie pancréatique. Ann. Chir. **20**, 465—472 (1966).

HERNANDEZ, C.: La radiologie vasculaire des tumeurs du foie. Vie méd. Specialité **48**, 1171—1186 (1967).

HERNANDEZ, C.: Angiographie pancréatique: intérêt et limites, à propos de 800 examens. Arch. Mal. Appar. dig. **59**, 687—696 (1970).

HERNANDEZ, C., CACHIN, M.: Méthodes morphologiques d'étude de la circulation hépatique. Artériographie sélective, portographie et cavographie. Rev. int. Hépat. **17**, 719—752 (1967).

HERNANDEZ, C., HÉLÉNON, CH.: Les tumeurs pancréatique langerhansiennes. Exploration vasculaire. J. Radiol. Électrol. **48**, 339—346 (1967).

HERNANDEZ, C., MORIN, G., ECARLAT, B.: L'embol pulsé en artériographie sélective digestive. Presse méd. **73**, 2889—2894 (1965).

HERNANDEZ, C., NATALIE, J.: Die Angiographie des Verdauungstraktes. In: Angiographie und ihre Leistungen, hrsg. von K. L. LOOSE, S. 123. Stuttgart: Thieme 1968.

HERNANDEZ, CL., BELLIN, A.: Angiographie digéstive et chirurgie abdominale. Ann. Radiol. **11**, 792—800 (1968).

HERNANDEZ, CL., ECARLAT, B., BISMUTH, V.: L'artérioportographie des affections pancréatique. J. Radiol. Électrol. **48**, 327—338 (1967).

HERRMANN, H.: Über die erste Arteriographie. Eine angiologische Reminiszenz zum 70. Jahrestag der Entdekkung der Röntgenstrahlen. Münch. med. Wschr. **107**, 2259—2260 (1965).

HERSCHMAN, A., BLUM, R., LEE, Y. C.: Angiographic findings in polyarteritis nodosa. Radiology **94**, 147—148 (1970).

HETTLER, M.: Angiographische Probleme und Möglichkeiten. I. Fortschr. Röntgenstr. **92**, 97—106 (1960).

HETTLER, M.: Angiographische Probleme und Möglichkeiten. II. Der perkutane Arterienkatheterismus an der Spitze verschlossener Katheter als Grundlage der Etagen-Aortographie. Fortschr. Röntgenstr. **92**, 198—206 (1960).

HETTLER, M.: Angiographische Probleme und Möglichkeiten. III. Fortschr. Röntgenstr. **92**, 420—433 (1960).

HETTLER, M.: Die Stereoangiographie. Ein Beitrag zur Situation der Röntgenstereoskopie. Fortschr. Röntgenstr. **95**, 482—492 (1961).

HETTLER, M. G.: Die differenzierte Angiographie der Aorta und ihrer Äste. Abh. IX. Int. Congr. Radiol. München 1959. **1**, 520 (1961).

HETTLER, M. G.: Die percutane Kathetermethode nach Hettler. Fortschritte in Technik und Instrumentarium — Ergebnisse. Fortschr. Röntgenstr. **110**, 553—563 (1969).

HEUCK, F.: Der Beitrag der Röntgendiagnostik zur Früherkennung von Pankreastumoren. Dtsch. Röntgenkongr. **45**, 160—163, 1964 (1965). Fortschr. Röntgenstr., Beih.

HIERONYMI, G.: Angiometrische Untersuchungen venöser und arterieller Gefäße verschiedenen Lebensalters. Frankfurt. Z. Path. **69**, 18—36 (1958).

HILLER, H. G.: Pediatric hepatic arteriography. Ann. Radiol. **11**, 30—33 (1967).

HÖHMANN, H., GEBHARDT, E., WAGNER, H. E.: Primärer bösartiger Milztumor. Zbl. Chir. **95**, 497—503 (1970).

HOLSTEN, D. R., ALEXANDER, K.: Zum Mesenteric-Steal-Syndrom. Fortschr. Röntgenstr. **108**, 253—255 (1968).

HONDA, K., KOSEKI, M., HOSHINO, S.: Significance of the left gastric arteriogram in stomach diseases. Surg. Ther. (Osaka) **18**, 247—253 (1968).

HONJO, I., SUZUKI, T., YOSHITOMI, G.: L'artériographie pancréatique. Sa valeur dans les cancers du pancréas. Lyon chir. **64**, 587—595 (1968).

HOPF, M. A., FUCHS, W. A.: Die Lymphographie, Cavographie und Urographie als Kombinationsuntersuchung. Radiologe **10**, 280—288 (1970).

HORNYKIEWYTSCH, TH., BARGON, G.: Die Gefahren und Schäden bei der modernen röntgenologischen Diagnostik und Strahlentherapie. Internist **3**, 487—498 (1962).

HUARD, P., DO XUAN-HOP: La ponction transhépatique des caneaux biliaires. Bull. Soc. méd.-chir. Indochine **15**, 1090—1100 (1937).

HUGHES, J. T., BROWNELL, B.: Paraplegia following retrograde abdominal aortography. An example of toxic myelitis. Arch. Neurol. (Chic.) **12**, 650—657 (1965).

HURWITT, E. S., SEIDENBERG, B.: The nonoperative management of two cases of catheter perforation of the aorta. Amer. J. Surg. **110**, 452—455 (1965).

ICHIKAWA (1936) aus: TASAKA, A.: Selective angiography. Tokio: Igaku Shoin Ltd. 1967.

IDEZUKI, Y., SUGIURA, M., HATANO, S., KIMOTO, S.: Hepatography for detection of small tumor masses in liver: experience with oily contrast medium. Surgery **60**, 565—572 (1966).

IMBERT, P., MERCIER, CL., JUHAN, CL., LENA, A.: Les accidents du cathétérisme artériel rétrograde. Ann. Radiol. **13**, 45—47 (1970).

IMPERATI, L., TOMMASEO, T.: Chirurgia della arteria mesenteriche. Roma: Edizione mediche e scientifiche 1960.

ISHIKAWA, H., KATSUBE, Y.: Catheterization needle for pediatric angiography. Rinshô Hôsha **13**, 549—542 (1968).

ISHIKAWA, H., KATSUBE, Y., NISHIO, T.: Experiences with abdominal aortography in children. Rinshô Hôsha **13**, 914—919 (1968).

JACOB, A., MEYERHÖFER, H.: Unsere Erfahrungen mit der percutanen transhepatischen Cholangiographie kombiniert mit der hypotonen Duodenographie (140 Fälle). Abstr. Int. Congr. Radiol. **12**, 250 (1969).

JACOBS, J. B., HAMMOND, W. G., DOPPMANN, J. L.: Arteriographic localization of suprahepatic abscesses. Radiology **93**, 1299—1300 (1969).

JACOBSSON, B., BERGENTZ, S. E., LJUNGQVIST, M.: Platelet adhesion and thrombus formation on vascular catheters in dogs. Acta radiol. (Diagn.) **8**, 221—227 (1969).

JACOBSSON, B., PAULIN, S., SCHLOSSMAN, D.: Thromboembolism of the leg following percutaneous catheterization of the femoral artery for arteriography: Symptomes and signs. Acta radiol. (Diagn.) **8**, 97—108 (1969).

JACOBSSON, B., SCHLOSSMAN, D.: Angiographic investigation of formation of thrombi on vascular catheters. Radiology **93**, 355—359 (1969).

JACOBSSON, B., SCHLOSSMAN, D.: Thromboemblism of leg following percutaneous catheterisation of femoral artery for angiography. Predisposing factors. Acta radiol. (Diagn.) **8**, 109—118 (1969).

JAFFÉ, B. F., YONKER, J. E., MARGULIS, A. R.: Aortographic localization of controlled gastrointestinal hemorrhage in dogs. Surgery **58**, 984—988 (1965).

JOHNSSON, K.-Å.: Abdominal aortography via the axillary arteries. Indications, technique and complications. Abstr. Int. Congr. Radiol. **12**, 255 (1969).

JONES, F. A., READ, A. E., STUBBE, J. L.: Alimentary bleeding of obscure origin. Brit. med. J. **1**, 1138—1142 (1959).

JONES, H. V., HARLEY, H. R. S.: Traumatic cyst of the liver. Brit. J. Surg. **57**, 468—470 (1970).

JUDKINS, M. P., KIDD, H. J., FRISCHE, L. H., DOTTER, C. T.: Lumenfollowing safety J-guide for catheterization of tortuous vessels. Radiology **88**, 1127—1130 (1967).

JÜRGENS, J.: Diskussion. In: Gefäßthrombosen und Katheterangiographie. Hrsg. ZEITLER, E. (Aktuelle Probleme in der Angiologie. Bd. 10.) Bern-Stuttgart-Wien: Huber 1970.

JUNGHANNS, K., WENZ, W., KOLIG, G., BEDUHN, D.: Percutane transhepatische Cholangiographie. Ihre Bedeutung für die Diagnostik des Verschlußikterus. Dtsch. med. Wschr. **94**, 24—27 (1969).

JUST, O.: Behandlung und Prophylaxe von Kontrastmittelzwischenfällen. Röntgenpraxis (1972) (im Druck).

KAHN, P. C.: Selective angiography of the inferior phrenic arteries. Radiology **88**, 1—8 (1967).

KAHN, P. C.: Contrast-vasoconstrictor mixtures in angiography. Amer. J. Roentgenol. **105**, 772—776 (1969).

KAHN, P. C., ABRAMS, H. L.: Inferior mesenteric arterial patterns. An angiographic study. Radiology **82**, 429—442 (1964).

KAHN, P. C., ALEXANDER, F. K.: Total hepatic angiography and vascular dynamics in liver disease. Amer. J. Gastroent. **52**, 317—325 (1969).

KAHN, P. C., CALLOW, A.: Selective vasodilatation as an aid to angiography. Amer. J. Roentgenol. **94**, 213—220 (1965).

KAHN, P. C., CALLOW, A. D.: Catheter arteriography in the evaluation of abdominal aortic aneurysms. Amer. J. Roentgenol. **98**, 879—887 (1966).

KAHN, P. C., FRATES, R. E.: The value of angiography of the small branches of the abdominal aorta. Amer. J. Roentgenol. **102**, 407—417 (1968).

KAHN, P. C., FRATES, W. J., PAUL, R. E., Jr.: The epinephrine effect in angiography of gastrointestinal tract tumours. Radiology **88**, 686—690 (1967).

KAHN, P. C., O'HALLORAN, J. F., PAUL, R. E.: Improved portography by delayed postepinephrine celiac and mesenteric arteriography. Radiology **92**, 86—89 (1969).

KAHN, P. C., WISE, H. M.: Simulation of renal tumor response to epinephrine by inflammatory disease. Radiology **89**, 1062—1064 (1967).

KAICK, G. VAN, WENZ, W., BEDUHN, D.: Die angiographische Diagnostik der Milzruptur. Fortschr. Röntgenstr. **112**, 633—640 (1970).

KAMMERER, V., DEINIGER, H.-K., PIEPGRAS, U.: Passagerer vollständiger Verschluß einer Nierenhauptarterie im Verlauf einer Arteriographie. Fortschr. Röntgenstr. **114**, 843—846 (1971).

KANTNER, J. E., SCHWARZT, A. J., FLEMING, R. J.: Localisation of bleeding point in chronic and acute gastrointestinal hemorrhage by means of selective visceral arteriography. Amer. J. Roentgenol. **103**, 386—399 (1968).

KAPPERT, A.: Lehrbuch und Atlas der Angiologie, 5. Aufl. Bern-Stuttgart-Wien: Huber 1970.

KATER, R. M. H.: Takayashu's disease with gastro-intestinal symptoms. Aust. Ann. Med. **16**, 80 (1967).

KATZ, A. M.: Hemorrhagic duodenitis in myocardial infarction. Ann. intern. Med. **51**, 212 (1959).

KATZ, D., DOUVERS, P., WEISBERG, H., CHARM, R., MCKINNON, W.: Sources of bleeding in upper gastrointestinal hemorrhage: A re-evaluation. Amer. J. dig. Dis. **9**, 447 (1964).

KATZ, M. C., MENG, C.-H.: Angiographic evaluation of traumatic intrahepatic pseudoaneurysm and hemobilia. Radiology **94**, 95—99 (1970).

KATZ, N., STRENGE, W. VON: Untersuchungen über die arteriovenösen Anastomosen des Mesenterialkreislaufes. Arch. klin. Chir. **191**, 618—631 (1938).

KAUDE, J.: Angiographischer Nachweis eines Insuloms und einer akzessorischen Milz. Fortschr. Röntgenstr. **111**, 130—131 (1969).

KAUDE, J. V., WEIDENMIER, C. H., AGEE, O. F.: Decompression of bile ducts with the percutaneous transhepatic technic. Radiology **93**, 69—71 (1969).

KEISER, D. VON, MÜLLER, H.: Die Cavographie und Phlebographie der Venae iliacae in der Diagnostik maligner Tumoren und deren Metastasen. Fortschr. Med. **81**, 847—852 (1963).

KAISER, D. VON, WENZ, W., BEDUHN, D.: Die Bedeutung der Katheterangiographie der Bauchaorta und ihrer Äste für die chirurg. Abdominaldiagnostik. Langenbecks Arch. klin. Chir. **311**, 191—208 (1965).

KELLEY, H. G., GRANT, G. N., ELLIOT, D. W.: Massive gastroduodenal hemorrhage. Arch. Surg. **87**, 6 (1963).

KERK, L., MÜLLER, H.: Beitrag zur Angiographie der Nierentumoren im Kindesalter. Z. Kinderchir., Suppl.-Bd. **6**, 153—165 (1969).

KETTLER, L.-H.: Die Leber. In: Lehrbuch der speziellen und pathologischen Anatomie. Hrsg. von E. KAUFMANN, M. STAEMMLER. Bd. 2, T. 2, S. 913—1260. Berlin: de Gruyter 1958.

KIDO, C., SASAKI, T., KANEKO, M.: Hepatic angiography in metastatic cancer of the liver. Rinshô Hôsha **13**, 173—180 (1968).

KIDO, C., SASAKI, T., KANEKO, M.: Hepatic angiography in primary liver neoplasms. Rinshô Hôsha **13**, 289—292 (1968).

KILLEN, D. A., FOSTER, J. H.: Spinal cord injury as a complication of contrast angiography. Surgery **59**, 969—981 (1966).

KING, E. G., MILLER, J. D. R.: Celiac scintiangiography. Amer. J. Med. **46**, 394—400 (1969).

KING, M. C., GLICK, W., FREED, A.: The diagnosis of splenic cysts. Surg. Gynec. Obstet. **127**, 509—512 (1968).

KINMOUTH, J. B.: Lymphography in man. Clin. Sci. **11**, 13—20 (1952).

KITTREDGE, R. D., COLAIACE, W. M., KANIK, V., FINBY, N.: Angiography in hemorrhage. Amer. J. Roentgenol. **107**, 181—190 (1969).

KLEIN, H. J., ALFIDI, R. J., MEANEY, T. F., POIRIER, V. C.: Angiography in the diagnosis of chronic gastrointestinal bleeding. Radiology **98**, 83—91 (1971).

KLEINERT, H. E., ROMERO, J.: Blunt abdominal trauma. Review of cases admitted to a general hospital over a 10 year period. J. Trauma **1**, 226—240 (1961).

KLOSTER, F. E., BRISTOW, J. D., GRISWOLD, H. E.: Femoral artery occlusion following percutaneous catheterization. Amer. Heart J. **79**, 175—180 (1970).

KLÜKEN, N.: (Hrsg.) Ergebnisse der Angiologie. Jahrestag der Dtsch. Ges. Angiologie Düsseldorf. Bd. 2. Stuttgart-New York: Schattauer 1968.

KÖHLER, P. R., SALMON, R. B.: Angiographic localization of unknown acute gastrointestinal bleeding sites. Radiology **89**, 244—249 (1967).

KOIKKALAINEN, K.: Haemodynamically significant stenosis in the coeliac and superior mesenteric arteries. An experimental study. Ann. Chir. Gynaec. Fenn. **60**, 25—30 (1971).

KOLLATH, J., SPITZ, P.: Probleme der Kontrastmittelverteilung bei Anwendung der Kathederhochdruckangiographie. Fortschr. Röntgenstr. **109**, 81—92 (1968).

KOTTKE, B. A., FAIRBAIRN, J. F., DAVIS, G. D.: Complications of aortography. Circulation **30**, 843—847 (1964).

KREEL, L., FRESTON, J. W., CLAIN, D.: Vascular radiology in the Budd-Chiari syndrome. Brit. J. Radiol. **40**, 755—759 (1967).

KREEL, L., JONES, E. A., TAVILL, A. S.: A comparative study of arteriography and scintillation scanning in space-occupying lesions of the liver. Brit. J. Radiol. **41**, 401—411 (1968).

KRIESSMANN, A.: Die Eingeweidearterien und ihre Kollateralen. Dtsch. Röntgenkongr. **48**, 51—53, 1967 (1968) (Fortschr. Röntgenstr. Beih.).

KRUSZEWSKI, S.: Experimental studies on development of collateral circulation in stenosis or occlusion of the inferior vena cava. [Polnisch, mit engl. Zusammenfassung.] Rozpr. Wydz. Nauk med. pol. Akad. Nauk **8**, 293—315 (1963).

KUNNEN, M.: Kleurradiografie, Kleurcineradiografie, Kleurbeeldversterkerfotografie. Gent: Rijksuniv. Gent, Lab. Röntgendiagn. 1969 (Proefschrift).

LAGERGREN, C., LINDERBOM, A., SODBERG, G.: Hypervascularisation in chronic inflammation demonstrated by angiography. Acta radiol. (Stockh.) **49**, 441—452 (1958).

LAMESCH, A.: Die Bedeutung der Angiographie bei Nierenruptur. Langenbecks Arch. klin. Chir. **305**, 168—173 (1964).

LANG, E. K.: A survey of the complications of percutaneous retrograde arteriography: Seldinger technic. Radiology **81**, 257—263 (1963).

LANG, E. K.: Prevention and treatment of complications following arteriography. Radiology **88**, 950—956 (1967).

LAOVIC, P., FERREIRA, V., LÉGARÉ, A., VIALLET, A.: Phlébographie sélective splénique, mésentérique ou portale par voie ombilicale. Presse méd. **74**, 2607—2608 (1966).

LAUBACH, K.: Noteingriff beim akuten Visceralarterienverschluß. Therapiewoche **21**, 3277—3283 (1971).

LAUFMAN, H., BERGGREN, R. E., FINLEY, T., ANSON, B. J.: Anatomical studies of the lumbar arteries: with reference to the safety to translumbar aortography. Ann. Surg. **152**, 621—634 (1960).

LAWSON, T. L., STEWART, E. T., RAMBO, O., GOMEZ, J., MARGULIS, A. R.: Canine ulcerating colitis, a radiographic and pathologic correlation. Abstr. Int. Congr. Radiol. **12**, 246 (1969).

LECHNER, G., POKIESER, H., ZAUNBAUER, K., BRÜCKE, P.: Zur angiographischen Diagnose des Pankreaskarzinoms. Fortschr. Röntgenstr. **113**, 340—348 (1971).

LEGER, L.: Splenoportographie. Paris: Masson 1955.

LEGER, L.: La cholangiographie et drainage biliare par ponction transpaneto-hépatique. Chirurgie du Pancréas. Paris: Masson 1956.

LEGER, L., CHALMEAU, M., BROU, R., MOULLÉ, P., CHAPUIS, Y., LEMAIGRE, G.: Sténose ostiale de l'artère hépatique. Syndrome clinique, cure chirurgicale. Presse méd. **75**, 1283—1288 (1967).

LEGER, L., MOUKTAR, M.: Angiomégalies portales. Presse méd. **72**, 1859—1864 (1964).

LEGER, L., PRÉMONT, M., ALPÉROVITCH, R.: Ruptures spléniques aprés spléno-portographie. Étude d'une série personnelle de 2000 examens. J. Chir. (Paris) **87**, 107—121 (1964).

LEGER, L., PRÉMONT, M., LEFORT, J.: Phlébographie sus-hépatique par injection dans le parenchyme hépatique. Presse méd. **70**, 1855—1857 (1962).

LEGRÉ, J., CLÉMENT, J.-P., GUIEN, C., PIETRI, H.: Circulation de suppléance dans deux cas de thrombose ostiale des branches digestives de l'aorte abdominale. Ann. Radiol. **13**, 49—54 (1970).

LEMAITRE, G., RÉINY, J., HERMINÉ, C. L., DIONNET, J. L.: Étude de la vésicule biliaire au cours de l'artériographie hépatique. J. Radiol. Électrol. **50**, 837—840 (1969).

LENZ, H., DÜX, A.: Diagnosis of arteriomesenteric duodenal compression by means of hypotonic duodenography, angiography of the superior mesenteric artery, and cineradiography. Surg. Dig. **6**, 25 (1971).

LEPASOON, J., OLIN, T.: Angiographic diagnosis of splenic lesions following blunt abdominal trauma. Acta radiol. (Diagn.) **11**, 257—273 (1971).

LINDBOM, A.: Venographie der Vena cava inferior. In: Ergebnisse der medizinischen Strahlenforschung, Bd. I. Hrsg. SCHINZ, H. R., GLAUNER, R., RÜTTIMANN, A. Stuttgart: Thieme 1964.

LINDER, F., GRÖZINGER, K.-H., WAWERSIK, J., WENZ, W.: Fortschritte in der Diagnostik chirurgischer Krankheitsbilder. Langenbecks Arch. klin. Chir. **327**, 13—48 (1970).

LINDER, F., VOLLMAR, J., KRUMHAAR, D.: Die arterio-venösen Fisteln des Pfortadergebiets. Langenbecks Arch. klin. Chir. **320**, 50—63 (1968).

LINDGREN, A. G. H.: Vascular supply of tumors with special reference to capillary angioarchitecture. Acta path. microbiol. Scand. **22**, 493—521 (1945).

LIPCHIK, E. O., ROB, C. G., SCHWARTZBERG, S.: Obstruction of the abdominal aorta above the level of the renal arteries. Radiology **82**, 443—446 (1964).

LIPSHUTZ, B.: A composite study of the coeliac axis artery. Ann. Surg. **65**, 159—169 (1917).

LÖHR, E., GÖBBELER, T.: Über das Verhalten des Aortentracks bei angiographischen Untersuchungen. Fortschr. Röntgenstr. **109**, 156—163 (1968).

LÖHR, E., HALLER, J.: Angiographische Darstellung von Aortenaneurysmen. Fortschr. Röntgenstr. **110**, 71—78 (1969).

LOOSE, K. E. (Hrsg.): Angiographie. Methoden — Indikation — Ergebnisse. Vorträge der Angiographietagung 18.—20. November 1965 in Baden-Baden. Stuttgart: Thieme 1966.

LOVE, L., GREENFIELD, G. B., BRAUN, T. W., MONCADO, R., FREEARK, R. J., BAKER, R. J.: Arteriography of splenic trauma. Radiology **91**, 96—102 (1968).

LUBARSCH, O.: Pathologische Anatomie der Milz. In: Handbuch der speziellen pathologischen Anatomie und Histologie, hrsg. von F. HENKE, O. LUBARSCH. Bd. I/2, S. 406. Berlin: Springer 1927.

LUDIN, H.: Zur Pancreasangiographie. Schweiz. med. Wschr. **98**, 283—284 (1968).

LUDIN, H.: Arteriographische Lokalisation der Blutungsquelle bei postoperativen Hämorrhagien nach Nephrektomie. Dtsch. Röntgenkongr. **48**, 55, 1967 (1968) (Fortschr. Röntgenstr. Beih.).

LUDIN, H., ELKE, M.: Bemerkungen zur Technik der femoralen Rückstrom-Aortographie. Fortschr. Röntgenstr. **103**, 606—609 (1965).

LUDIN, H., ELKE, M.: Abdominale Aortenkoarktation. Aortographische Diagnose in einem Fall. Fortschr. Röntgenstr. **104**, 34—39 (1966).

LUDIN, H., ENDERLIN, F., FAHRLÄNDER, H. J., SCHEIDEGGER, S.: Failure to diagnose Zollinger-Ellison syndrome by pancreatic arteriography. Brit. J. Radiol. **39**, 494—497 (1966).

LUDIN, H., FAHRLÄNDER, H. J., RENGGLI, I.: Zur Darstellung von Karzinoid-Lebermetastasen mittels visceraler Arteriographie. Schweiz. med. Wschr. **96**, 1642—1648 (1966).

LUDIN, H., KÜNZLI, H. F.: Resolution of angiography in detecting liver metastases. Brit. J. Radiol. **42**, 145—151 (1969).

LUDIN, H., FERNEX, M., WAIBEL, P.: Aortographic demonstration of intrathoracic para-aortic pheochromocytoma. Acta radiol. (Diagn.) **3**, 465—474 (1965).

LUKE, J., MCGRAW, J. Y.: Complications following catheter angiography. Arch. Surg. **86**, 414—418 (1963).

LUNDERQUIST, A.: Angiography in carcinoma of the pancreas. Acta radiol. (Stockh.), Suppl. **235** (1965).

LUNDERQUIST, A.: Arterial segmental supply of the liver. An angiographic study. Acta radiol. (Stockh.), Suppl. **272** (1967).

LUNDERQUIST, A., LUNDERQUIST, A.: Angiography in ulcerative colitis. Amer. J. Roentgenol. **99**, 18—23 (1967).

LUNDERQUIST, A., LUNDERQUIST, A., HOLMDAHL, K. H., CLEMENS, F.: Selective superior mesenteric arteriography in recticulum-cell sarcoma of the small bowel. Radiology **98**, 113—115 (1971).

LUNDERQUIST, A., LUNDERQUIST, A., KNUTSON, H.: Angiography in Crohn's disease of small bowel and colon. Amer. J. Roentgenol. **101**, 338—344 (1967).

LUNDERQUIST, A., LUNDERQUIST, A., NOMMESEN, N.: Angiographic changes during digestion. Amer. J. Roentgenol. **107**, 191—197 (1969).

LUNDSTRÖM, B.: Angiographic demonstration of rupture of the spleen. Acta radiol. (Diagn.) **10**, 145—150 (1970).

LUTZ, H., WENZ, W., WINKLER, J., HEILMANN, F.: Röntgenkontrastdarstellungen des Gefäßsystems in Allgemeinanaesthesie. Dtsch. med. Wschr. **93**, 291—295 (1968).

MADSEN, B.: Demonstration of pancreatic insulomas by angiography. Brit. J. Radiol. **39**, 488—493 (1966).

MADSEN, B., HANSEN, E. S.: Correlation between angiographic diagnosis and histology of pancreatic insulomas. Brit. J. Radiol. **43**, 185—192 (1970).

MALLET-GUY, P., JACQUEMET, P., MURAT, J., EJAZI, M.: Notre expérience des techniques radiologiques modernes dans les affections pancréatiques. Ann. Radiol. **11**, 857—863 (1968).

MARGOLIS, G., YERASIMIDES, T. G.: Vasopressor potentiation of neurotoxicity in experimental aortography. Implications regarding pathogenesis of contrast medium injury. Acta radiol. (Diagn.) **5**, 388—412 (1966).

MARGULIS, A. R.: Arteriography of tumors: difficulties in interpretation and the need for magnification. Radiol. Clin. N. Amer. **2**, 543—562 (1964).

MARGULIS, A. R., HEINBECKER, P.: Mesenteric arteriography. Amer. J. Roentgenol. **86**, 103—113 (1961).

MARSTON, A.: Patterns of intestinal ischemia. Ann. roy. Coll. Surg. Engl. **35**, 150—181 (1964).

MARTELLA, M., ROSTAGNO, R., SALVIDEA, J.: Angiografia y centellografia de la hidatidosis hepatica. Pren. med. argent. **55**, 1372—1373 (1968).

MARTINEK, H., PIZA, F.: Pankreatitis als seltene Komplikation nach lumbaler Aortographie. Acta chir. Austr. **2**, 105—106 (1970).

MARTINI, G. A.: Erkrankungen der Leber und der Gallenwege. In: Lehrbuch der Inneren Medizin, hrsg. von R. GROSS u.a., S. 525. Stuttgart-New York: Schattauer 1970.

MARYNOWSKI, A.: Entzündlicher Tumor des großen Netzes, radiologisch diagnostiziert (Vasographie). Zbl. Gynäk. **90**, 831—834 (1968).

MATEEV, B., WIRBATZ, W., KIESSLING, J., WITTBRODT, S., EICHHORN, H.-J.: Die Katheterisierung der vena portae über die V. umbilicalis (transumbilikale Portohepatographie). Fortschr. Röntgenstr. **110**, 178—191 (1969).

MATTSON, O.: Practical photographic problems in radiography. Acta radiol. (Stockh.) Suppl. **120** (1955).

MAURER, H.-J., IRMER, W., RINGLER, W., JUNGBLUT, R.: Röntgenbefund und Operationsindikation bei Verschlüssen der Bauchaorta und der Beckenarterien. Dtsch. Röntgenkongr. **48**, 56—59, 1967 (1968) (Fortschr. Röntgenstr. Beih.).

MAY, R., NISSL, R.: Gefäßverschlüsse nach Angiographien. Fortschr. Röntgenstr. **110**, 64—71 (1969).

MAYALL, G. F.: Arterial waves. Clin. Radiol. **15**, 355—357 (1964).

MCAFEE, J. G.: A survey of complications of abdominal aortography. Radiology **68**, 825 (1957).

MCCONNEL, F., THOMPSON, A. G., KISS, J.: Selective celiac and superior mesenteric arteriography. Canad. J. Surg. **9**, 15—23 (1966).

MCCORT, J. J.: Infarction of the descending colon due to vascular occlusion. New Engl. J. Med. **262**, 168—172 (1960).

MCDONALD, P.: Hepatic tumors in childhood. Clin. Radiol. **18**, 74—82 (1967).

MCDONALD, P., HILLER, H. G.: Angiography in abdominal tumours in childhood with particular reference to neuroblastome and Wilm's tumour. Clin. Radiol. **19**, 1—18 (1968).

MCLOUGHLIN, M. J., HOBBS, B. B.: Selective angiography in the diagnosis of hydatid disease of the liver. Canad. med. Ass. J. **104**, 1147 (1971).

MCNULTY, J. G.: Angiographic manifestations of hydatid disease of the liver. A report of two cases. Amer. J. Roentgenol. **102**, 380—383 (1968).

MCNULTY, J. G.: High dose percutaneous transsplenic portal venography. Brit. J. Radiol. **41**, 55—58 (1968).

MEANEY, T. E., BUONOCORE, E.: Selective arteriography as a localizing and provocative test in the diagnosis of pheocromocytoma. Radiology **87**, 309—314 (1966).

MEISEL, P., FLÖTE, F.: Fehlermöglichkeiten und Zwischenfälle bei der perkutanen transfemoralen Aortographie. Röntgenpraxis **18**, 49—58 (1965).

MERCADIER, M., CLOT, J. P., MELLIÈRE, D.: Valeur de l'arteriographic sélective dans le diagnostic des tumeurs langerhansiennes hypoglycémiantes. A propos de 3 observations. Sem. Hôp. Paris **44**, 1875—1878 (1968).

MERCIER, R., VANNENVILLE, G.: Anatomie radiologique de l'aorte abdominale et ses branches. Paris: L'Expansion Scientifique 1968.

MERKLIN, R. J., MICHELS, N. A.: The variant renal and suprarenal blood supply with data in the inferior phrenic, ureteral and gonadal arteries. Statistical analysis based on 185 dissections and review of literature. J. int. Coll. Surg. **29**, 41—47 (1958).

MEYERS, M. A.: Paraduodenal hernias: radiologic and arteriographic diagnosis. Radiology **95**, 29—37 (1970).

MEYERS, M. A., KING, M. C.: Leiomyosarcoma of the duodenum: angiographic findings and report of a case. Radiology **91**, 788—790 (1968).

MICHEL, J.-R., MOREAU, J.-F., JAPHET, Y.: L'artériographie dans la transplantation rénale. Ann. Radiol. **16**, 361–374 (1973).

MICHELS, N. A.: Blood supply of upper abdominal organs with a descriptive atlas. Philadelphia-Montreal: Lippincott 1955.

MIKKELSEN, W. P.: Intestinal angina. Its surgical significance. Amer. J. Surg. **94**, 262 (1957).

MIKKELSEN, W. P., BERNE, C. J.: Intestinal angina. Med. Clin. N. Amer. **42**, 1321—1328 (1962).

MILLER, J. D., HOWIE, P. W.: Traumatic rupture of the diaphragm after blunt injury. Brit. J. Surg. **55**, 423—428 (1968).

MILLER, W. J., REUTER, S. R., REDMAN, H. C.: Epinephrime effect in angiography of colonic carcinoma (An inconsistent aid in diagnosis). Invest. Radiol. **4**, 246—251 (1969).

MILLER, W. T., SCOTT, J., ROSATO, E. F., ROSATO, F. E., CROW, H.: Ischemic colitis with gangrene. Radiology **94**, 291—297 (1970).

MING, S. C., LEVITAN, R.: Acute hemorrhagic necrosis of the gastrointestinal tract. New Engl. J. Med. **263**, 59—65 (1960).

MONIZ, E.: (1928) entnommen aus: SAVORY, P. B.: Arteriography: Principles and techniques. Illinois med. J. **138**, 215—221 (1970).

MONIZ DE BETTENCOURT, J., RATO, J. A., SILVA CARVALHO, J.: Recherches sur l'artère hépatique. VII. L'anatomie et de débit de l'artère hépatique chez l'homme normal et dans la cirrhose du foie (étude artériographique). Arch. port. Sci. biol. **15**, 13—30 (1965).

MONTERO, V. F.: Contribución al estudio de la portografia transumbilical. Arch. Fac. Med. Zaragoza **15**, 537—561 (1967).

MORDEKHAI, M.: Unusual clinical manifestations and angiographic findings in patients with Zollinger-Ellison syndrome. Ann. intern. Med. **71**, 1133—1140 (1969).

MORINO, F.: Die Arteriographie der Arteria hepatica. In: Röntgendiagnostik der Leber. Hrsg. H. ANACKER u.a. Berlin-Göttingen-Heidelberg: Springer 1959.

MORINO, F., OLIVERO, S., ROSSI, L., PAGANELLI, F., LA VILLA, G., DECUNTIS, G.: Neoplasie primitive e metastatiche: possibilita diagnostiche dei metodi arteriografici. Minerva med. **58**, 819—840 (1967).

MORINO, F., TARQUINI, A.: Cateterismo attraverso l'arteria omerale per l'arteriografia dei rami collaterali dell'aorta addominale. Minerva med. **47**, 935—944 (1956).

MORRISH, F. H.: Color-additive subtraction. Radiology **92**, 1211—1215 (1969).

MÜNSTER, W., MÜLLER, J. A. H.: Angiographische Diagnostik chronischer abdominaler Durchblutungsstörungen. Radiol. diagn. (Berl.) **8**, 545—555 (1967).

MUSSGANG, G., PORTMANN, J.: Beckenangiographie zur präoperativen Diagnostik von Sigma-Rectum-Prozessen. Chirurg **36**, 500—504 (1965).

NEBESAR, R. A., FLEISCHLI, D. J., POLLARD, J. J., GRISCOM, N. T.: Arteriography in infants and children with emphasis on the Seldinger technique and abdominal diseases. Amer. J. Roentgenol. **106**, 81—91 (1969).

NEBESAR, R. A., KORNBLITH, P. L., POLLARD, J. J., MICHELS, N. A.: Celiac and superior mesenteric arteries. A correlation of angiograms with dissections. Boston: Little, Brown & Comp. 1969.

NEBESAR, R. A., POLLARD, J. J.: Portal venography by selective arterial catheterization. Amer. J. Roentgenol. **97**, 477—487 (1966).

NEBESAR, R. A., POLLARD, J. J.: A curved-tip guide for thoracic and abdominal angiography. Amer. J. Roentgenol. **97**, 508—510 (1966).

NEBESAR, R. A., POLLARD, J. J.: A critical evaluation of selective celiac and superior mesenteric angiography in the diagnosis of pancreatic diseases, particularly malignant tumor: facts and "artefacts". Radiology **89**, 1017—1027 (1967).

NEBESAR, R. A., POLLARD, J. J.: Catheter recoil and whipping aortography. A potentially serious hazard. Radiology **89**, 845—847 (1967).

NEBESAR, R. A., POLLARD, J. J., STONE, D. L.: Angiographic diagnosis of malignant disease of the liver. Radiology **86**, 284—292 (1966).

NEBESAR, R. A., TEFFT, M., COLODNY, A. H.: Angiography of liver abscess in granulomatous disease of childhood. A case report. Amer. J. Roentgenol. **108**, 628—631 (1970).

NEBESAR, R. A., TEFFT, M., FILLER, R. A.: Correlation of angiography and isotope scanning in abdominal disease of children. Amer. J. Roentgenol. **109**, 323—340 (1970).

NEUER, A.: Das angiographische Bild des arteriellen Aneurysmas. Med. Diss. Heidelberg 1972.

NEY, H. R.: Röntgenologischer Nachweis portovenöser und intervenöser Nebenschlüsse in der Leber. Acta radiol. (Stockh.) **49**, 227—232 (1958).

NIKOLAUS, S.: Angiographie beim stumpfen Bauchtrauma. Med. Diss. Heidelberg 1972.

NORDENSTRÖM, B.: Baloon catheters for percutaneous insertion into the vascular system. Acta radiol. (Stockh.) **57**, 411—416 (1962).

NORDENSTRÖM, B.: Percutaneous baloon-occlusion of the aorta. Acta radiol. (Diagn.) **4**, 365—374 (1966).

NORDENSTRÖM, B., TÖRNELL, G.: Possibilities of angiography during temporary occlusion of the aorta in man. Acta radiol. (Diagn.) **4**, 321—330 (1966).

NORELL, H. G.: Traumatic rupture of the spleen diagnosed by abdominal aortography. Report of a case. Acta radiol. (Stockh.) **48**, 449—452 (1957).

NUSBAUM, M., BAUM, S.: Radiographic demonstration of unknown sites of gastrointestinal bleeding. Surg. Forum **14**, 374—375 (1963).

NUSBAUM, M., BAUM, S., BLAKEMORE, W.S., FINKELSTEIN, A. K.: Demonstration of intra-abdominal bleeding by selective arteriography. J. Amer. med. Ass. **191**, 389—390 (1965).

NUSBAUM, M., BAUM, S., BLAKEMORE, W. S.: Clinical experience with the diagnosis and management of gastrointestinal hemorrhage by selective mesenteric catheterization. Ann. Surg. **170**, 506—514 (1969).

NUSBAUM, M., BAUM, S., KURODA, K., BLAKEMORE, W. S.: Control of portal hypertension by selective mesenteric arterial drug infusion. Arch. Surg. **97**, 1005—1013 (1968).

NYLANDER, G.: Vascular response to vasopressin as reflected in angiography. An experimental study in the dog. Acta radiol. (Stockh.), Suppl. **266** (1967).

ÖDMAN, P.: Percutaneous selective angiography of the main branches of the aorta. Preliminary report. Acta radiol. (Stockh.) **45**, 1—14 (1956).

ÖDMAN, P.: Percutaneous selective angiography of the coeliac artery. Acta radiol. (Stockh.), Suppl. **159** (1958).

ÖDMAN, P.: Percutaneous selective angiography of the superior mesenteric artery. Acta radiol. (Stockh.) **51**, 25—32 (1959).

O'HALLORAN, J. F., Jr., KAHN, P. C.: Concomitant aortography and inferior vena cavography in patients with abdominal masses. Arch. Surg. **98**, 341—343 (1969).

OI, I., KOBAYASHI, S., KONDO, T.: Endoscopic pancreatocholangiography. Endoscopy **2**, 103—107 (1970).

OLSSON, O.: Angiographic diagnosis of an islet cell tumor of the pancreas. Acta chir. scand. **126**, 346—351 (1963).

OLSSON, O.: Coeliacography. In: Progress in Angiography. Springfield, Ill.: Thomas 1964.

OLSSON, O.: Die Frühdiagnose von Tumoren im Abdomen mit Hilfe der Angiographie. Dtsch. Röntgenkongr. **45**, 73—74, 1964 (1965). (Fortschr. Röntgenstr. Beih.)

OLSSON, O.: Angiographie bei Pankreastumoren. Radiologe **5**, 281—285 (1965).

OLSSON, O.: Viszerale Angiographie. In: Erkrankungen der Aorta und ihrer Äste. Hrsg. von F. DEUCHER u. a. (Bibl. gastroent. Fasc. 8, S. 127—139.) Basel-New York: Karger 1965.

OLSSON, O.: Angiographie in drei Fällen von Insuloma Pankreatis. Radiologe **5**, 286—297 (1965).

OOSTERKAMP, W., VANT'T HOF, A., SCHEREN, W.: Röntgenfarbbilder: neue Möglichkeiten der Subtraktion durch die Fernsehtechnik. Dtsch. Röntgenkongr. **47**, 168—170, 1966 (1967). (Fortschr. Röntgenstr. Beih.)

OTTO, K.: Das venöse Gefäßsystem der Gallenblase. Fortschr. Med. **89**, 437—440 (1971).

PALUBINSKAS, A. J., BALDWIN, J., MCCORMACK, K. R.: Liver-cell adenoma. Angiographic findings and report of a case. Radiology **89**, 444—447 (1967).

PALUBINSKAS, A. J., RIPLEY, H. R.: Fibromuscular hyperplasia in extrarenal arteries. Radiology **82**, 451 (1964).

PATURET, G.: Traité d'anatomie humaine. Paris: Masson 1951/59.

PAUL, R. E., Jr., MILLER, H. H., KAHN, P. C., CALLOW, A. D., EDWARDS, T. L., Jr., PATTERSON, J. F.: Pancreatic angiography with application of subselective angiography of the celiac or superior mesenteric artery to the diagnosis of carcinoma of the pancreas. New Engl. J. Med. **272**, 283—287 (1965).

PAULIN, S., JACOBSSEN, B., SCHLOSSMAN, D.: Thrombembolische Komplikationen bei perkutaner Arterienkatheterung. In: Angiographie und ihre Leistungen, S. 108—114. Hrsg. LOOSE, K. E. Stuttgart: Thieme 1968.

PEIRCE, E. C.: Percutaneous arterial catheterization in dogs with special reference to aortography. Ann. Surg. **133**, 544—547 (1951).

PERNKOPF, E.: Topographische Anatomie des Menschen Bd. 2,1. Berlin-Wien: Urban & Schwarzenberg 1941.

PICCONE, V. A., LEVEEN, H. H., WHITE, J. J., SKINNER, G. B., MACLEAN, L. D.: Transumbilical portal hepatography, a significant adjunct in the investigation of liver disease. Surgery **61**, 333—346 (1967).

PINTO, R. S., ZAUSNER, J., BERANBAUM, E. R.: Gastric tuberculosis. Report of a case with discussion of angiographic findings. Amer. J. Roentgenol. **110**, 808—812 (1970).

PLEWE, B.: Indikationen nach Komplikationen der direkten und indirekten Aortographie. Med. Diss. Heidelberg 1966.

POKIESER, H.: Angiographie bei Pankreaserkrankungen. Röntgen-Bl. **24**, 281—288 (1971).

POLLARD, J. J., NEBESAR, R. A.: Catheterization of the splenic artery for portal venography. New Engl. J. Med. **271**, 234—237 (1964).

POLLARD, J. J., NEBESAR, R. A.: Altered hemodynamics in the Budd-Chiari syndrome demonstrated by selective hepatic and selective splenic angiography. Radiology **89**, 236—243 (1967).

POLLARD, J. J., NEBESAR, R. A.: Abdominal angiography. New Engl. J. Med. **279**, 1035—1042, 1093—1100, 1148—1152 (1968).

POLLARD, J. J., NEBESAR, R. A., MATTOSO, L. F.: Angiographic diagnosis of benign diseases of the liver. Radiology **86**, 276—283 (1966).

POLLER, S., WHOLEY, M. H.: Splenic cysts: confirmation by selective visceral angiography. Amer. J. Roentgenol. **96**, 418—420 (1966).

POPPER, H., ELIAS, H., PETTY, D. E.: Vascular pattern of the cirrhotic liver. Amer. J. clin. Path. **22**, 717—729 (1952).

POPPER, H., SCHAFFNER, F.: Die Leber. Struktur und Funktion. Stuttgart: Thieme 1961.

PORSTMANN, W.: Angiographic examinations of children and especially of infants and young children. Ann. Radiol. **11**, 411—421 (1968).

POTEMPA, J., WENZ, W.: Die Indikationsstellung zur konservativen und operativen Behandlung geschlossener Nierenverletzungen. Langenbecks Arch. klin. Chir. **321**, 149—170 (1968).

PREGER, L.: Hepatic arteriovenous fistula after percutanous liver biopsy. Amer. J. Roentgenol. **101**, 619—620 (1967).

PRÉVÔT, R., LASSRICH, M.: Röntgendiagnostik des Magen-Darm-Kanals. Stuttgart: Thieme 1959.

PUGEDA, F., HINSHAW, J. R.: Preoperative diagnosis and treatment of a splenic artery aneurysm ruptured into the stomach. Amer. Surg. **36**, 473—476 (1970).

PYRAH, L. N., COWIE, J. W.: Two unusual aortograms. J. Fac. Radiol. (Lond.) **8**, 416—420 (1957).

RALL, E.: Die Milzarterie im Angiogramm. Med. Diss. Heidelberg 1971.

RANNIGER, K., MENGUY, R., KITTLE, C. F., ABRAMS, E.: Angiographic diagnosis of an intrahepatic aneurysm as a cause of unexplained bleeding. Radiology **90**, 507—509 (1968).

RANNIGER, K., ÖDMAN, P.: Angiographischer Nachweis multipler arteriovenöser Anastomosen in der Leber bei einem Patienten mit familiärer Teleangiektasie. Fortschr. Röntgenstr. **98**, 768—769 (1963).

RASTELLI, G. C., MAGNANI, L., BOCCHIALINI, C.: L'impiego dell'arteriografia nella diagnostica delle emorragie del tobo digerente. Minerva chir. **14**, 1188—1194 (1959).

RAUBER, A., KOPSCH, F.: Lehrbuch und Atlas der Anatomie des Menschen, Bd. II, 19. Aufl. Stuttgart: Thieme 1955.

REDMAN, H. C., REUTER, S. R.: Angiographic demonstration of surgically important vascular variations. Surg. Gynec. Obstet. **129**, 33—39 (1969).

REDMAN, H. C., REUTER, R. S.: Angiographic demonstration of portocaval and other decompressive liver shunts. Radiology **92**, 788—792 (1969).

REDMAN, H. C., REUTER, S. R., BOOKSTEIN, J.-J.: Angiography in abdominal trauma. Ann. Surg. **169**, 57—66 (1969).

REDMAN, H. C., REUTER, S. R., MILLER, W. J.: Improvement of superior mesenteric and portal vein visualization with tolazoline. Invest. Radiol. **4**, 24—27 (1969).

REIFFERSCHEID, A.: Chirurgie der Leber. Klinik und Technik. Stuttgart: Thieme 1957.

RESCHKE, H.: Die selective Angiographie der A. phrenica ascendens. Fortschr. Röntgenstr. **107**, 200—205 (1967).

REUTER, S. R.: Superselective pancreatic angiography. Radiology **92**, 74—85 (1969).

REUTER, S. R.: Modification of pancreatic blood flow with ballon catheters; a new approach to pancreatic angiography. Radiology **95**, 57—63 (1970).

REUTER, S. R., BOIJSEN, E.: Angiographic findings in two ileal carcinoid tumors. Radiology **87**, 836 (1966).

REUTER, S. R., KANTER, I. E., REDMAN, H. C.: Angiography in reversible colonic ischemia. Radiology **97**, 371—375 (1970).

REUTER, S. R., OLIN, T.: Stenosis of the celiac artery. Radiology **85**, 617—627 (1965).

REUTER, S. R., REDMAN, H. C.: Gastrointestinal angiography. Philadelphia-London-Toronto: W. B. Saunders Co. 1972.

REUTER, S. R., REDMAN, H. C., BOOKSTEIN, J. J.: Differential problems in angiographic diagnosis of carcinoma of pancreas. Radiology **96**, 93—99 (1970).

REUTER, S. R., REDMAN, H. C., JOSEPH, R. R.: Angiographic findings in pancreatitis. Amer. J. Roentgenol. **107**, 56—64 (1969).

REUTER, S. R., REDMAN, H. C., SIDERS, P. B.: The spectrum of angiographic findings in hepatoma. Radiology **94**, 89—94 (1970).

RIGLER, L. G., OLFELT, P. C., KRUMBACH, R. W.: Roentgen hepatography by injection of a contrast medium into the aorta. Radiology **60**, 363—367 (1953).

RIPLEY, H. R., LEVIN, S. M.: Abdominal angina associated with fibromuscular hyperplasia of the celiac and superior mesenteric arteries. Angiology **17**, 297—310 (1966).

ROB, CH.: Vascular diseases of the intestine. In: Modern trends in gastroentgenology. S. 252. Eds. CARD, W. J., CREAMER, B.: London: Butterworth 1970.

ROCKOFF, S. D., DOPPMAN, J., BLOCK, J. B., KETCHAM, A.: Variable response of tumor vessels to intraarterial epinephrine: an angiographic study in man. Invest. Radiol. **1**, 205—213 (1966).

RÖSCH, J.: Die Rolle der Splenoportographie in der Diagnostik der Epigastriumgeschwülste. Fortschr. Röntgenstr. **90**, 415—434 (1959).

RÖSCH, J.: Lebertumoren und Leberabszesse im Splenportogramm. In: Röntgendiagnostik der Leber. Hrsg. von H. ANACKER u.a., S. 33—56. Berlin-Göttingen-Heidelberg: Springer 1959.

RÖSCH, J.: Splenoportographie. In: Ergebnisse der medizinischen Strahlenforschung, N.F. 1, S. 143—200. Stuttgart: Thieme 1964.

RÖSCH, J.: Röntgenuntersuchungen und Einsatz der Methoden bei Pankreaserkrankungen. Radiologe **5**, 257—268 (1965).

RÖSCH, J.: Roentgenologic possibilities in spleen diagnosis. Amer. J. Roentgenol. **94**, 453—461 (1965).

RÖSCH, J.: Tumours of the spleen. The value of selective arteriography. Clin. Radiol. **17**, 183—190 (1966).

RÖSCH, J.: Roentgenology of the spleen and pancreas. Springfield, Ill.: Thomas 1967.

RÖSCH, J.: Roentgenologic diagnosis of pancreatic disease. Amer. J. Roentgenol. **100**, 664—672 (1967).

RÖSCH, J., BRET, J.: Unsere Erfahrungen mit der Milzarteriographie in der Diagnostik der Milzerkrankungen. Fortschr. Röntgenstr. **97**, 239—255 (1962).

RÖSCH, J., BRET, J.: Arteriography of the pancreas. Amer. J. Roentgenol. **94**, 182—193 (1965).

RÖSCH, J., BRET, J.: Angiographie in der Diagnostik der Epigastriumgeschwülste. Dtsch. Röntgenkongr. **45**, 81—87, 1964 (1956). (Fortschr. Röntgenstr. Beih.)

RÖSCH, J., DOTTER, CH. T.: Extrahepatic portal obstruction in childhood and its angiographic diagnosis. Amer. J. Roentgenol. **112**, 143—149 (1971).

RÖSCH, J., DOTTER, C. T., ROSE, R. W.: Röntgenologische Kontrolle akuter Magen-Darm-Blutungen. Fortschr. Röntgenstr. **114**, 729—740 (1971).

RÖSCH, J., GROLLMAN, J. H., Jr.: Superselective arteriography in the diagnosis of abdominal pathology: Technical considerations. Radiology **92**, 1008—1013 (1969).

RÖSCH, J., GROLLMANN, J. H., STECKEL, R.J.: Arteriography in the diagnosis of gallbladder disease. Radiology **92**, 1485—1491 (1969).

ROESCH, W., OTTENJANN, R.: Gastric erosions. Endoscopy **2**, 93—99 (1970).

ROSENBUSCH, G., CEN, M.: Zöliakographie mit Sekretin. Möglichkeiten der Pharmakoangiographie in der Pankreasdiagnostik. Fortschr. Röntgenstr. **110**, 639—651 (1969).

ROSENBUSCH, G., CEN, M., DIHLMANN, W.: Indirekte Portographie mit Bradykinin bei Zustand nach Splenektomie. (Möglichkeiten der Pharmakoangiographie.) Fortschr. Röntgenstr. **111**, 805—809 (1969).

ROSSI, P., GOULD, H. R.: Angiography and scanning in liver disease. Radiology **96**, 553—562 (1970).

ROSSI, P., RUZICKA, F. F.: Differentiation of intrahepatic and extrahepatic masses by arteriography. Radiology **93**, 771—780 (1969).

ROSSI, P., YOUNG, J., PANKE, W.: Techniques, usefulness and hazards of arteriography of pheochromocytoma. Review of 99 cases. J. Amer. med. Ass. **205**, 547—553 (1968).

ROTH, F.-J., HORBASCHEK, H., WENZ, W.: Farbige Röntgenbilder. Fortschr. Röntgenstr. **115**, 705—717 (1971).

ROTH, F.-J., WENZ, W.: Das Farbröntgenbild. Erste Erfahrungen mit der elektronisch-photographischen Methode. Visum **13**, 119—121, 132—134 (1969).

ROTH, F.-J., WENZ, W., KRAMER, H.: Elektronische Verbesserung von Röntgenaufnahmen. Dtsch. med. Wschr. **94**, 1483—1485 (1969).

ROURKE, J., BOSNIAK, M., FERRIS, E.: Hepatic angiography in "alcoholic hepatitis". Radiology **91**, 290—296 (1968).

ROZMAN, C., PADRÓS-ARCHS, W., MARTINEZ-MUÑOZ, A.: Quiste hidatidico de bazo, diagnosticado por arteriografia. Med. clín. (Barcelona) **39**, 85—88 (1962).

RÜTTIMANN, A., BEELER, E.: 3. Diagnostik-Kurs, Kursunterlagen. Davos 1971.

RÜTTIMANN, A., PRETER, B., BIRCHER, J.: Zur percutanen transhepatischen Cholangiographie. Schweiz. med. Wschr. **98**, 278—279 (1968).

RÜTTIMANN, A., WIRTH, W.: Möglichkeiten und Grenzen der Lymphographie mit öligen Kontrastmittel. Radiologe **8**, 140—149 (1968).

RUZICKA, F. F., Jr.: Percutaneous splenography. In: Vascular roentgenology, p. 588—607. Eds. SCHOBINGER, R. A., RUZICKA, F. F., Jr. New York: MacMillan 1964.

RUZICKA, F. F., Jr., BRADLEY, E. G., ROUSSELOT, L. M.: Two-phase opacification of the liver in cirrhosis. Ann. N.Y. Acad. Sci. **78**, 819—828 (1959).

RUZICKA, F. F., Jr., ROSSI, P.: Arterial portography: Pattern of venous flow. Radiology **92**, 777—787 (1969).

RUZICKA, F. F., Jr., ROSSI, P., ABRAMS, R. E., TRACHT, D. G.: Anomalous and parasitic arterial blood supply in the abdomen. Radiology **96**, 261—268 (1970).

RUZICKA, F. F., Jr., SANCHEZ-UBEDA, R.: Percutanous transhepatic cholangiography. N.Y. St. J. Med. **68**, 3034—3039 (1968).

SAKUMA, S., IKEDA, H., AYAKAWA, Y., TANAKA, Y., TAKAHASHI, S.: Angiography with direct fourfold magnification. Invest. Radiol. **4**, 310—316 (1969).

SAMMONS, B. P., NEAL, M. P., Jr., ARMSTRONG, R. H., Jr., HAGER, H. G.: Ten years experience with celiac and upper abdominal superior mesenteric arteriography. Amer. J. Roentgenol. **101**, 345—360 (1967).

SANDBLOM, P.: Hemorrhage into biliary tract following trauma: "Traumatic hemobilia". Surgery **24**, 571—586 (1948).

SANDBLOM, PH.: Gastrointestinal hemorrhage through the pancreatic duct. Ann. Surg. **171**, 61—66 (1970).

SATO, T., KOYAMA, K., SAITO, Y.: Angiography in surgical liver diseases with special reference to its diagnostic value. [Jap.] Rinshô Hôsha **13**, 163—172 (1968).

SATO, T., WATANABE, K., SAITOH, Y., KOYAMA, K., SUDA, Y.: Selective arteriography for gallbladder diseases. Evaluation with references to carcinoma of the gallbladder. Arch. Surg. **99**, 598—605 (1969).

SAUR, H, TH.: Ein Überblick über die Komplikationen bei der indirekten (perkutanen Katheter-)Methode der Aortographie. Z. Kreisl.-Forsch. **53**, 314—321 (1964).

SAVORY, P. B.: Arteriography: Principles and techniques. Illinois med. J. **138**, 215—221 (1970).

SCHEININ, T. M., VÄNTTINEN: Aneurysms of the splenic artery in portal hypertension. Ann. Clin. Res. **1**, 165—168 (1969).

SCHIMANSKI, K., SCHMIDT, H.: Klinische Erscheinungsformen der Viszeralarterieninsuffizienz. Z. Gastroent. **9**, 11—22 (1971).

SCHMIDT, H., SCHIMANSKI, K.: Die Stenose der Arteria coelica — ihre Diagnose und klinische Bedeutung. Fortschr. Röntgenstr. **106**, 1—12 (1967).

SCHMIDT, H., SCHIMANSKI, K.: Klinik und Diagnose der Angina abdominalis. In: Angiographie und ihre Leistungen. Hrsg. von K. E. LOOSE, S. 125—129. Stuttgart: Thieme 1968.

SCHMITZ, W., WENZ, W., KRUMHAAR, D.: Erfolgreiche Operation einer 52 Jahre bestehenden arteriovenösen Fistel. Langenbecks Arch. klin. Chir. **318**, 126—133 (1967).

SCHOEN, D.: Über die Gefahren bei der intravasalen Anwendung jodhaltiger Kontrastmittel. Med. Welt. **52**, 200—209 (1962).

SCHOENMACKERS, J., VIETEN, H.: Atlas postmortaler Angiogramme. Stuttgart: Thieme 1967.

SCHORN, J., STONDER, H., VOEGT, H.: Untersuchungen über die arterielle Strombahn der Leber. Langenbecks Arch. klin. Chir. **286**, 187—194 (1957).

SCHREIBER, H.W.: Indikationen zur Splenoportographie. Dtsch. med. Wschr. **90**, 1439—1440 (1965).

SCHREIBER, H.W., ACKEREN, H. VAN: Die akute Blutung aus Magen und Darm. Med. Welt 793—797 (1965).

SCHREIBER, M.H., WOLMA, F.J., MANSKE, A.O., MOORE, C.H.: Experimental visceral arteriography in blunt abdominal trauma. Amer. J. Roentgenol. **104**, 732—755 (1968).

SCHRÖDER, K.: Das akute und das chronische Verschlußsyndrom der Eingeweideschlagadern. Med Diss. Heidelberg 1966.

SCHULTE-BRINKMANN, W.: Zur Röntgendiagnostik der Milzzysten. Dtsch. med. Wschr. **93**, 1906—1910 (1968).

SCHWARTZ, S., BOLEY, S.J., ROBINSON, K., KRIEGER, H., SCHULTZ, L., ALLAN, A.C.: Roentgenologic features of vascular disorders of the intestines. Radiol. Clin. N. Amer. **2**, 71—87 (1964).

SELDINGER, S.I.: Catheter replacement of the needle in percutaneous arteriography; a new technique. Acta radiol. (Stockh.) **39**, 368—376 (1953).

SELKE, A.C., CORNELL, S.H.: Infantile hepatic hemangioendothelioma. Amer. J. Roentgenol. **106**, 200—203 (1969).

SENN, A.: Die chirurgische Behandlung der akuten und chronischen arteriellen Verschlüsse. Bern: Huber 1963.

SERVELLO, M.: L'angiographie du foie pour la mise en évidence de son système artériel, portal et sus-hépatique. Ann. Radiol. **3**, 31—71 (1960).

SHANNON, R.: Ischemic necrosis of the left colon following artery occlusion. Brit. J. Surg. **50**, 533—534 (1962).

SHANNON, R.: Ischemic necrosis of the left colon following resection of a ruptured abdominal aortic aneurysm. Med. J. Aust. **2**, 756 (1962).

SHIBATA, S., IWASAKI, N.: Angiographic findings in diseases of the stomach. Amer. J. Roentgenol. **110**, 322—331 (1970).

SHIBATA, S., IWASAKI, N., MITO, M., KASAI, Y.: Radiological findings in tumor of the liver. Abstr. Int. Congr. Radiol. **12**, 254 (1969).

SHUFORD, W.W., SYBERS, R,G., WEENS, H.S.: Problems in the aortographic diagnosis of dissecting aneurysm of the aorta. New Engl. J. Med. **280**, 225—231 (1969).

SIEGELMANN, S.S., CAPLAN, L., ANNES, G.: Complications of catheter angiography. Study with oscillometry and "pollout" angiograms. Radiology **91**, 251—253 (1968).

SIELAFF, H.J.: Die radiologische Diagnostik der Dünndarmerkrankungen. Therapiewoche **20**, 3207—3215 (1970).

SMITH, G.W., WESTGAARD, I., BJÖRN-HANSEN, R.: Hepatic venous angiography in the evaluation of cirrhosis of the liver. Ann. Surg. **173**, 469 (1971).

SMITH, R.B., STONE, H.H.: Traumatic arteriovenous fistulas involving the portal venous system. Amer. J. Surg. **119**, 570—573 (1970).

SOBOTTA, J., BECHER, H.: Atlas der deskriptiven Anatomie des Menschen. 15. Aufl., T. 2. München-Berlin: Urban & Schwarzenberg 1960.

SOLHEIM, K.: Acute intestinal infarction. Acute mesenteric vascular occlusion. Acta chir. scand. **126**, 133—143 (1963).

SOLHEIM, K.: Angiography in the surgery of trauma. Norsk Laegeforen **88**, 346—347 (1968).

SPÄH, K.: Oszillographische Kontrolluntersuchungen nach transfemoralen Katheterangiographien. Med. Diss. Heidelberg 1971.

SPALTEHOLZ, W.: Gefäßbaum und Organbildung. Arch. Entwickl.-Mech. Org. **52—97**, 480—531 (1923).

SPENCER, R.: Gastrointestinal hemorrhage in infancy and childhood: 476 cases. Surgery **55**, 718—734 (1964).

SPJUT, H.J., MARGULIS, A.R.: Micro-angiographic patterns of chronic ulcerative colitis. Dis. Colon Rect. **8**, 215—221 (1965).

SPJUT, H.J., MARGULIS, A.R., MCALISTER, W.H.: Microangiographic study of gastrointestinal lesions. Amer. J. Roentgenol. **92**, 1173—1187 (1964).

STACHENFELD, R.A., GORDIMER, H., FRIEDENBERG, R.M., LOPEZ, F.A.: Aneurysm of the left gastric artery: preoperative angiographic diagnosis. Radiology **83**, 1026—1028 (1964).

STAUBESAND, J.: ArteriovenöseAnastomosen. In: Die arteriovenösen Anastomosen. Hrsg. von F. HAMMERSEN, D. GROSS. Aktuelle Probleme in der Angiologie. Bd. 2, S. 11. Bern: Huber 1968.

STECKEL, R.J., ROSCH, J., ROSS, G., GROLLMAN, J.H.: New developments in pharmacoangiography (and arterial pharmacotherapy) of the gastrointestinal tract. Invest. Radiol. **6**, 199—211 (1971).

STECKEL, R.J., ROSS, G., GROLLMAN, J.H.: A potent drug combination for producing constriction of the superior mesenteric artery and its branches. Radiology **91**, 579—581 (1968).

STECKENMESSER, R., BAYINDIR, S., HEGER, N., RISTIG, W., SCHIEMER, H.: Die Leistungsfähigkeit der selectiven Arteriographie bei raumfordernden Prozessen der Leber. Bericht über 117 Untersuchungen. Fortschr. Röntgenstr. **114**, 58—74 (1971).

STEIN, H.L.: The diagnosis of traumatic laceration of the spleen by selective arteriography, direct serial magnification angiography and intraarterial epinephrine. Radiology **93**, 367—372 (1969).

STEIN, H.L., STEINBERG, J.: Selective aortography, the definitive technique for diagnosis of dissecting aneurysm of the aorta. Amer. J. Roentgenol. **102**, 333—348 (1968).

STEINBERG, I., FINBY, N., EVANS, J.A.: A safe and practical intravenous method for abdominal aortography, peripheral arteriography, and cerebral angiography. Amer. J. Roentgenol. **82**, 758—772 (1959).

STOCKS, L.O., HALPERN, M., TURNER, A.F.: Complete translumbar aortography. The teflon sleeve technique. Amer. J. Roentgenol. **107**, 835—839 (1969).

STOOPEN, M., CASAL, R., ELIZANDO, L., LAUDA, L.: Angiographic alterations in hepatic amebic abscesses: A study of 60 cases. Rev. mex. Radiol. **23**, 9—22 (1969).

STREICHER, H.J.: Chirurgie der Milz. Berlin-Göttingen-Heidelberg: Springer 1961.

STRICKLAND, B.: Localisation using physical divices, radioisotopes and radiographic methods. IV. The place of arteriography in tumor localisation. Brit. J. Radiol. **34**, 555—562 (1961).

STULBERG, H.J., BIERMAN, H.R.: Selective hepatic arteriography. Normal anatomy, anatomic variations and pathological conditions. Radiology **85**, 46—55 (1965).

SUNDGREN, R.: Selective angiography of the left gastric artery. Acta radiol. (Stockh.) Suppl. **299** (1970).

SWANSON, G. E.: A case of cystadenoma of the pancreas studied by selective angiography. Radiology **81**, 592—595 (1963).

SWART, B.: Die Röntgenuntersuchung des Pankreas. Fortschr. Röntgenstr. **95**, 809—820 (1961).

SWART, B.: Die Röntgendiagnostik der akuten und chronischen Pancreatitis. Dtsch. med. J. **14**, 784—787 (1963).

SWART, B., DINGENDORF, W.: Die Potenz der röntgendiagnostischen Untersuchungsmethoden bei Abflußstörungen an den Gallenwegen mit und ohne Ikterus. I. Suprapankreatische Gallenwege. Radiologe **8**, 84—90 (1968).

SWART, B., MANI, M.: Zur verbesserten angiographischen Darstellung der peripheren Nierengefäße mit Hilfe der direkten Röntgenvergrößerung. Radiologe **8**, 6—10 (1968).

TAMAO, H.: Experimental and clinical studies on the intrahepatic vascular changes in chronic liver injury. II. Radiological observations in chronic hepatitis and liver cirrhosis. Jap. Circulat. J. **30**, 297—308 (1966).

TANK, E. S., ERAKLIS, A. J., GROSS, R. E.: Blunt abdominal trauma in infancy and childhood. J. Trauma **8**, 439—448 (1968).

TASAKA, A.: Selective Angiography. Tokio: Igaku Shoin Ltd. 1967.

TAVERNIER, J., DELORME, G., LAFITTE, J., TESSIER, J., BELLET, M.: Apports de l'angiographic cœliaque et mésentérique à la radiographie pancréatique. J. Radiol. Électrol. **50**, 867 (1969).

TAVERNIER, J., DELORME, G., FAGOLA, M.: L'arteriographie «super-sélective» du pancreas. Ann. Radiol. **14**, 55—566 (1971).

TERNBERG, J. L., KOEHLER, P. R.: The use of arteriography in the diagnosis of the origin of acute gastrointestinal hemorrhage in children. Surgery **63**, 686—689 (1968).

TESCHENDORF, W.: Lehrbuch der röntgenologischen Differentialdiagnostik, 4. Aufl., Bd. 2: Erkrankungen der Bauchorgane. Stuttgart: Thieme 1964.

THOMAS, R. L., ROBINSON, A. E., JOHNSRUDE, I. S., GOODRICH, J. K., LESTER, R. G.: The demonstration of an insulin and gastrin producing pancreatic tumor by angiography and pancreatic scanning. Amer. J. Roentgenol. **104**, 64—651 (1968).

TIEDEMANN, F.: Von der Verengung und Schließung der Pulsadern in Krankheiten. Heidelberg: Groos 1843.

TILLANDER, H.: Magnetic guidance of a catheter with articulated steel tip. Acta radiol. (Stockh.) **35**, 62 (1951).

TILLANDER, H.: Selective angiography of the abdominal aorta with a guided catheter. Acta radiol. (Stockh.) **45**, 21 (1956).

TJENG, K.-L.: Angiographische Darstellung der Gallenblase bei der Coeliacographie. Med. Diss. Heidelberg 1971.

TOMCHIK, F. S., WITTENBERG, J., OTTINGER, L. W.: The roentgenographic spectrum of bowel infarction. Radiology **96**, 249—260 (1970).

TREDE, M.: Gefäßchirurg. Noteingriffe: Die Verletzung der peripheren Gefäße. Mittelrhein. Chirurgenvereinigung. Karlsruhe 1971. Bruns' Beitr. klin. Chir. (im Druck).

TRINEZ, G., ROZAN, R., PIETRI, J., PETIT, PH., GENTIT, F., DESCOMBES, PH.: Fistule hépatico-portale spontanée avec syndrome d'ischémie mésentérique. Étude angiographique. Ann. Radiol. **16**, 349–360 (1973).

UDÉN, R.: Effect of secretin in celiac and superior mesenteric angiography. Acta radiol. Diagn. **8**, 497—513 (1969).

VERDURON, J., BAUDOUX, M., GAILLARD, J., HERNANDEZ, C., ROUGEULLE, J.: L'éiomyome de grêle découvert par artériographie. Sem. Hôp. Paris **45**, 1194—1196 (1969).

VIAMONTE, M.: Gastrointestinal angiography. Amer. J. Gastroent. **46**, 187—211 (1966).

VIAMONTE, M., Jr., GILSON, A.: Angioscanography. Radiology **87**, 351—352 (1966).

VIAMONTE, M., Jr., MARTINEZ, L., PARKS, R. E., WARREN, W. D., FOMON, J.: Liver shunts. Amer. J. Roentgenol. **102**, 773—775 (1968).

VIAMONTE, M., Jr., PARKS, R. E.: Progress in angiography. XII, 562 p. Springfield, Ill.: Ch. C. Thomas 1964.

VIAMONTE, M., Jr., STEVENS, R. C.: Guided angiography. Amer. J. Roentgenol. **94**, 30—39 (1965).

VIAMONTE, M., Jr., WARREN, W. D., FOMON, J. J., MARTINEZ, L. O.: Angiographic investigations in portal hypertension. Surg. Gynec. Obstet. **130**, 37—53 (1970).

VOEGELI, E.: Die Vergrößerungstechnik, klinische Anwendung. In: Röntgendiagnostik. Hrsg. FUCHS, W. A., VOEGELI. (Aktuelle Probleme der Röntgendiagnostik. Bd. 1, S. 24—31.) Bern: Huber 1971.

VOGLER, E.: Aorta abdominalis und ihre großen Äste. In: Handbuch der medizinischen Radiologie. Hrsg. von L. DIETHELM, O. OLSSON u. a. Bd. X, 3, S. 259—309. Berlin-Göttingen-Heidelberg: Springer 1964.

VOLLMAR, J.: Traumatische arteriovenöse Fisteln. Zbl. Chir. **89**, 1930—1939 (1964).

VOLLMAR, J.: Rekonstruktive Chirurgie der Arterien. Stuttgart: Thieme 1967.

VOLLMAR, J.: Steal-Syndrome. Münch. med. Wschr. **113**, 501—506 (1971).

VOLLMAR, J., HARTERT, H., HASSE, H. M., SCHRÖDER, K., COERPER, H. G.: Das chronische Verschlußsyndrom der Eingeweideschlagadern (A. coeliaca, mesenterica sup. et inf.). Angina abdominalis (BACCELLI); Dysphragia intermittens angiosclerotica (ORTHNER); Mesenteric arterial insufficiency (DERRICK); Angina intestinalis (MIKKELSEN); Syndrome d'ischémie intestinale paroxystique (LEYMARIOS). Langenbecks Arch. klin. Chir. **305**, 473—490 (1964).

WAGNER, A., WENZ, W.: Enterales Proteinverlustsyndrom bei einem Patienten mit generalisierter Dickdarmpolypose und essentiellen Teleangiektasien. Schweiz. med. Wschr. **99**, 777—781 (1969).

WAGNER, E., SCHULTIS, K., BAYINDIR, S.: Erfahrungen mit der Angiographie bei Abdominaltumoren. In: Aktuelle Gastroenterologie. Hrsg. von H. BARTELHEIMER, N. HEISIG. Stuttgart: Thieme 1968.

WALDRON, R. L., TEIXIDOR, H., MACKEN, K. L.: Celiac pancreatography. A preliminary report. Radiology **93**, 932—934 (1969).

WANKE, E.: Zit. nach HELLNER, NISSEN, VOSSSCHULTE: Lehrbuch der Chirurgie. Stuttgart: Thieme 1957.

WANNAGAT, L.: Die laparaskopische Splenographie. Klin. Wschr. **33**, 750—758 (1955).

WANNAGAT, L.: Das intrahepatische Splenoportogramm bei der Hepatitis. Med. Klin. **57**, 853—857 u. Bild. 843—845 (1962).

WANNAGAT, L.: Die direkte Cholezysto-Cholangiographie und Cholangiographie in der Differentialdiagnose des Ikterus. Aus: Der Ikterus, hrsg. von K. BECK. Stuttgart-New York: Schattauer 1968.

WARREN, I. A., BERK, J. E.: The etiology of chronic nonspecific ulcerative colitis. Gastroenterology **33**, 395—422 (1957).

WARREN, S., SOMMERS, S. C.: Pathogenesis of ulcerative colitis. Amer. J. Path. **25**, 657 (1949).

WARTER, J., STORCK, D., KIENY, R., TONGIO, J.: Sténosis congénitales du tronc coeliaque. Arch. Mal. Appar. dig. **59**, 765—780 (1970).

WATZKA, M.: Über Gefäßsperren und arteriovenöse Anastomosen. Z. mikr.-anat. Forsch. **39**, 521—544 (1936).

WEAVER, D. H., FLEMING, R. J., BARNES, W. A.: Aneurysm of the hepatic artery: The value of arteriography in surgical management. Surgery **64**, 891—896 (1968).

WEHLING, H.: Zur Frühdiagnose von Pankreastumoren. Untersuchungen zur angiographischen Darstellung des Pankreas unter Verwendung vasoaktiver Stoffe. Fortschr. Med. **89**, 1008—1011 (1971).

WEIDNER, W., FOX, P., JAMES, B. A., BROOKS, W., VINIK, M.: The roentgenographic diagnosis of aneurysms of the superior mesenteric artery. Amer. J. Roentgenol. **109**, 138—142 (1970).

WEIGERT, C.: In die Milzvene geborstenes Aneurysma einer Milzarterie. Virchows Arch. path. Anat. **104**, 26 (1886).

WEIL, F., GISSELBRECHT, P., BONNEVILLE, J. F., RICATTE, J. P., PREVOTAT, N.: Plaidoyer pour l'angiography première au cours des héinatéméses massives. Ann. Radiol. **13**, 353—361 (1970).

WEISSLEDER, H., BAUMEISTER, L., FISCHER, P., RENEMANN, H.: Die selektive Darstellung der Arteria coeliaca und mesenterica superior in der abdominalen Diagnostik. Fortschr. Röntgenstr. **104**, 137—149 (1966).

WEISSLEDER, H., RÄDEKER, U., NIEMANN, H., EMMRICH, J.: Pankreasdiagnostik durch selektive Angiographie. Röntgen-Bl. **20**, 501—511 (1967).

WELLAUER, J.: Radiologie der Aorta und der großen Gefäße. Schweiz. med. Wschr. **95**, 1640—1647 (1965).

WENZ, W.: Thorotrasttumoren. Quantitative Untersuchungen über das Dosis-Wirkungs-Problem bei der Thorotrastose. Ergebn. Chir. **46**, 81—166 (1964).

WENZ, W.: Selektive Arteriographie der Oberbauchorgane. Dtsch. med. Wschr. **90**, 643—646 (1965).

WENZ, W.: Darstellung der Vena portae über die Arteria coeliaca und Arteria mesenterica superior. Dtsch. Röntgenkongr. **46**, 70—74 (1966). (Fortschr. Röntgenstr. Beih.)

WENZ, W.: Angiographische Darstellung der Gallenblasenarterien. Fortschr. Röntgenstr. **106**, 387—392 (1967).

WENZ, W.: Die perkutane transhepatische Cholangiographie. Röntgenpraxis **20**, 66—75 (1967).

WENZ, W.: Die Röntgendiagnostik der akuten gastrointestinalen Blutung. Chirurg **40**, 100—105 (1969).

WENZ, W.: Radiographic technics in diagnosis of vascular disease. In: American College of Surgeons. Dtsche Ges. für Chirurgie. Joint meeting. Munich 1968. S. 22—31. Ed. by H. BÜRKLE DE LA CAMP, F. LINDER, M. TREDE. Berlin-Heidelberg-New York: Springer 1969.

WENZ, W.: Bedeutung der Angiographie in einem traumatologischen Zentrum. Abstr. 2nd. Congr. Europ. Assoc. Radiol. Amsterdam 1971. p. 234—235. Amsterdam: Excerpta Medica 1971.

WENZ, W., BECKENBACH, H., DAUM, R.: Die kindliche Pfortader bei Erkrankungen der Oberbauchorgane. Z. Kinderchir. **9**, 354—362 (1971).

WENZ, W., BEDUHN, D., OEFTERING, T.: Viscerale Durchblutungsstörungen. Röntgen-Bl. **24**, 423—432 (1971).

WENZ, W., BEDUHN, D., ROTH, F.-J., VAN KAICK, G., CZEMBIREK, H.: Abdominale Angiographie: Technik, Pathomorphologie, Indikationen. Röntgenpraxis **23**, 97—124 (1970).

WENZ, W., BEDUHN, D., WAWERSIK, J., VAN KAICK, G., LOHÖLTER, H.: Die Wertigkeit der Angiographie in der abdominalen Tumordiagnostik. In: Diagnostische und therapeutische Fortschritte in der Krebschirurgie. Hrsg. LINDER, F., OTT, G., RUDOLPH, H. Berlin-Heidelberg-New York: Springer 1971.

WENZ, W., KAICK, G. VAN, CZEMBIREK, H., GRUSS, J. D.: Angiogramme de rupture de rate. Signification et limites. Ann. Radiol. **14**, 883—894 (1971).

WENZ, W., KAICK, G. VAN, WEGENER, K.: Kritisches zur angiographischen „Tumoranfärbung". Fortschr. Röntgenstr. **115**, 180—185 (1971).

WENZ, W., KOLIG, G.: Fehler und Gefahren der perkutanen, transhepatischen Cholangiographie. Fortschr. Röntgenstr. **103**, 713—725 (1965).

WENZ, W., KREBS, H.: Angiographischer Nachweis eines blutenden Dünndarmneurinoms. Dtsch. med. Wschr. **92**, 2264—2267 (1967).

WENZ, W., OTT, G.: Aktuelle Thorotrastprobleme: Ein Lebersarkom mit intraperitonealer Blutung. Strahlentherapie **127**, 463—469 (1965).

WENZ, W., ROTH, F.-J., BRÜCKNER, U.: Die Angiographie bei der akuten Gastrointestinalblutung. Experimentelle Voraussetzungen und klinische Ergebnisse. Fortschr. Röntgenstr. **110**, 616—629 (1969).

WENZ, W., SPÄH, U.: Kontrolluntersuchungen nach Katheterangiographie. In: Die Gefäßthrombosen nach Katheterangiographie. Hrsg. ZEITLER, E. (Aktuelle Probleme in der Angiologie. Bd. 10, S. 20—22.) Bern-Stuttgart-Wien: Huber 1970.

WEXLER, L., ABRAMS, H. L.: Hamartoma of the spleen. Angiographic observations. Amer. J. Roentgenol. **92**, 1150—1155 (1964).

WEYER, K. H. VAN DE, KÖSSLING, F. K., HABIGHORST, L. V., ALBERS, P. B.: Experimentelle Untersuchungen zur Technik und Risiko der Pankreasangiographie. Fortschr. Röntgenstr. **108**, 733—740 (1968).

WEYER, K. H. VAN DE, MAPPES, G.: Präoperative angiographische Darstellung eines Aneurysmas der Arteria gastro-duodenalis. Fortschr. Röntgenstr. **108**, 740—745 (1968).

WHIPPLE, A. O.: Problems of portal hypertension in relation to hepatosplenopathies. Ann. Surg. **122**, 449—475 (1945).

WHOLEY, M. H., BRON, K. M., HALLER, J. D.: Selective angiography of the colon (Symposium). Surg. Clin. N. Amer. **45**, 1283—1291 (1965).

WHOLEY, M. H., JACKMAN, V.: A new instrument: controllable guide for angiography. Amer. J. Roentgenol. **97**, 500—503 (1966).

WHOLEY, M. H., STOCKDALE, R., HUNG, T. K.: A percutaneous ballon catheter for the immediate control of hemorrhage. Radiology **95**, 65—71 (1970).

WIRBATZ, W.: Der transumbilikale Katheterismus der Vena portae und seine Bedeutung für die Onkologie. (Diagnostik und Therapie von Lebermetastasen.) Med. Habil.-Schr. Humboldt-Univ. Berlin 1971.

WISE, L. K., GANSON, J.: Subtraction technic. Video and color methode. Radiology **86**, 814—821 (1966).

WITT, H., KOURIK, W.: Gemeinsame Versorgung des Gastrointestinaltraktes sowie der Leber und Milz durch erweiterte, schleifenförmig verlaufende A. mesenterica caudalis. Fortschr. Röntgenstr. **111**, 92—95 (1969).

WOODRUFF, J. H., OTTOMAN, R. E., SIMONTON, J. H., AVERBROOK, B. D.: The radiological differential diagnosis of abdominal trauma. Radiology **72**, 641—650 (1959).

YATES, L. N., CLAUSEN, E. G.: Simple nonspecific ulcers of the sigmoid colon. Arch. Surg. **81**, 535—541 (1960).

YOUNG, J. R., BRITTON, R. C., DE WOLFE, V. G., HUMPHRIES, A. W.: Intestinal ischemic necrosis following abdominal aortic surgery. Surg. Gynec. Obstet. **115**, 615—620 (1962).

YÜ, C.: Primary carcinoma of the liver (hepatoma). Its diagnosis by selective celiac arteriography. Amer. J. Roentgenol. **99**, 142—149 (1967).

ZAHN, D. G. H., GOERTTLER, KL.: Über die Sklerose der Eingeweidearterien. Pathomorphologische Befunde, Lokalisation und Häufigkeit. Arch. Kreisl.-Forsch. **64**, 235—272 (1971).

ZEITLER, E.: (Hrsg.) Die Gefäßthrombosen nach Katheterangiographie. (Aktuelle Probleme in der Angiologie. Bd. 10.) Stuttgart-Wien: Huber 1970.

ZENKER, R., BEDACHT, R., ZIMMERMANN, H.: Die Bedeutung der Angiographie für die Therapie bei Inselzellgeschwülsten. Münch. med. Wschr. **108**, 1691—1696 (1966).

ZEPPA, R., PETROU, H. D., WOMACK, N. A.: Collateral circulation to the liver: a case of mycotic aneurysm of the celiac artery. Ann. Surg. **163**, 233—236 (1966).

ZIEDSES LES PLANTES, B. G.: Subtraktion. Fortschr. Röntgenstr. **52**, 69—79 (1935).

ZOLLINGER, R. M., ELLISON, E. N.: Primary pectic ulcerations of the jejunum associated with islet-cell tumors of the pancreas. Ann. Surg. **142**, 709—728 (1955).

ZSEBÖK, Z. B., SZLÁRY, P. L.: Über die EKG-Veränderungen, die bei der Verabreichung von angiographischen Kontrastmittelinjektionen zu registrieren sind. Fortschr. Röntgenstr. **102**, 42—48 (1965).

ZUM WINKEL, K., KEISER, D. VON: Kombinierte Metastasensuche im Bauchraum mit der Szintigraphie des Lymphsystems und der Cavographie. Fortschr. Röntgenstr. **100**, 90—99 (1964).

IX Subject Index

Plain numerals refer to page numbers in text, italicized page numbers to the Plates

GPSR Compliance

The European Union's (EU) General Product Safety Regulation (GPSR) is a set of rules that requires consumer products to be safe and our obligations to ensure this.

If you have any concerns about our products, you can contact us on ProductSafety@springernature.com

In case Publisher is established outside the EU, the EU authorized representative is:

Springer Nature Customer Service Center GmbH
Europaplatz 3
69115 Heidelberg, Germany

Batch number: 10615099

Printed by Printforce, the Netherlands